Behavioral Health in Primary Care: A Guide for Clinical Integration

Behavioral Health in Primary Care: A Guide for Clinical Integration

Editors

Nicholas A. Cummings, Ph.D., Sc.D.
Janet L. Cummings, Psy.D.
John N. Johnson, M.D.

Contributors

Neil J. Baker, M.D.
Mick Braddick, M.B., Ch.B.
Matthew A. Budd, M.D.
Simon H. Budman, Ph.D.
Stephen F. Butler, Ph.D.
Steven Cole, M.D.
Janet L.Cummings, Psy.D.
Nicholas A. Cummings, Ph.D., Sc.D.
Barbara Gawinski, Ph.D.
James H. Gordon, M.D.
Malcolm Gordon, M.D.
William B. Gunn, Jr., Ph.D.
Matthew R. Handley, M.D.
Steven C. Hayes, Ph.D.
Deborah L. Heggie, Ph.D.
John N. Johnson, M.D.
Jaylene Kent, Ph.D.
Jeremy Kisch, Ph.D.
Alan Lorenz, M.D.

Steven F. Lucas, M.D.
Larry B. Mauksch, M.Ed.
Caroline McLeod, Ph.D.
Bruce Meltzer, M.D.
James R. Moon, Ph.D., M.B.A.
C. J. Peek, Ph.D.
H. Edmund Pigott, Ph.D.
Patricia Robinson, Ph.D.
Stephen M. Saravay, M.D.
David Seaburn, M.S.
Gregory E. Simon, M.D., M.P.H.
James D. Slay, Jr., Rel.D.
Maurice D. Steinberg, M.D.
Kirk Strosahl, Ph.D.
Michael E. Stuart, M.D.
Michael VonKorff, Sc.D.
Steven Walerstein, M.D.
Redford B. Williams, M.D.
Virginia P. Williams, Ph.D.

PSYCHOSOCIAL PRESS
Madison   Connecticut

Library of Congress Cataloging-in-Publication Data

Behavioral health in primary care : a guide for clinical integration /
    editors, Nicholas A. Cummings, Janet L. Cummings, John N. Johnson ;
    contributors, Neil J. Baker . . . [et al.].
        p.   cm.
    Includes bibliographical references and index.
    ISBN 1-887841-10-5
    1. Mental health services—United States. 2. Integrated delivery
of health care—United States.   I. Cummings, Nicholas A.
II. Cummings, Janet L. III. Johnson, John N. IV. Baker, Neil J.
    [DNLM: 1. Primary Health Care—organization & administration-
-United States. 2. Behavioral Medicine—organization &
administration—United States. 3. Delivery of Health Care,
Integrated—methods—United States.   W 84.6 B419 1997]
RC465.6.B44   1997
362.2'0973—dc21
DNLM/DLC
for Library of Congress   97-19722
                                                             CIP

Manufactured in the United States of America

Contents

Part VI. The Epilogue

About the Authors

Neil J. Baker, M.D. Administrative and Clinical Director, Seattle area mental health services for Group Health Cooperative of Puget Sound. Team leader for the development and implementation of an evidence-based guideline and clinical pathway for the primary care treatment of depression. Formerly Associate Professor of Psychiatry, University of Colorado Health Sciences Center, where he developed alternatives to traditional psychiatric hospitalization in collaboration with Denver businesses and managed care companies. Doctor of Medicine, Stanford, 1977.

Mick Braddick, M.B., Ch.B. Clinical epidemiologist, Group Health Cooperative of Puget Sound. Graduated University of Manchester, England, 1981.

Matthew A. Budd, M.D. President, H.S.C. Associates, Inc., Assistant Professor of Medicine, Harvard Medical School. Formerly internist, Harvard Pilgrim Health Care. Formerly Founder and Chief, Department of Behavioral Medicine, Harvard Pilgrim Health Care. Developer of the Ways to Wellness program, and the Personal Health Improvement program, both ways of managing somatization in primary care. Developer of training programs for medical students, medical residents, and practicing physicians in the doctor–patient relationship.

Simon H. Budman, Ph.D. President, Innovative Training Systems, Inc. Assistant Professor of Psychology, Department of Psychiatry, Harvard Medical School, and Director of Mental Health Research, Training and Development, Harvard Community Health Plan. Former Associate Director, Institute for Health Research, Harvard Community Health Plan. Post-Doctoral Fellow and Instructor in Psychiatry, Strong Memorial Hospital, University of Rochester (New York) Medical Center. Doctorate, University of Pittsburgh, 1971.

Stephen F. Butler, Ph.D. Vice President, Innovative Training Systems, Inc. Former Director of Psychology, Northeast Psychiatric Associates/Brookside Hospital, Nashua, New Hampshire. Former Director of Mental Health Research, National Medical Enterprises. Former Assistant Professor, Medical College of Virginia and Director, University Center for Addictive Behaviors, Richmond, Virginia. Previously Research Assistant Professor, Vanderbilt University and Director, Center for Psychotherapy Research Clinic. Doctorate, Emory University, 1981. NIMH Post-Doctoral Fellow, Vanderbilt University.

Steven Cole, M.D. Professor of Psychiatry, Albert Einstein College of Medicine, and Director, Managed Care and Service System Development, Hillside Hospital, Long Island Jewish Medical Center. Dr. Cole is a consultation-liaison and geriatric psychiatrist whose book, *The Medical Interview: The Three Function Approach,* is required reading in 22 U.S. medical schools. Doctor of Medicine and M.A. in Sociology, both in 1974, Duke University.

Janet L. Cummings, Psy.D. President, The Nicholas & Dorothy Cummings Foundation, Inc. Former staff psychologist, American Biodyne (MedCo, now Merit Behavioral Care). Doctorate, School of Professional Psychology, Wright State University, 1992.

Nicholas A. Cummings, Ph.D., Sc.D. President, Foundation for Behavioral Health and Chairman, The Nicholas & Dorothy Cummings Foundation, Inc. Founding CEO, American Biodyne (MedCo, now Merit Behavioral Care). Former President, American Psychological Association. Founder of the four campuses of the California School of Professional Psychology. Chief Psychologist (Retired), Kaiser Permanente. Founder, National Academies of Practice, Washington, DC. Founder, American Managed Behavioral Healthcare Association. Former Executive Director, Mental Research Institute, Palo Alto. Founder, National Council of Schools of Professional Psychology. Currently Distinguished Professor, University of Nevada, Reno. Doctorate 1958, Adelphi University.

Barbara Gawinski, Ph.D. Assistant Professor of Family Medicine and Psychiatry, and Director of the Family Medicine Internship, University of Rochester. Also Assistant Director of Pre-Doctoral Education and Associate Director of Mental Health Services, Highland Hospital Family Medicine program. Doctorate in Family Therapy, Texas Technical University.

James H. Gordon, M.D. Associate Attending Psychiatrist in Consultation–Liaison Psychiatry, Department of Psychiatry, Hillside Hospital and Long Island Jewish Medical Center. Clinical Assistant Professor of Psychiatry, Albert Einstein College of Medicine. Doctor of Medicine, Harvard Medical School, 1966.

Malcolm Gordon, M.D. Assistant Chief of Adult Medicine, Kaiser Permanente Medical Center, San Jose, California, where he is also Chief of Quality Assurance and a member of the Department of Behavioral Medicine and the Spine Unit. Staff physician, Santa Teresa Community Hospital. Doctor of Medicine, University of Southern California, 1978.

William B. Gunn, Jr., Ph.D. Director of Faculty Development and Family Studies, Cabarrus Family Medicine Residency Program, Concord, North Carolina. Formerly Director of Behavioral Medicine in family medicine residencies in Roanoke (Virginia), Fort Collins (Colorado), and the Duke University Medical Center. Member of the advisory board, Family Health Care Coalition, and the steering committee for the Group on the Family. Doctorate in Family Therapy, Virginia Polytechnic, 1986.

Matthew R. Handley, M.D. Associate Director of Provider Education and Guideline Development, Group Health Cooperative of Puget Sound. Doctor of Medicine, University of California, Davis, 1984.

Steven C. Hayes, Ph.D. Nevada Foundation Professor, Chair of the Department of Psychology, and formerly Director of Clinical Training at the University of Nevada, Reno. Previously Associate Professor and Director of the Psychological Services

Center at the University of North Carolina, Greensboro. President-Elect, Association for the Advancement of Behavior Therapy. Past-President, American Association of Applied and Preventive Psychology. Past-President, Division 25 of the American Psychological Association. Listed in 1992 by the Institute of Scientific Information as the 30th "highest impact" psychologist in the world based on the citation impact of his writings. Doctorate in Clinical Psychology, West Virginia University, 1977.

Deborah L. Heggie, Ph.D. Director of Operations, Greenspring Health Services. Former Director of Managed Care, Capitol Region Mental Health Center, State of Connecticut Department of Mental Health and Addiction Services. Former Director of Outpatient Services, PATH, P.C. Previously, Director of Psychology Training; staff psychologist, Mt. Sinai Hospital, Hartford, Connecticut. Doctorate 1986, Fuller Graduate School of Psychology, Pasadena, California.

John N. Johnson, M.D. Medical Director, Director of Behavioral Health, and Director of Clinical Programs and Professional Development, HealthCare Partners, Ltd., Los Angeles. Former President, Medical Group, Torrance, California. A lifelong practicing gastroenterologist. Doctor of Medicine, University of California College of Medicine, 1964.

Jaylene Kent, Ph.D. Chief, Department of Behavioral Medicine, member of the Department of Adult Medicine, Consultant to the Spine Unit, and staff psychologist at Santa Teresa Community Hospital, California. Founding President and Past-President, Kaiser Regional Psychological Society. Fellowship in Health Psychology, University of California, San Francisco. Doctorate, University of Colorado at Boulder, 1988.

Jeremy Kisch, Ph.D. Director of Behavioral Health Services, Blue Cross Blue Shield of Connecticut. Lecturer in the Department of Psychiatry, Yale School of Medicine. Formerly Chief of Mental Health Services for Community Health Care Plan, Connecticut's first HMO. Previously Chief of Psychology,

Rockland Psychiatric Center, and Assistant Professor, New York Medical College. Formerly Assistant Attending Psychologist, New York Hospital, and Assistant Professor, Cornell University School of Medicine. Doctorate in Psychology, University of Michigan, 1967.

Alan Lorenz, M.D., is one of a handful of professionals with dual training in family medicine and family therapy. His family residency and Postgraduate Family Therapy Training were both at University of Rochester, New York. He currently practices in Palmyra, New York, and teaches at the University of Rochester. He has established a model collaborative practice in Palmyra.

Steven F. Lucas, M.D. Chief, Department of Family Practice at HealthPartners, Minneapolis. Dr. Lucas has practiced family medicine in this setting for the past 17 years, and has practiced in a primary care clinic with integrated on-site health clinicians for the past 2 years. His 60% full-time practice is full-range, including OB, pediatrics, and geriatrics. He is a participant on the evaluation and development team for a collaborative care model. Doctor of Medicine, University of Minnesota, 1975.

Larry B. Mauksch, M.Ed. Clinical Associate Professor of Family Medicine at the University of Washington where he is also the Coordinator of the Behavioral Science Curriculum and the Director of the Mental Health Internship in Collaborative Care. Member, board of directors of the Collaborative Family Health Care Coalition, and 1997 Program Chair for its conference.

Caroline McLeod, Ph.D. Collaborative Care Researcher, HealthCare Partners, Ltd., Los Angeles. Formerly Director of Quality Assurance for the Personal Health Improvement Program, Harvard Pilgrim Health Care, Boston. Dr. McLeod has conducted research in psychological factors associated with effectiveness of behavioral medicine programs in various programs in the Boston area. Doctorate, Boston University, 1995.

Bruce Meltzer, M.D. Assistant Professor of Psychiatry, Pediatrics and Emergency Medicine, University of Pittsburgh Medical Center, and Medical Director of Emergency Psychiatry and Telemedicine, Western Psychiatric Institute. Doctor of Medicine, Tufts University, 1987.

James R. Moon, Ph.D., M.B.A. Director of Clinical Operations, Behavioral Health Division, Winter Haven Hospital, Florida. Formerly Tampa/St. Petersburg Center Director, staff psychologist, American Biodyna (MedCo, now Merit Behavioral Care). Formerly Program Director, Substance Abuse Treatment Program, Veterans Administration Medical Center, Erie, Pennsylvania. Previously staff psychologist, Human Development Center of Pasco County, Florida, and Assistant Professor and Director, Residential Aging Program, Florida Mental Health Institute, University of South Florida, Tampa. Doctorate, Virginia Polytechnic Institute, 1982. Masters of Business Administration, Nova Southeastern University, Fort Lauderdale, Florida, 1997.

C. J. Peek, Ph.D. Consulting Psychologist for Medical Management Development, HealthPartners, Minneapolis. Internal consultant in areas of clinician manager development, care system change processes, and the integration of medical and psychosocial healthcare. Formerly Director of Health Psychology and Integrated Care within the Mental Health Department, HealthPartners. Doctorate in Clinical Psychology, University of Colorado, 1976.

H. Edmund Pigott, Ph.D. President, Pathware, Inc., Hartford, Connecticut. Previously Founder and President, Positive Alternatives to Hospitalization, P.C. Former President, Pathwise Behavioral Health. Doctorate, Fuller Graduate School of Psychology, Pasadena, California, 1986.

Patricia Robinson, Ph.D. Clinical and Research Psychologist, Mental Health Service, Group Health Cooperative of Puget

Sound. Behavioral Health Consultant, Health at Work Programs, Center for Health Promotion. Former Research Psychologist, National Institute of Mental Health. Doctorate, Texas Women's University, 1976.

Stephen M. Saravay, M.D. Chief, Consultation-Liaison Psychiatry, Department of Psychiatry, Hillside Hospital and Long Island Jewish Medical Center. Associate Clinical Professor of Psychiatry, Albert Einstein College of Medicine. Doctor of Medicine, State University of New York, Downstate Medical Center, 1962.

David Seaburn, M.S. Assistant Professor of Psychiatry and Family Medicine, University of Rochester, New York, where he is also the Director of the Postgraduate Family Therapy Training Program. Teaches in the Highland Hospital Family Medicine Residency Program. Co-author (with McDaniel and Campbell) of the widely used textbook, *Family Oriented Primary Care*. Masters in Counseling, State University of New York, Brockport. Ph.D. candidate, Union Institute.

Gregory E. Simon, M.D., M.P.H. Investigator, Center for Health Studies, and psychiatrist, Mental Health Services, Group Health Cooperative of Puget Sound. Research Assistant Professor in Psychiatry and Behavioral Sciences, University of Washington, Seattle. Doctor of Medicine, University of North Carolina, 1982. Masters of Public Health, University of Washington, 1990.

James D. Slay, Jr., Rel.D. Director of Behavioral Services, and Director of Collaborative Care Development, HealthCare Partners, Ltd., Los Angeles. Formerly the Director of Behavioral Health and Professional Development, Bay Shores Medical Group, where he was also in charge of the Health Care Integration Task Force. He is Co-chair of the Behavioral Health Managers Committee for the American Medical Groups Association. Doctorate, Claremont School of Theology, Claremont, California, 1973.

Maurice D. Steinberg, M.D. Associate Director, Consultation-Liaison Psychiatry, and Director, Consultation-Liaison Fellowship Program, Department of Psychiatry, Hillside Hospital/Long Island Jewish Medical Center. Clinical Assistant Professor of Psychiatry, Albert Einstein College of Medicine. Doctor of Medicine, University of Manitoba, Canada, 1962.

Kirk Strosahl, Ph.D. Research Evaluation Coordinator and staff psychologist, Mental Health Service, Group Health Cooperative of Puget Sound. Pioneering advocate of the integration of behavioral health services with primary care. Doctorate in Clinical Psychology, Purdue University, 1981.

Michael E. Stuart, M.D. Director, Provider Education and Guideline Development, Group Health Cooperative of Puget Sound. Doctor of Medicine, University of Washington, Seattle, 1971.

Michael VonKorff, Sc.D. Investigator, Center for Health Studies, Group Health Cooperative of Puget Sound. Affiliate Professor in Health Services, in Psychiatry, and in Behavioral Sciences, University of Washington, Seattle. Doctorate, Johns Hopkins University School of Public Health, 1978.

Steven Walerstein, M.D. Director, Medicine Residency Program, Hillside Hospital/Long Island Jewish Medical Center. Assistant Professor of Medicine, Albert Einstein College of Medicine. Doctor of Medicine, Albany Medical College, New York, 1979.

Redford B. Williams, M.D. Professor of Psychiatry and Behavioral Sciences, Professor of Psychology, Associate Professor of Medicine, and Director of the Behavioral Medicine Research Center, Duke University. Adjunct Professor of Epidemiology, School of Public Health, University of North Carolina, Chapel Hill. CEO of LifeSkills, Inc. Author of the best-selling *Anger Kills*. Doctor of Medicine, Yale University, 1967.

Virginia P. Williams, Ph.D. President, LifeSkills, Inc. Former Chair, Department of History, Amity Regional High School, Woodbridge, Connecticut. Coauthor of *Anger Kills*. Doctorate, Duke University, 1978.

Foreword

John N. Johnson, M.D.

Health care professionals, such as physicians and psychologists, who have never worked together in a true collaborative sense, are now being asked to unite in a mutual effort to improve both the design and quality of the American health care delivery system. Accepting these newfound roles has been difficult since we are the same professionals who were trained in separate and distinct environments that emphasized professional independence rather than mutual interdependence. This long-established tradition has contributed to the fragmented care of the patient as two separate entities: one physiological and the other psychological. Our success in correcting this approach inherent in our education and practice will be contingent on the acquisition and adaptation of new skills and organizational behaviors.

The changing climate of health care is not new to me. As I have observed the evolution of medical care over the last 30 years, I have witnessed many appropriate and rational clinical theories that have been transformed into high degrees of sophistication and application only to vanish with little fanfare. I can recall from my training days as a gastroenterologist embracing a compelling treatment approach that surfaced, disappeared, and suddenly reemerged all within a decade or two while other concepts simply endured. I have always wondered what guided this cyclical phenomenon of sound ideas that faded as suddenly as they bloomed while others persevered. There are probably many explanations; however, I believe that each had a key element in common: the skill and dedication of one committed individual who espoused a focused doctrine. In fact, I believe that concepts that prevail have the luxury of a determined leader and the benefit of strong and sustained organizational support. In this book, you will be introduced to the advocates and their institutions responsible for initiating and driving this important transition from a fragmented mode to an integrated and collaborative health care approach.

As we approach the millennium, the current environment of increasing competition in health care is exerting formidable external pressure on all aspects of the American health delivery system. This profound effect can be evaluated by exploring three interrelated issues.

First, the intensifying penetration of managed care into our health delivery system has created significant practice changes, including the coalescence of individual practitioners, small group practices, and independent physician associations (IPAs) into large, multispecialty medical groups. One may assume the focus of this recent enthusiasm for newfound relationships is based strictly on economic survival.

Second, the advent of capitation, an alternative compensation system of managed care, has been shown to have great potential for stimulating collaboration and innovation in the way we deliver health care services. To meet this challenge, multispecialty groups must create integrated delivery systems to both maintain and improve the physical and emotional health status of their populations through health education, health promotion, and disease prevention.

Finally, in order to support this endeavor, medical groups must also develop a reliable information infrastructure to furnish the health care providers with timely population-based information to assist them with analyzing treatment modalities and outcomes. Such data would also serve to validate the organization's accountability to its providers, consumers, and the payors of health care services.

How an organization responds to these challenges will reflect more on the organization than on the external demands. Successful groups will recognize the opportunities that await them and seize the occasion to develop organizations poised for the future by investing in the philosophical, managerial, and economic changes essential to properly implement the collaborative care model. The advocacy for such change can be supported and then applied by utilizing the concepts, knowledge, and information found in this book. By adopting the collaborative care approach, health care providers are now able to integrate the physical and the psychological aspects of health care into one single process. Innovative and committed organizations can create a clinical environment where the quality and ethics of practice dictate that patients will receive care that addresses all their biopsychosocial health care needs.

This book is about the rediscovery of a vital vision for health care. The authors of this text are the pioneers who will prove that the collaborative care model will be an efficient delivery system as well as a major contributor to the quality and cost effectiveness of health care.

Introduction

The integration of behavior health with primary care has commanded much recent attention. Yet few fully comprehend the medical, social, and economic forces that are mandating this next step in the evolution of health care. Equally confusing are the forces arrayed against this change, ranging from the traditional manner in which health care is dispensed, to more recent innovations in health care delivery that are struggling to find a place before their time passes in a swiftly moving current of change. This book is written by pioneers in the area of integration, and it is intended for practitioners, administrators, health economists, educators, program planners, and the purchasers of health care who want to understand the nature of the next wave in the rapid evolution in health care.

The integration of behavioral health with primary care is in its infancy. There is a babble of terms and an even greater confusion of concepts. Small now, it is on the same threshold of explosive growth that characterized managed care 15 years ago. Many at that time scoffed, only to be amazed at how seemingly overnight managed care went from 5 to 80% of the insured market. That no one is scoffing at the predictions regarding the growth of integration reflects the fact that it is a concept whose time has come. Those traditionalists who oppose integration pay lip-service to the concept, all the while looking for ways to strengthen the lines demarcating the medical specialties, and stiffening the caste-system that differentiates the various disciplines. But the integration of behavioral health with primary care will happen for three reasons: it is an effective and efficient treatment, it is sound economically, and it benefits the overwhelming majority of patients whose distressing emotions and faulty life-styles impede their health and well-being.

Recent years have seen several national conferences devoted solely to the subject of the integration of behavioral health with primary care. The most frequently asked question among the attendees has been, "What *is* integration, anyway?" Part I of this volume demystifies the concept and separates the real efforts from those that are merely cosmetic.

In the first chapter, Dr. Nicholas Cummings, who four decades ago with his colleagues at Kaiser Permanente, discovered the medical cost-offset phenomenon, presents the economic foundation that makes integration not only feasible but also mandatory. He replaced the term *hypochondria,* common in the medical parlance of the time, with the word *somatization,* stripping the condition of its unfortunately pejorative tone. He demonstrated that behavioral interventions dramatically reduce medical and surgical overutilization, a finding since replicated scores of times. In this chapter, Dr. Cummings traces three generations of medical cost offset research and delineates the conditions under which savings occur or do not occur.

Concluding that cost savings are best demonstrated in organized settings where behavioral health is permitted to impact on primary care, Dr. Cummings discusses in the second chapter the factors favoring integration and those opposing it. Perhaps the greatest advocates are primary care physicians whose ubiquitous experiences in the trenches have convinced them that up to 80 and 90% of their patients' conditions are complicated by psychological factors rather than the 60% estimated in most research. Suggestions for the enhancement of incentives and the amelioration of opposition are integral to the speed with which integration will occur.

Throughout the medical cost-offset literature, the number of physician visits needing behavioral health services varies from 50 to 90%. This disparity reflects differences in health delivery systems with varying effectiveness of reporting, as well as wide variations in the populations being served. For example, adolescents and older adults are at greater risk. Additionally, there are surprising geographic differences, with depression occurring more frequently in North Dakota than in the sunbelt. The most frequently cited figure, and the one which would reflect the greatest agreement, is 60%.

Dr. Kirk Strosahl, who was actively working toward integrated settings long before it became fashionable, gives the reader a "road map" in chapter 3. He lays out critical issues and directions for building effective integrated systems and conceptualizes a set of "report card" parameters on how real integrated products can be differentiated from fake ones. Unless there is some early understanding as to what constitutes effective integration, health care is destined to meander unnecessarily.

Part II details specific models of integration, all exemplifying varying stages of the fulfillment of Dr. Strosahl's criteria as to what constitutes a fully integrated behavioral health/primary care system. In the first of these (chapter 4), Drs. Kirk Strosahl and Neil Baker, along with their colleagues, describe the Group Health Cooperative model of integrated care developed over many years of research and field testing. They conclude with a nine-part differentiation of the characteristics of specialty mental health care versus primary mental health care, and a description of the key attributes of the twelve most frequently requested services in primary mental health care.

In most settings, a leap toward integration is not feasible as chapter 5 indicates. Dr. Matthew Budd, Assistant Professor at the Harvard Medical School and formerly of the Harvard Pilgrim Care Plan, and now heading his own company, describes products available for those settings which are prepared to accept and see the importance of holistic as well as behavioral intervention. Such settings will dramatically change the way in which medicine is practiced.

Drs. Jaylene Kent and Malcolm Gordon (chapter 6) trace the rediscovery of collaborative care in their Kaiser Permanente Medical Center (San Jose) and the internal steps taken toward integrating behavioral health in primary care. They describe a number of integrated programs, cutting across traditional specialties, all of which can be transplanted to other settings, providing that a serious commitment toward integration has been fostered. The authors' successes belie the difficulty of a task that required all the king's horses and all the king's men to put Humpty Dumpty together again.

Charged with the integration of behavioral health with primary care at HealthCare Partners, Dr. James Slay, along with his colleague, Dr. Caroline McLeod, in chapter 7 walks the reader through the arduous task that begins with the vision, evolves a mission, obtains the commitment and cooperation of the entire group, and no matter how well or how amicably these steps have gone, eventually must grapple with the ultimate test: financing the plan of integration. Their description of the process, which includes the resolution of unavoidable conflicts, is a map for those who have yet to walk the road to integration.

As absorbing as the clinical aspects of integration are, no health care system can exist without appropriate research and training, topics addressed in Part III. Drs. Gregory Simon and Michael VonKorff at the Center for Health Studies of the Group Health Cooperative of Puget Sound tackle the ultimate question head-on when they ask if integration is worth the effort. In chapter 8, they review the evidence, ever mindful that systems of integration must be evidence-based if they are to succeed. They conclude that the data reflect a number of conclusions that are supportive of the integration of behavioral health with primary care.

Training the primary care physician for the integrated delivery system has occupied much of the time of Dr. Steven Cole (chapter 9) and his colleagues at Hillside Hospital/The Long Island Jewish Medical Center and the Albert Einstein College of Medicine. Working with both residents and practicing physicians in the community, Dr. Cole concludes that such training is vital, and that the new skills are described as invaluable by the physicians.

Theory and research are interdependent, and Drs. Patricia Robinson and Steven Hayes proffer in chapter 10 a theoretical model for guiding integration of behavioral health with primary care service. This theoretical model is at once profound and practical and can point the way for educators who develop programs for professionals, and providers who develop clinical programs for specific populations. Acceptance and commitment strategies may empower patients to live well under difficult circumstances and providers to work successfully within the limits of modern day medicine.

Epidemiological research over the past two decades reveals that several psychosocial factors impact negatively on the development, course, and cost of a wide range of medical illnesses.

In chapter 11 Drs. Redford and Virginia Williams describe how the provision of skills training for patients can ameliorate the impact of these psychosocial factors, and they detail one model intervention, the Life Skills Workshop, that is adaptable for use in a variety of health settings, either by trained internal staff, or by outside providers.

The Lilly Family Depression Project, presented by Drs. Simon Budman and Stephen Butler, in chapter 12, not only underscores the importance of population based programs, but stresses the importance of the kind of early intervention that behavioral health within a primary care setting can maximally provide. Their use of cutting-edge technology is startling: the interactive video provides early intervention and prevention in the children of depressed parents.

Even though most practitioners wince at the mention of the word, health care is still a business. Furthermore, the business that was once a cottage industry has now been industrialized, and can no longer succeed without sophisticated informatics and an equally sophisticated understanding of finance. Both are the topics of Part IV. Dr. H. Edmund Pigott and his colleagues, in chapter 13, give the reader the benefit of their years of developing medical and behavioral care informatics, and stress the critical role of electronic data and communication systems in the success of integrative efforts. The last two years has seen the availability of excellent systems adaptable to most settings, all of which will impact on the totality of health care.

Dr. Jeremy Kisch, who directs mental health services for Blue Cross/Blue Shield of Connecticut, and has also served as head of a successful provider group, addresses the complicated world of financial structures, especially that of capitation, in chapter 14. He describes in practical, understandable terms how financial arrangements can enhance or hamper integration, further elucidating workable modifications to avoid difficulties. Professionals, often resistant to discussions of finance, will learn much from this clear presentation.

The integration of behavioral health with primary care cannot proceed without the understanding, cooperation, and knowledge of the practitioners, the importance of which commands an entire section: Part V. Dr. William Gunn, formerly of Duke University, and his colleagues, enunciate the features of a collaborative model in action. Chapter 15 is directed primarily at the mental health providers, pointing to the key strategies available in striving for a collaborative relationship in the future delivery system. Several intermediary positions leading to eventual full integration will illuminate the transitions needed of this mental health practitioner.

In chapter 16, Dr. James Moon, who learned the managed care carveout as an executive for American Biodyne and was inspired to go back to school to obtain his M.B.A., admonishes practitioners to move meticulously, but deliberately, into integrated models in which collaborating specialties acknowledge the leadership role of the primary care provider. As director of clinical operations at Winter Haven (Florida) Hospital, he describes his experiences on the road to integration in a manner useful to those contemplating such an endeavor.

It is predicted that the psychotherapy of the future will be only 25% individual, 25% time-limited groups, while 50% or more will be targeted behavioral modules in protocol form. Drs. Nicholas and Janet Cummings comment in chapter 17 on the design, utility, and efficacy of such protocols in the future integrated delivery system. This is a role familiar to health psychologists, but drastically different from that for which most mental health professionals were trained.

The integrated behavioral care system, in its emphasis on prevention and wellness, makes use of alternative medicine. In chapter 18, Drs. Janet and Nicholas Cummings, recognizing that this valuable resource is riddled with junk science and pop psychology, help clarify for the reader what is verified or verifiable, as opposed to that which is fanciful and speculative. Special importance is placed on the placebo effect of a belief system, resulting in fanciful potions and procedures yielding improbably positive results, along with a discussion of the professional's role when confronted with patients who claim benefits from the ostensibly impossible.

Finally, in the Epilogue (Part VI), a primary care physician discusses his own first-hand experience with the integration of behavioral health care. In an interview format conducted by a behavioral care specialist, Dr. C. J. Peek, a lifelong primary care physician, Dr. Steven Lucas, describes his practice in both a traditional system and a newer, integrated model. Primary care physicians will resonate to Dr. Lucas' responses, and behavioral care practitioners can gain new insights as to how to serve in a collaborative capacity.

The Editors

PART I

Integration: Why? What? How?

1.

Behavioral Health in Primary Care: Dollars and Sense

Nicholas A. Cummings, Ph.D., Sc.D.

Ever since the medical cost-offset was discovered over 35 years ago (Cummings, Kahn, & Sparkman, 1962) at the Kaiser Permanente health maintenance organization (HMO), the most important argument for the inclusion of behavioral health in primary care has been that it saves medical and surgical costs, and reduces inappropriate physical utilization. Since the seminal research (Cummings & Follette, 1968; Follette & Cummings, 1967) there have been scores of studies, many of which elicited the medical cost offset effect, while others did not. In order to be meaningful, the savings in medical utilization must exceed the costs of providing the behavioral health interventions. Some studies have shown a negative effect, painfully demonstrating that traditional mental health services cannot be parachuted into a traditional medical delivery system without incurring disappointing results.

A recently reported study (Fraser, 1996) reveals just how disastrous the results can be. A managed care organization (MCO) obtained an important delivery contract on the basis of promising medical cost savings. The negotiations were market driven in conjunction with misguided clinicians who bypassed the experts in medical cost offset. Neither knowing how to

3

conduct medical cost-offset research nor having the ability to deliver the necessary and appropriate interventions, no medical–surgical savings were realized and the contract was canceled by the client. In contrast, one Blue Cross/Blue Shield organization revealed that in a year when most health plans were raising their premiums they did not have to do so because of the medical cost-offset realized.

This chapter will focus on how and when behavioral health interventions produce the medical cost-offset effect and when they do not. In order to do so, it will review three generations of medical cost-offset research, and conclude with the most recent findings as to what circumstances enhance the effect, and what circumstances depress the potential effect.

THE DISCOVERY OF SOMATIZATION

In the 1950s the physicians at the Kaiser Permanente Health Plan, the prototype of the modern HMO, found to their surprise that 60% of physician visits were by patients who had no physical disease (Cummings & VandenBos, 1981). These patients were "diagnosed" in their medical charts as hypochondriacs in keeping with the parlance of the time. This unfortunate term was subsequently changed to that of *somatizer*, reflecting their *somatization*, a newly coined word in the medical nomenclature. It must be emphasized that this term has no relationship to the diagnosis of Somatiform Disorder in the current DSM-IV (American Psychiatric Association, 1994). Rather, it is defined as follows: Somatization is the translation of emotional problems into physical symptoms, or the exacerbation of a disease by emotional factors or stress.

Somatization inevitably results in the overutilization of health care, overloading the system. Originally it was erroneously believed that it was the function of the HMO in that when all barriers to access of health care are removed, patients will somaticize. Currently it is a generally accepted figure that between 60 and 70% of all physician visits are by somaticizers, and when one adds the visits resulting from faulty or unhealthy life-styles, the figure approaches 90% (Mechanic, 1966, 1991). The reason it was first discovered in an HMO setting is because capitated physicians were not compelled to declare a diagnosis where there was none, while fee-for-service physicians had to enter a diagnosis on the insurance form, even if preliminary, in order to be reimbursed. Consequently, the factor of somatization was obscured and even inadvertently hidden.

MEDICAL COST OFFSET

The history of medical cost offset can be roughly divided into three generations, each with its own set of discoveries and constellation of problems. It parallels the evolution of health care delivery, and as the system moved steadily and swiftly from fee-for-service to managed care, so did the challenges for medical cost offset investigations. It has been extensively described (Cummings, 1991b, 1993, 1996a) and will only be summarized here.

The First Generation: 1960–1980

Medical cost offset research was catapulted into the scientific literature following the discovery at Kaiser Permanente that 60% of physician visits were by somatizers and the seminal research by Cummings and his colleagues (Cummings & Follette, 1968, 1976; Cummings, Kahn, & Sparkman, 1962; Follette & Cummings, 1967) that medical utilization typically is reduced by 62% over 5 years following the application of behavioral interventions, and that the reduction in costs substantially exceeds the cost of providing the behavioral health services. Furthermore, without any additional behavioral care services, the utilization of medicine and surgery, both outpatient and inpatient, steadily declined to an ultimate level and stayed down, as compared to a comparison group of high utilizers who did not receive any behavioral health services. The typical Cummings and Follette effect is shown in Figure 1.1.

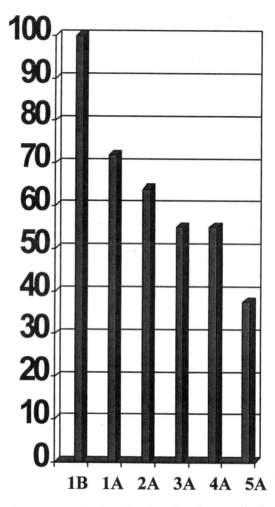

Figure 1.1. Average medical utilization for the year before (1B) and the 5 years after (1A, 2A, 3A, 4A and 5A) behavioral intervention (from Follette & Cummings, 1967).

During these decades the National Institute of Mental Health (NIMH) sponsored a number of investigations, and the Alcohol, Drug Abuse, and Mental Health Administration (ADAMHA) summarized 28 medical cost offset studies (Jones & Vischi, 1979), all but one of which showed the effect. The end of the decade was marked by the Bethesda Consensus

Conference in 1980 which concluded not only that medical cost offset was real, but the array of studies varied from savings that were highly significant to those that were not sufficient to cover even the cost of providing the behavioral health services. It further noted the methodological difficulties inherent in the retrospective design of these studies, with the recommendation that future research be prospective with a control group even if this meant that those in the control group would be denied services. In spite of the difficulties reflected in this first generation of studies, the Bethesda Conference concluded that the health system is burdened by patients with no real physical disease whose symptoms are caused by stress. Without psychotherapy, it was believed these persons would suffer needlessly.

The report of the Bethesda Consensus Conference (Jones & Vischi, 1980) was never widely disseminated because it appeared only a few weeks before the end of the Carter Administration and the scientists who convened it left government service when the next administration took office. That report noted that medical cost offset is more likely to occur in organized settings, and it was recommended that future research determine what factors increase medical–surgical cost savings and what factors mitigate such savings. To overcome the limitations of past studies it was recommended that a way be found to conduct controlled experiments and to address the problem of how medical cost offset research could aid in program planning and in clinical delivery (Jones & Vischi, 1980).

In regard to the integration of behavioral health into primary care, the era ended with two very significant events in the Kaiser Permanente Health Plan where the medical cost-offset effect was first discovered. The first of these was the design and implementation of the nation's first comprehensive prepaid psychotherapy benefit. Prior to this monumental event, the conventional wisdom in health care was that psychotherapy could not feasibly be covered as an insurance benefit, because it had the potential to bankrupt the system. The conclusion at Kaiser Permanente was that because of the overloading of the medical–surgical system by the somatizer, no comprehensive health delivery system could operate without psychotherapeutic interventions. Within these conclusions was the finding that the treatment of choice for 85% of the somatizers was brief, focused psychotherapy. The 15% of patients who needed and received longer term psychotherapy tended to substitute psychotherapy visits for physician visits, and therefore did not demonstrate any overall cost savings except in the reduction of medical–surgical hospitalization.

Advocates for the inclusion of psychotherapy, and especially of long-term psychotherapy in health insurance, overlooked the fact that medical cost offset was the result of interventions of brief therapy of the type later to be known as "HMO Therapy." This led to the first series of studies that embarrassingly did not result in enough medical cost savings to offset the unnecessary expenditures of long-term therapy. Although this generation of research revealed a minority of patients need longer term psychotherapy, this should be determined by the patient's condition, not therapist bias or ineptitude. The lesson learned is that if 85% of patients can benefit from brief therapy (average 6–7 sessions), then the longer term treatment of those who really need it can be successfully financed.

The second event in regard to the integration of behavioral health into primary care was a series of demonstration projects, early and noble experiments, indeed, in which this integration was actually accomplished. These will be described in the next chapter.

The Second Generation: 1980–1990

This second generation of studies numbers about 80, and along with merely replicating previous findings, the majority of researchers turned to addressing the concerns and issues discussed at the Bethesda Conference. But as momentum was building, suddenly all activity stopped as managed behavioral care "carve-outs" sought to tether out-of-control psychiatric and chemical dependency treatment costs by removing behavioral care from the medical–surgical delivery system. In addition, mental health costs were so high that their provision would more than swallow up any medical cost offset effect. Integration all but came to an abrupt halt.

As unfortunate as this turn of events seems in retrospect, the carve-outs actually saved the mental health benefit from extinction. Congress' enactment of Diagnosis Related Groups (DRGs) had dramatically tethered medical–surgical costs, but inadvertently encouraged the hospital industry's survival tactic of turning thousands of empty hospital beds into psychiatric (and especially adolescent psychiatric) and chemical dependency treatment services. Faced with the fact that this was now driving the double-digit inflation in health care, third party payors began to drop the mental health/chemical dependency (MH/CD) benefit from their coverage. By curtailing the accelerating inflation rate of MH/CD, the managed behavioral care industry prevented the extinction of the benefit, an accomplishment for which sufficient credit has not been accorded the carve-outs. Nonetheless, carving out behavioral care is the very antithesis of integration. When Cummings (1986) defined the parameters of the carve-outs, he pointed out that their necessity was solely economic and for about a 10-year period, a fact overlooked and resisted by the carve-out industry which now fears its own extinction inasmuch as it has outlived its usefulness. As important as the carve-outs were in their time, we are now confronted with the task of carving back in.

This second generation of medical cost offset research enunciated very clearly the methodological difficulties involved, and charted a course for the future. The first and foremost difficulty was that most health care settings did not possess the information systems needed to conduct such research. The carve-out arrangement only exacerbated the problem; if the informatics was deficient within a health plan, that between it and its carve-out was virtually nonexistent. Embarrassed by this, actuaries found it easier to ignore the medical cost offset phenomenon than to acknowledge their data processing shortcomings. The current emphasis (third generation) on outcomes research and accompanying drives toward sophisticated medical informatics has heralded a brighter future for researchers.

A second major difficulty in conducting medical offset research stems from practice disparity among psychotherapists.

Psychotherapists display a seemingly infinite number of competing and warring approaches to treatment, and most research employs a "lumping" of practitioners who may be canceling each other out. The emergence of organized settings is more likely to result in more homogeneity among psychotherapists. For example, in HMOs in which practitioners are trained and monitored in effective short-term psychotherapy, significant medical cost offset is usually elicited (Cummings & Follette, 1968, 1976; Goldberg, Krantz, & Locke, 1970, 1979), while in a fee-for-service setting in which practitioners characteristically practice longer term therapy, a dosage effect seems to prevail (Schlesinger, Mumford, Glass, Patrick, & Sharfstein, 1983). In the latter study, the greatest savings occurred with hospitalization, inasmuch as the higher costs of longer term therapy subtracted from the potential savings in ambulatory health care. Thus, there needs to be greater specificity in selecting providers and treatment.

Most somatizers are not referred for psychotherapy because the nonpsychiatric physicians who see them recognize less than one-fourth of those with emotional distress or chemical dependency (Glazer, 1993; Glazer & Bell, 1993). The problem is greater in fee-for-service settings where incentives for referral are absent. In a study by the RAND Corporation (1987), physicians who were capitated were more likely to refer patients for psychotherapy than were fee-for-service physicians, and the likelihood of referrals markedly decreased in geographical areas where there was a surplus of physicians resulting in the "patient scarcity" phenomenon. Some studies have sought to train nonpsychiatric physicians to recognize the somatizer and to appropriately refer him or her for psychotherapy. Even screening with computer printouts to primary care physicians has been utilized with mixed results (Cummings, 1985a). However, to maximize referral to a psychotherapist, in addition to increasing physician cooperation, an outreach program directed at the somatizer may be necessary.

Medical offset studies need to be prospective and controlled, in contrast to most previous studies, which relied on retrospective data and multiple regression analysis. Such studies are subject to selection bias and do not answer the question of whether so-called positive results are a statistical regression to the mean (Fiedler & Wight, 1989). Further, they would have to include a randomly selected group of somatizers who do not receive psychotherapy. The denial of services is not generally contractually permitted by the third party payor and constitutes an ethical dilemma for the practitioner. One way of addressing the problem is by a phase-in of a new psychotherapy benefit. A random phase-in could include the required control group, at least until the implementation of psychotherapy benefits. It remained for the next (third) generation of medical cost offset research to adequately address this problem. While the concentration of effort to control MH/CD costs all but curtailed medical cost offset research, a large number of second generation studies helped to clarify the role of stress and unhealthy life-styles in relation to medical utilization and to identify and promote issues of wellness. This body of literature is extensive, and somatization as a life-style has been reviewed by Ford (1983) and Pelletier (1993). The relationship between stress and somatization, which was not well understood when Kaiser Permanente dealt with this problem in the 1950s, will continue to occupy a significant sector of the health field. Medical overutilization can be affected by programs designed to promote healthy life-styles (Ford, 1983, 1986).

The Third Generation: 1990 to the Present

The unprecedented growth of managed behavioral health care plans over the past decade has provided large organized settings that have shown a revitalized interest in medical cost offset research. These companies are under considerable pressure to empirically demonstrate claims of quality, efficiency, and effectiveness. Outcomes research is experiencing a surge of activity, with contract research organizations springing up to meet the demand. Today, most of the unnecessary costs in delivering behavioral health care have been eliminated, and managed care organizations are turning to answer whether, how, and when such services can have an effect on unnecessary medical and surgical costs.

The forerunner and prototype of this new medical cost offset research is the Hawaii Medicaid Study (Cummings, Dorken, Pallak, & Henke, 1993; Pallak, Cummings, Dorken, & Henke, 1994), conducted over a period of 7 years with the entire Medicaid population of the Island of Oahu (Honolulu) and in a managed behavioral care setting specifically organized for that purpose under the auspices of the federal Health Care Financing Administration (HCFA). The study was designed to meet the several scientific criticisms delineated in the second generation of medical cost offset research.

The Hawaii Medicaid Study was (1) prospective in design with (2) all Medicaid eligibles (N = 36,000) randomly assigned to experimental and control groups, keeping families intact. It was in a specially created (3) organized setting that accorded (4) standardization of psychotherapists by 6 months of prior training and perpetual monitoring and case management in a staff (salaried) model. All practitioners were half-time, and 15% of their time was spent in quality assurance and adherence to the (5) empirically derived treatment protocols in which they were trained. (6) Access was enhanced by a series of satellite centers in high-density Medicaid areas, as well as a main center placed at the Ala Moana Shopping Mall where all Oahu public transportation converges. Housecalls were routine for those who could not come to any center. (7) An aggressive outreach program was coupled with (8) programs designed to encourage physician, social work, agency, and community participation. Every month the top 15% of users of health services as defined by frequency, who accounted for 80% of Medicaid costs, were outreached by mail, telephone, and for patients that responded to neither of these, by house call from a registered nurse dressed in full regalia and carrying a black bag. In contrast to the psychotherapists who very seldom were invited into the house, the registered nurses were never refused entrance.

Interestingly, this controlled prospective study confirmed years of retrospectively derived results. The cost of creating the behavioral health care system was recovered by medical–surgical savings within 18 months, and the significant reduction in medical utilization continued thereafter with no additional behavioral health care required to maintain the cost savings. These were estimated to be $8 million per year in constant dollars, with the greatest savings attributed to the group with a chronic medical diagnosis. This group consisted of high utilizers who suffered from diabetes, hypertension, chronic airway and respiratory diseases, ischemic heart disease, and rheumatoid arthritis, and who account for 40% of all Medicaid costs in Hawaii.

In contrast, the control group, which was seen in the fee-for-service private sector for psychotherapy, revealed a 17% increase in medical–surgical utilization, which was not statistically different from the 27% increase in control group patients who received no MH/CD services whatsoever. These results are found in Figures 1.2 and 1.3.

Hawaii was chosen as the site for this study because of its liberal Medicaid benefit of up to 52 sessions per year and renewable every year with any psychiatrist or psychologist in the community of the patient's own choosing. This permitted a direct comparison of the effectiveness and efficiency of empirically derived protocols delivered in a standardized setting versus traditional psychotherapy delivered in a laissez-faire private sector. The superiority of focused interventions designed and targeted to specific conditions, often in group psychoeducational format, was demonstrated in this and other settings (Goleman & Gurin, 1993) and may indicate that such protocols may be the psychotherapeutic wave of the future. These programs will be described in detail in a subsequent chapter in the volume.

Finally, the third generation of medical cost offset research indicates the importance of this methodology in program planning (Cummings, 1994). Results are in hard data, such as measurable reductions in units of medicine and surgery delivered, as compared to soft variables known as patient satisfaction, reported happiness, well-being or adjustment, and other rather difficult to quantify responses. Perhaps even more importantly, and as reluctant as health care practitioners may be to admit it, the results impinge on that almighty "bottom line" which, in this era of diminishing resources, is the ultimate determiner.

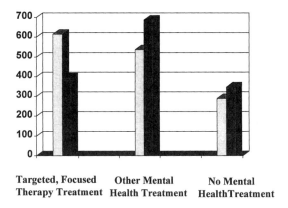

Figure 1.2.   Nonchronic group. Average medical utilization in constant dollars for the Hawaii Project Nonchronic Group for the year before (lightly shaded columns) for those receiving targeted and focused treatment, other mental health treatment in the private practice community, and no mental health treatment (from Cummings, Dorken, Pallak, & Henke, 1993).

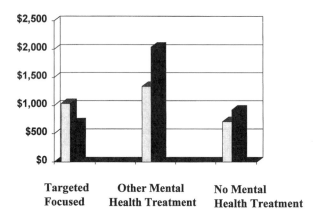

Figure 1.3.   Chronically ill group. Average medical utilization in constant dollars for the Hawaii project chronically ill group for the year before (lightly shaded columns) and the year after (darkly shaded columns) for those receiving targeted and focused treatment in the private practice community, and no mental health treatment (from Cummings, Dorken, Pallak, & Henke, 1993).

Now that managed care covers 70% of America's insured, some believe it is no longer possible to demonstrate medical cost offset as there is very little fat left. Nothing could be farther from the truth. Although managed care has reduced the acceleration of the inflationary spiral, it has not reversed it. There is still considerable waste and duplication in the system, and medical–surgical savings through behavioral health interventions have yet to more than scratch the surface. Two examples will be described. The first is a demonstration of how medical cost offset research must adapt to managed care realities, and the second demonstrates how dramatic savings can be realized in an efficient and effective managed care setting by a simple, heretofore untried behavioral health intervention.

The Reverse Medical Offset Threat

When the medical cost offset phenomenon was first demonstrated, a frequent criticism from traditional psychotherapists was that psychological or other physical symptoms would replace the physical symptoms in remission (symptom substitution). However, an 8-year follow-up study showed otherwise: not only had the somatizing abated, but patients had actually resolved the underlying stress that had resulted in their original symptomatology (Cummings & Follette, 1976). This finding seemed to put an end to the criticism called *transfer of equivalence* by more traditional psychotherapists. Less clear was the relationship between medical and psychiatric hospitalization.

Several studies have shown that hospitalized medical patients with psychiatric comorbidity have longer hospital stays and that psychotherapeutic consultation in the hospital can reduce the length of stay (Fulop, Strain, & Fahs, 1989; Hengeveld, Ancion, & Rooihans, 1988; Levenson, Hamer, & Silverman, 1986). However, what is the fate of a patient who presents for psychiatric hospitalization and is denied admission? Does that patient subsequently have a greater incidence of medical hospitalization? Such a finding would clearly be a *reverse* medical cost offset effect.

To investigate this question, Pallak and Cummings (1992) followed for one year every patient who presented for psychiatric hospitalization within a 6-month period in a managed care program and who was either admitted to a psychiatric hospital or was diverted to outpatient psychotherapy. They were interested in whether patients who presented for psychiatric hospitalization and were denied admission were more likely to be admitted for medical and surgical hospitalization for an ostensibly nonpsychiatric diagnosis. Patients who accepted outpatient psychotherapy either in lieu of psychiatric hospitalization or subsequent to discharge from a psychiatric unit, whether they were diverted or hospitalized psychiatrically, were not likely to be admitted to a medical or surgical unit. Both psychiatrically diverted *and* hospitalized patients who did not accept outpatient psychotherapy were more likely to be medically or surgically hospitalized during the subsequent year. The critical variable determining hospitalization was whether patients received outpatient psychotherapy.

The Managed Medicare Bereavement Program

It has long been recognized that in the first year or two following the death of a spouse, the surviving widow or widower demonstrates a significant and often startling increase in medical utilization. Cummings (in press) studied a group of 140,000 older adults who were receiving their Medicare benefits through a large managed care company. These retirees living in Florida were yielding about 20 widows and widowers every day, most of whom reduced medical utilization the year before the spouse died, ostensibly because they were too busy caring for the ill and dying spouse to attend to their own health care needs, only to strikingly increase medical utilization the year following the death of the spouse.

An aggressive but sensitive and compassionate outreach program contacted the survivor shortly after the death of the spouse and screened each one for signs of depression (reflecting unresolved issues with the deceased that would hamper bereavement) and those who were essentially in mourning with often severe sadness, but not pathological depression. The former were referred to psychotherapy for depression, while the latter were referred to a group program for bereavement. Because this older generation is characteristically respectful of the doctor and compliant with medical advice, acceptance of referrals was high.

The bereavement program consisted of 5 to 8 mourners in each group depending on patient traffic. There were 14 sessions of 2 hours duration each, spaced as follows: 4 semi-weekly sessions, followed by 6 weekly sessions, and concluding with 4 monthly sessions for a total treatment period of $6^1/_2$ months. The program was psychoeducational in nature, imparting information about the process of mourning, encouraging the patient to experience it as painful healing, and providing relaxation techniques and guided imagery to help them over the most stressful periods. A "buddy system" paired patients for mutual support and accessibility as needed. Patients were encouraged to discontinue antidepressant medication or use it sparingly as this may reduce the sadness but interferes with the natural healing process and prolongs it. The thrust of the program was to enhance self-efficacy, reduce learned helplessness, and restore a sense of coherence, all of which are described in greater detail in a subsequent chapter.

The medical utilization of 323 patients in this experimental group was compared with that of 278 widowed older adults in a nearby center of the same managed care company where the bereavement program had not been implemented. All patients were followed for 2 years except for a small number that did not live the entire 2 years following participation in the bereavement program. As is seen in Figure 1.4, following the death of the spouse the medical utilization of the bereavement program group rises somewhat higher than is expected of this age group, but then declines the second year after. The group not receiving the bereavement program demonstrated a sharp increase in medical utilization the first year after, with the increase being twice that of the bereavement program group. And although average medical utilization was considerably reduced in the second year after, it remains 40% higher than

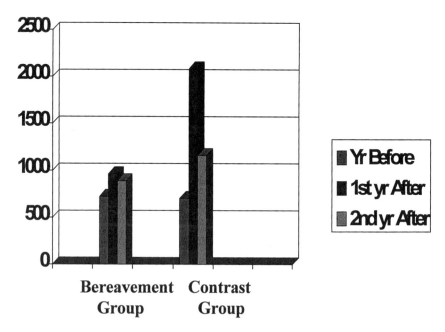

Figure 1.4. Average medical utilization for the year before and each of the two years after beginning the program, and for the same period for the contrast group that did not receive bereavement counseling. Amounts are in 1988–1992 dollars (from Cummings, in press).

that of the bereavement program participants. The savings in medical utilization of the experimental group over the control group was $1,400 per patient for the 2 years. Extrapolated to the older adult population in this 140,000 Medicare cohort alone, this amount translates potentially to several million dollars. But even more importantly, it spared these widowed older adults 2 years of avoidable suffering from physical symptoms and psychologically-induced ill health.

WHERE'S THE BEEF?

Considering the overwhelming evidence, this author has maintained that traditional services cannot be parachuted into a traditional setting with the expectation of finding medical cost offset. A recent project known as the Fort Bragg Study has demonstrated that *improved* traditional behavioral health care services cannot be injected into an *improved* traditional setting to obtain medical cost offset (Bickman, 1996). After spending $80 million to greatly increase access and to provide longer psychotherapy to more people, costs significantly increased, leading the researchers to conclude that more is not necessarily better. As is the subject of a later chapter in this volume, some of the least costly nontraditional behavioral health care services are the most efficacious in ameliorating patient pain, anxiety, and depression, in enhancing disease management, and in promoting prevention.

The cost containment that can be realized in MH/CD pales by comparison with the cost containment that lies potentially in medicine and surgery. Dollar amounts tend to obscure the importance of the comparison inasmuch as practitioners, like the general public, have become inured to large monetary sums being bandied about. Figure 1.5 is startling in that it dramatically shows the difference for 5, 10, and 15% cost savings in MH/CD (the first three columns) versus the same percentages in total health care (last three columns). All are in billions of dollars, and the 5, 10, and 15% reduction figures are modest estimates when most medical cost offset research demonstrates 15 to 60% savings. This figure graphically reveals that a 10% savings in medicine and surgery far exceeds the entire MH/CD budget of the United States!

The health care costs that might be saved through behavioral interventions, especially in a cutting-edge integrated program, have not begun to realize their potential.

SUMMARY

Over 35 years of medical cost offset research, spanning 3 generations of activity, reveal that the cost offset is greater (1) in organized settings where (2) behavioral health and primary care are somehow integrated, and where (3) the behavioral

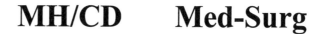

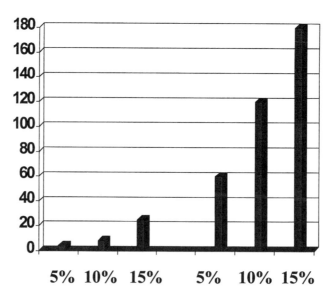

Figure 1.5. Reduction in billions of dollars potentially at the 5, 10, and 15% levels for the nation's mental health/chemical dependency budget (first three columns) and these percentages for the nation's medical/ surgical budget.

health interventions and the delivery system are cutting edge rather than traditional. Furthermore, it is enhanced by (4) standardized treatment procedures involving nontraditional modalities with (5) psychotherapists who have been standardized through training and subsequent monitoring. (6) The latest in informatics is critical, and the referrals of somatizers (7) are increased by capitation and suppressed by fee-for-service financial arrangements. (8) Controlled prospective studies are needed, but where they have been conducted they tend to confirm findings from years of less scientific retrospective research.

    For years the medical cost offset has been blurred by methodological, delivery, and informatics problems, but there is emerging a set of clear conditions under which significant savings can be demonstrated. For years advocates of psychotherapy, and particularly of long-term psychotherapy in health insurance, have confused the issue by misusing the medical cost offset literature as "proof" that traditional psychotherapeutic services should be included in every health plan. To the contrary, the evidence now points to innovation in both behavioral health interventions and primary care delivery systems as the crucial factor.

2

Pioneering Integrated Systems: Lessons Learned, Forgotten, and Relearned

Nicholas A. Cummings, Ph.D., Sc.D.

The incentives for integration of behavioral care with medicine are many. Health delivery is inundated with somatizers, the worried well, depressed, and anxious patients, stress related problems, faulty and unhealthy life-styles, chronic pain and learned helplessness among the chronically ill, increasing chemical dependency (both illegal and iatrogenic), and legions of chronically mentally ill. The primary care physician who has addressed the problem realizes 60 to 70% of patient visits are comprised of these patients, while seeing 35 to 40 patients a day makes it impossible to respond effectively to the need. So it is not surprising that over three dozen national conferences and seminars made integration their theme in 1996.

Why, then, with integration being discussed all around us, does it not move ahead with dispatch? Why are there only a handful of settings that are seriously and speedily moving toward the inclusion of behavioral care as an integral, indistinguishable part of the health delivery system, many of which are discussed in subsequent chapters of this volume? The impediments to integration surfaced with a vengeance 35 years ago during the implementation of a series of projects in integration. An historical perspective of these resistances reveals that most, if not all, continue to exist.

THE EARLY NOBLE EXPERIMENT

In 1962 one of the 19 medical–hospital centers in existence in the Kaiser Permanente health system at the time decided to have a psychologist or social worker physically present in every clinic during its hours of operation, be it an appointment clinic, a drop-in clinic, or the emergency service. Because none of the salaried mental health practitioners wanted a full-time assignment to one of the medical clinics, a schedule of rotating coverage was implemented that proved satisfactory in providing total coverage on the premises of each clinic.

There were obvious reasons why Kaiser Permanente would be the first to undertake such a project. As the forerunner of the modern health maintenance organization (HMO), it operated as a capitated staff model, so the physicians had no incentive not to refer somatizers as often happens in a fee-for-service setting. On the contrary, the primary care physicians were aware that they were inundated by patients who were translating stress into physical symptoms, often necessitating working long hours with no additional compensation. Also, the time was right inasmuch as a chief of medicine who had been consistently and openly disdainful of psychiatry had just been replaced. The founder of the Kaiser health system, Sidney Garfield, M.D., had for several years envisaged a strong primary care role for behavioral health, and especially since the discovery that 60% of physician visits in the Kaiser system were by patients who had no physical disease, or whose physical disease was being exacerbated by psychological factors. He agreed the project should move forward in advance of financial arrangements, which would be decided later. Garfield believed the main impediment, antagonism between medicine and psychiatry, had been mitigated, and the lesser problem of financial arrangements should not prevent the seizing of the moment.

During a 6-month trial period psychologists and social workers were rotated by schedule through all of the primary care clinics so that each was actually on the premises. A primary care physician (PCP) who wanted to involve a behavioral health practitioner only had to explain the reasons to the patient and both would walk a few feet to the psychologist's or social worker's office. Then, instead of merely leaving the patient, the physician remained and was involved in the subsequent examination and disposition. The behavioral care practitioners wore white coats along with the physicians, and a number of other deliberate steps were taken to blur the line of demarcation between medicine and behavioral health toward a unified primary care.

The PCPs made full use of the arrangement, involving a surprisingly large percentage of patients, and learning by participation in the behavioral care process. Weekly clinical case conferences attended by all involved reviewed the interventions and course of the most difficult cases. At the end of the 6-month trial period the PCPs had nothing but praise for the arrangement and enthusiastically wanted it continued. The psychologists and social workers, however, were lukewarm and expressed a preference that the project be discontinued. The PCPs were insistent, and the arrangement was extended 6 months at the end of which the psychologists and social workers all but mutinied in their refusal to continue. The project collapsed.

The resistance on the part of the mental health practitioners was surprising and unexpected. Attempts during the second 6 months of the project to address and ameliorate some of their concerns were unsuccessful, and at the end of the year they were adamant in their opposition. In retrospect, this outcome might have been anticipated when these same practitioners initially expressed reluctance to spend more than 2 hours a day on rotation in the primary care clinics. The major lesson learned was that most mental health practitioners are unsuited to participating in primary care, and the selection of psychologists and social workers must be carefully made.

The objections voiced by the mental health workers were deep seated, but sometimes ludicrous. They resented wearing white coats, complaining that this contributed to a loss of identity. All were insistent that a separate mental health clinic was like a temple, whose awesome presence resulted in the patient being half cured by merely walking through its portals. This esoteric and perhaps amusing version of the placebo effect was proffered with all sincerity, underscoring how far the participating psychologists and social workers would go to avoid conceptualizing anything even remotely like primary care. But the most outspoken opposition had to do with the issue of confidentiality. The argument that the confidentiality belongs to the patient, that it can and often must involve a team of healers, and that in one year not a single patient complained or even expressed concern about it, did nothing to mitigate the stridency of the mental health practitioners' stance. With considerable emotion and not a great deal of logic, they had unanimously concluded that the psychotherapeutic process had been violated.

Two subsequent successful integration projects learned from these early mistakes and did well. The first was an integration of pediatricians and behavioral health practitioners into a Teenage Clinic where patients from 13 to 18 could be treated, with parental consent or as emancipated minors, with the same consideration as would be accorded adult patients. The mental health practitioners (a psychiatrist, a psychologist, and three social workers) were hired for the expressed purpose of working full time in the Teenage Clinic with their counterparts in pediatrics, so none of the resistances seen in the first project were extant. A later project among an orthopedic surgeon, internist, and a behavioral care practitioner and named the Back Clinic also flourished in spite of unwarranted predictions to the contrary. It treated, among other problems, the very frequent and often somaticized symptom of low back pain.

BARRIERS TO INTEGRATION

The integration of behavioral health into primary care has suddenly been catapulted into prominence as reflected in the number of national conferences and publications addressing that topic in just the last year. Why, then, are there so many resistances to its accomplishment? Social policy moves slowly; health care policy moves even more slowly. We are confronted by centuries of tradition, attitudes, beliefs, and biases, and at least one century of modern medicine in which allopathics and the biomedical model have contributed enormously, along with public health, to our longevity, well-being, and quality of life. It is easy to improve on failure. Modern medicine has been a stellar success, and now manifests all of the entrenchment of a system that has served us well. But progress has brought us to the crossroads as evidence mounts that the biomedical and the psychosocial components are inseparable, and that the way we live is as important as what we were born with in regard to disease, immunity, longevity, vigor, and so forth. The question of which is the most important, the biomedical or the psychosocial, will soon become as arcane an inquiry as which is the most important to area, length or width? In the meantime, it is worthwhile to examine some of the major barriers to the implementation of that toward which most health practitioners are paying at least lip service.

René Descartes Lives

As Descartes admonished us nearly 500 years ago, the mind and the body are separate. Little did this 16th century philosopher and physician realize that at the dawning of the 21st Century the ultimate proof of his contention would be the existence today of separate departments of medicine and psychiatry. The lines of demarcation have spawned a necessary profession known as liaison psychiatry which attempts to bridge the gap between the two specialties. This is not to demean the valuable work of liaison psychiatry. This author has current experience with the system in the United Kingdom where six liaison psychiatrists serve the entire nation, leaving the GPs (as the PCPs are known) to plod along without this valuable service. But the existence of liaison psychiatry underscores the separation of mind and body. Turf interests are zealously guarded, and the blurring of the demarcation between medicine and psychiatry would threaten that liaison psychiatry itself would become obsolete.

Reductionism, which posits that disease can best be understood at the molecular level of biology and physiology is, along with the mind–body dualism, at the very heart of the medical culture and the basis for much of its past scientific progress. It has been more than half a century since Neal Miller ushered in medical psychology with his experiments on the interplay between behavior and the adrenal glands, bringing into serious question a simple cellular view of health and disease. Yet the molecular approach persists as perhaps the most characteristic feature of medical training and practice.

John B. Watson Also Lives

Psychology in the United States has never completely overcome the heritage given it by Watson who maintained that at birth a child is a blank slate and that the environment can make of that child a genius or a criminal. Biology was all but ignored by most American psychologists who are now reeling from the embarrassment of the genetic revolution. The ultimate psychosocial model no more wants to deal with DNA than the strict biomedical model can explain disease producing behavior.

The role of psychology as a health profession was won over several decades in bitter social, legislative, and judicial battles. Consequently, psychology is more zealous of preserving its turf than medicine which must worry only about losing its preeminence. For this reason issues of identity, arrogantly insisting the best way to practice is that which was initially learned, and the use of the important matter of confidentiality as a red herring, are unfortunate characteristics of a profession that continues to see itself as embattled.

The paradox, however, is that as health care is at the threshold of integration, there are responsible leaders within psychology who are advocating their profession opt out of the health care arena and become a strictly psychosocial endeavor paid for out-of-pocket by clients (not patients). Many of these same leaders oppose the profession's drive to gain prescription privileges, with all the training in the biological sciences that this would require. In part this is a response to psychology's opposition to managed care, but primarily it reflects an over-adherence to the psychosocial model which tends to be emulated by social work and counseling in general.

Not Out of My Budget

Financial barriers to integration are discussed in a later chapter of this volume and only a brief discussion follows here. As Melek (1996) has stated, medical offset savings are real and have been demonstrated clearly and repeatedly in a variety of settings. Yet:

> Little progress has been made in integrating behavioral and medical healthcare through the identification and risk-sharing of medical costs offsets from behavioral healthcare. This lack of progress is because of (1) the desire for fixed and isolated behavioral healthcare costs, (2) the difficulty of identifying and measuring such medical cost offsets, (3) the subjective nature of some behavioral healthcare, and (4) the natural cost savings within behavioral healthcare organizations from their own carve-outs when they are able to reduce their costs. (Melek, 1996, p. 40)

Very often integration moves forward when two to four different specialties pool resources from separate departments to form an innovative service, then figuring out the finances at a later date when the medical offset savings become apparent and measurable. This is the manner in which the Kaiser Permanente integrated programs evolved from small beginnings to over a dozen successful programs (see Kent and Gordon, chapter 6).

What, More Training?

More than half of all behavioral health care is delivered by PCPs who still miss as much as 80% of the patients who could benefit from such services. Clearly, PCPs need much more than the few hours of psychiatry lectures that are included in the 4-year medical school curriculum, and psychologists and social workers must be grounded in the biological sciences with further courses in neuroanatomy, neurology, and clinical medicine. Because of the already overloaded curriculum in both medical schools and graduate psychology and social work programs, there is tremendous opposition from academia, necessitating postgraduate training (see chapter 9).

There's No Time for Pandora and Her Box

No matter how extensive the PCP's training and skills, when that PCP is seeing 35 to 40 patients a day, mental, emotional, and chemical dependency problems are viewed as a potential Pandora's Box (Cole, 1996). Every PCP has had the experience of asking a small question and seeing the patient dissolve into tears and emotional turmoil while the waiting room is filled with patients both with and without appointments. A few painful experiences such as this will render most PCPs "gun shy," resulting in the unconscious overlooking of emotional signs.

Under current managed care arrangements, there is an even greater pressure on the PCP to see more and more patients. The primary care system is and will remain the "front line" in which behavioral care is required and delivered. Speaking as a business consultant, Melek (1996) argues that it is time some medical offset savings are reinvested in the PCPs' schedule, enabling them to use their skills. In this age of cost containment, very often derived medical offset savings are used to make possible a lower, more competitive capitation rate.

The One-on-One Complex

Traditional health care delivery, whether this be medical or behavioral, is based upon a one-on-one relationship and responsibility between doctor and patient. When referral is made it is to a specialist who replicates the one-on-one arrangement. The resistances to changing this to the more team oriented innovative and integrated therapies on the parts of both medicine and behavioral health are enormous. Arguments for the preservation of the system are couched in terms of the doctor–patient relationship and in confidentially, regardless of the fact that integrated services have demonstrated that patients readily extend the doctor–patient relationship to the treating team, and are comfortable in trusting the matter of confidentiality to the same team.

Within psychology there are two different thrusts toward treatment guidelines. One is in the interest of progress, facilitating treatment protocols based on empirical research and thereby moving away from traditional, unverified approaches. The second would intend through treatment guidelines to lock in the traditional one-on-one arrangement, with the possible exception of traditional group therapy which is often merely a number of individual patients seen together. As is discussed in chapter 18, the newer behavioral care interventions are group programs having a strong psychoeducational component, stressing disease management, and including prevention and self-efficacy. These programs not only are more likely to produce medical offset savings, but their delivery costs less than that of providing traditional services.

Both physicians and behavioral health practitioners need additional training for the integrated systems of the future (see chapter 9). One note of caution, however, is that many providers are unable to make the paradigm shifts necessary to overcome the one-on-one complex and other features of traditional practice. In addition to training, careful selection is also important. This is why new delivery systems have a golden opportunity to implement many of the innovations from the ground up rather than having to reform a system from the top down.

The Carve-Out and the Carve-In

As one of the pioneers who launched the behavioral carve-out industry, this author cited its necessity in the face of health care's inability to manage mental health and chemical dependency costs, and predicted its usefulness would be about 10 years (Cummings, 1986). Once the technology of tethering MH/CD costs was available to all, it would become an atavism holding back the progress toward integration. It is time for the industry, that is struggling to perpetuate itself beyond its usefulness, to now carve-in. This does not mean the acquisition of the carve-outs by large health conglomerates with the continuation from within of the carve-out concept. This is a frequent scenario in the current climate of consolidation, but here carve-in is defined as behavioral care becoming an integral part of the primary care system. As long as the carve-out arrangement exists, whether it is freestanding or part of a larger system, it will remain a barrier to true integration.

Patients Challenge the Frontiers of Medicine

Somatizers, through a complicated process involving learned behavior, manifest a constellation of symptoms that are both plausible and baffling. In their plausibility they appear consistent with what might be expected in a disease entity, but they are baffling in that they are not completely consistent with the plausible diagnosis. When this author first began his career nearly 50 years ago the most common somatized response came to be known as cardiac neurosis: it appeared as if it were cardiac disease but it was never confirmed by ECG, laboratory tests, sequelae, or morbidity. As cardiology became more sophisticated, neurotic heart became easily differentiated from actual heart disease and somatizers turned to other symptoms. For many years low back pain baffled physicians, but as orthopedics and back clinics increased their technology, lower back pain is giving way to carpal tunnel syndrome and multiple chemical sensitivity. For a short few years hypoglycemia and yeast conditions occupied much investigatory activity, and Epstein-Barr syndrome, chronic fatigue syndrome, and similar conditions are ever present in some form. Thirty-five years ago Icelandic disease was invoked to explain baffling symptoms, with subsequent severe embarrassment to the physicians who undertook to treat it.

Physicians are trained to find disease, and they fulfill their obligation well in fervent pursuit of a physical diagnosis. The patient, on the other hand, receives considerable attention and concern from a conscientious physician, all the while remaining in denial regarding the underlying psychological problem he or she wishes to avoid facing. To be certain, difficult-to-identify physical conditions exist, but for every actual such disease there are 10 or more somatizers. Carpal tunnel syndrome is an interesting example in that its sudden skyrocketing frequency is explained by use of computers. Yet the feather-touch of the modern PC as compared to the pounding necessary to use the old-fashioned typewriter suggests that the increased incidence may more parallel the decline of low back pain than the increased use of computers.

There is an optimal point at which the PCP can be confident the obligation to find physical disease has been fulfilled, and that to go beyond that reinforces the somatization and prevents the patient from addressing the real problems that will eventually bring relief. The degree of comfort and confidence required can occur only in an integrated system where the presence of behavioral health interventions are functional and successful. The physician who is skeptical regarding the influence of stress and emotions on physical symptoms will resist integration, while the physician who recognizes the connection will welcome behavioral health collaboration which will relieve much of the pressure on his or her busy practice.

Patients Challenge the Frontiers of Psychology

Similar to the somatizer who can display many plausible physical symptoms in the service of an underlying need for attention and caring is the *psycholyzer* who can mimic any emotional or mental condition. These patients are often aided by the psychological provider who is given to overly diagnosing, especially whatever may be the current psychological fad. Often such providers, with the help of the media, popularize tentative psychological findings into fads. When depression is redefined so as to encompass 60% of adults, or attention-deficit/hyperactivity disorder is said to affect 35% of all males in a grammar school, it is questionable whether these are any longer valid syndromes with pathognomonic features.

The mimicry of the psycholyzer of the latest psycho-fad can be dramatic, but it is preceded by a provider who inadvertently encourages the patient to mimic that condition. Borderline personality disorder is particularly vulnerable to becoming whatever the psychotherapist is looking for, and even more adept at mimicking it. Multiple personality disorder is far more iatrogenic than real, with the incidence closely allied to the number and location of practitioners who overly diagnose the "disorder" in their patients (Bloom, 1991). Similarly, the scandal of the false memory syndrome followed closely the overdiagnosis of childhood sexual abuse and the highly suspect satanic ritual abuse (Ceci & Bruck, 1995; Loftus, 1993). The many practitioners whose practices flourish by their promotion of questionable psychiatric syndromes are adamantly opposed to integration which would control such overzealousness. On the other hand, neither would an integrated system wish to have such providers in its ranks.

Well-Meaning Physician Empathy

A physician can so empathize with the patient's plight that the existence of depression, panic disorder, or even mental illness might be missed. "Physicians often explain away the emotional distress of mental disorders with an assertion like, 'You have *good reasons* to be depressed' " (Cole, 1996, p. 34). It is as if the physician identifies with the patient's loss of a job, a loved one, or a relationship and responds with what his or her own feelings would be under the circumstances. Such physicians consistently miss diagnosing emotional distress because of denial of intense feelings existing in their own lives. As an otherwise competent PCP only referred women alcoholics, but always for depression. He never saw the alcoholism, and when this was pointed out to him, his next referral was prefaced by, "For the first time I am referring a woman who is not an alcoholic." Of course, she was an alcoholic, and it is not surprising that this PCP had not recognized the alcoholism in his own spouse. PCPs who are in denial of their own feelings, or uncomfortable with emotional distress or mental disorder, rarely qualify for an integrated delivery system.

SUMMARY

The barriers that mitigate against the integration of behavioral health with primary care are formidable, and reflect centuries of tradition and over 100 years of modern practice patterns. Yet the need and efficacy of integration are widely accepted and heralded concepts, at least on the level of lip service. It can be anticipated that progress will be slow, with a few cutting-edge, practice-driven settings implementing the kinds of integrated systems that will differentiate them from the lookalike managed care organizations (MCOs) and health maintenance organizations (HMOs). This will accord them the competitive edge that eventually will be recognized and emulated.

3.

Building Primary Care Behavioral Health Systems that Work: A Compass and a Horizon

Kirk Strosahl, Ph.D.

Monumental changes are in the process of reshaping and reengineering both the health and mental health delivery systems in the United States. The advent of managed health care, with what many consider to be an excessive emphasis on supply side cost containment strategies, is simply a harbinger of even more fundamental change. As the health care reform process enters its second decade, two powerful industry themes are likely to emerge. First, there will be an intense focus on developing cost and quality oriented delivery systems, in response to increasing purchaser and customer dissatisfaction with the current overemphasis on cost containment. Second, redundancies in health care administrative and service delivery structures are likely to come under intense scrutiny, as market forces begin to favor

Acknowledgments. This chapter is the result of years of stimulating dialogue with my colleagues at Group Health, to whom I am eternally grateful. To Patricia Robinson, Ph.D., Greg Simon, M.D., and David Kanofsky, Ph.D., who have done so much to build the theory, research, and practice of integrated care. To David Brubakken, Ph.D., who had the temerity to launch the integration task force well before it was "politically correct" and Michael Quirk, Ph.D., who has been a staunch advocate of integrative services throughout the years.

systems that can consolidate delivery systems and capitalize on the economy of scale. This means that not only will delivery systems merge to achieve a national marketplace identity, but also the emphasis will be on *integrated services* (Cummings, 1995; Strosahl, 1994a, 1995, 1996a). Separated delivery systems will be merged as a way of reducing unnecessary administrative and infrastructure costs as well as addressing consumer preferences. Put simply, integrated delivery systems will emerge as a key cost, quality, and consumer satisfaction strategy.

Of the opportunities presented in the era of health care reform, none is more intriguing than the potential for integrating health and behavioral health services. As we have seen in the two prior chapters, the artificial separation of health and mental health services has had a destructive impact, not only upon the health of the general population, but also on the ability of each system to contain costs (Strosahl & Sobel, 1996). So pervasive is this growing impetus that most behavioral health companies are racing to put an integrated services product "on the shelf." While this is a welcome development, it also brings to mind the following Chinese saying: "If we don't decide where we're going, we're bound to end up where we're headed." Once we've accepted the compelling data pointing to the need for a behavioral health component in primary medical care, we are left with even more daunting questions. What exactly do we mean by integrated services? What should delivery system planners strive for? How will they know they have achieved it? What service delivery models will work the best and be the least costly? How will purchasers of integrated care products separate the "wheat from the chaff"? While many widely discussed obstacles will need to be overcome to achieve integration (i.e., culture clash, turf issues, financing, and benefit design), the most formidable and, ironically, least discussed challenge is to develop a framework for planning, implementing, and evaluating integrated care products.

At a very minimum, an acceptable framework should specify the mission of integrated services (something other than as a way to gain market share), how they should be organized to address the needs of the primary care population, the type(s) of services that need to be delivered, and how to evaluate specific integrated service programs both for delivery system coherency and potential population impact. Any successful framework should tell us what is required for full integration of systems. Much like a compass and a horizon, the behavioral health industry desperately needs a long-term direction, a set of mileposts, and a specific mechanism for finding its way. Otherwise, "we're bound to end up where we're headed," and, if the result is anything like what occurred in the public relations nightmare of generation 1 managed care, we will surely wish we had directed the integration movement differently.

The purpose of this chapter is to provide the reader with an overall framework that addresses the important dimensions involved in developing and evaluating integrated service programs. First, a population-based care framework will be introduced to help articulate the mission of integrated services. Two required, complementary integration models will be described which can satisfy the requirements of population-based care approach. Next, the reader will be exposed to the primary mental health care model as a specific approach to integrated services that has established clinical efficacy, produces high levels of customer and provider satisfaction, and can be implemented with a minimum of additional resources. Finally, the reader will be offered a framework for evaluating various integration products, many creative examples of which are presented in subsequent chapters.

DILEMMAS IN DEVELOPING INTEGRATED DELIVERY SYSTEMS

From a service delivery planning perspective, the task of building integrated behavioral health and primary care systems involves identifying and overcoming some major conceptual and logistical hurdles. Taken collectively, the nature of these hurdles demands that behavioral health planners think "out of the box" to be successful.

Reengineering, Not Reshaping

The core dilemma is best exemplified in population morbidity
data reported by the Epidemiological Catchment Area study
(Narrow, Regier, Rae, Manderscheid, & Locke, 1993; Regier et
al., 1993) and largely replicated in the National Co-morbidity
Study (Kessler et al., 1994). These large epidemiological studies
have revealed not only an astoundingly high annual onset rate
of mental disorders (18%), but also have demonstrated that
50% of all care for patients with mental disorders is delivered
solely by general medical practitioners. Equally intriguing is
that 50% of all patients with diagnosed mental disorders seek
no formal care at all. However, other service utilization studies
suggest that 70 to 80% of the general population will make at
least one primary care visit annually. The conclusion is that
approximately 65 to 70% of patients with mental disorders are
cycling through the general medical sector, whether they are
recognized and treated or not. These patients, as a rule, do not
seek specialty mental health care to address their behavioral
health needs. Note, in addition, that these data speak only to
patients with diagnosable mental disorders; there is an equally
large population of patients with psychosocial stresses and sub-
threshold symptom complaints circulating in primary care
(VonKorff et al., 1987; VonKorff & Simon, 1996). In toto, psychosocial distress and mental disorders are the basis for 70%
of all primary care visits. The service planning implication is
that many more patients with mental disorders and psychological problems will need services in an integrated system. The
capacity of this system would need to be twice that of the current mental health specialty system.

Current Service Delivery Models Won't Work

Obviously, the increased volume of eligible patients in primary
care would require an enormous expansion in the supply of
mental health providers, if integrated services are delivered
in a specialty mental health model of care. Simply relocating

existing mental health providers in primary care clinics and delivering traditional psychotherapy or medication services would completely outstrip the available behavioral health resources in this country. In this era of shrinking behavioral health resources, this seems highly unlikely to occur. Without some type of fundamental paradigm shift, we will be forced to implement isolated and unconnected services that have market appeal but little real impact on the lives of most primary care patients.

Incompatible Missions

Simply put, the mission of specialty mental health systems to a significant degree is inconsistent with the mission of primary health care (Strosahl, 1996a, 1996b). Whereas primary care providers are responsible for the health of an entire population and operate from a public health perspective, mental health providers typically attend only to the needs of patients who have already developed problems. Consequently, there are profound differences in perspective, how work is organized, and in the primary strategies that are employed to attend to health and/or mental health needs. This fact has implications for what types of behavioral health services will be acceptable to primary care providers and patients alike. It also raises important questions about the ability of mental health providers, trained in a specialty "office practice" model of care, to adapt to the realities of primary care medicine.

The Needs of the Primary Care Population Are Heterogeneous

Regardless of how well conceived, no single integrated behavioral health program can address the needs of all primary care patients. There are not only patients with mental disorders in primary care, but also a large group with psychosocial stresses, chronic disease burden, caregiving burden, social disenfranchisement, and so on. The obvious implication is that different models of care need to be integrated to address this diverse set of needs, yet in a way that does not breed redundant administrative–program costs.

Primary Care and Specialty Mental Health Patients: One Population or Two?

A particularly vexing question for program developers and administrators alike has to do with the degree of overlap between patients who receive mental health services from their primary care provider and those who elect to access the specialty mental health system. Is this the same cohort of patients seen by different systems at different points in the development of a mental disorder, or are these two unrelated populations? This question has massive cost and service implications. If there is an overlap between the two groups, one would expect integrated delivery systems to divert a certain percentage of patients away from specialty mental health care, where their problems could be resolved in toto in primary care. If the populations are largely unrelated, behavioral health systems will simply be adding a large piece of work to an already strained delivery system. This very likely is not a "black and white" question. In other words, there is probably a degree of overlap. Anecdotal experience at the Group Health Cooperative of Puget Sound suggests the overlap is in the range of 50%. However, this is a question yearning for a research-based answer, and in all likelihood, will have a direct impact on how integrated services are financed. If the overlap between primary care and specialty mental health populations is low, purchasers will have to pay increased premiums (either health or mental health) to subsidize the start up of the system. In this scenario, the ability to demonstrate significant medical cost offsets in integrated systems will be a critical parameter for purchasers (Strosahl & Sobel, 1996). If the overlap is high, there would be less financial pressure on existing delivery systems. In this scenario, a conceptual shift would be required among behavioral health system administrators to build systems that identify potential mental health specialty patients "upstream" in the early course of their disorder.

Naturally, primary care is the ideal venue for such early identification, aggressive intervention, and prevention initiatives.

POPULATION-BASED CARE: A FRAMEWORK FOR HEALTH AND BEHAVIORAL HEALTH INTEGRATION

In this author's opinion, the population-based care perspective provides an enormously flexible and powerful framework for sorting through and resolving the key issues in building an integrated delivery system that works. Population-based care is based on a public health view of service delivery planning. In this perspective, the service "mission" is not just to address the needs of the "sick" patient, but to think about similar patients in the population who may be at risk, or who are sick and do not seek care. A few examples of typical population-based service planning questions will illustrate this point: What percentage of the population has conditions like this? How many seek care? Where do they seek care? Are there variations in the way care is being provided for patients like this that result in differential clinical outcomes? Can we prevent the condition from occurring in patients who have similar risk factors?

When developing a framework for constructing integrated behavioral health services, the same approach can be used. For example, what types of behavioral health service needs exist in the population of patients served by this primary care team? What type of service delivery structure will allow maximum penetration into the whole population? What types of interventions will work with the "common causes" of psychological distress? What secondary, and more elaborate, interventions are appropriate for a primary care setting? At what level of complexity is a patient better treated in specialty mental health care? These are pivotal service delivery planning questions.

Figures 3.1 and 3.2 provide two different perspectives on population-based service planning. Figure 3.1 illustrates the types of behavioral health "need" within a hypothetical primary care population. These estimates are based upon recent

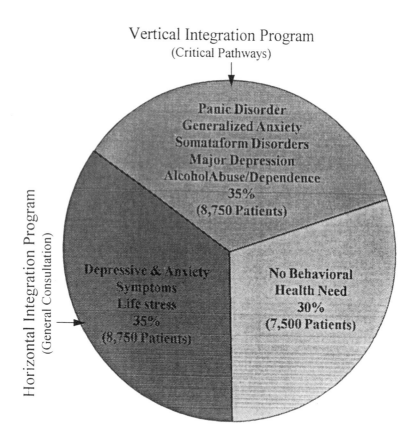

*Hypothetical Cohort of 25,000 patients

Figure 3.1. Analysis of behavioral health needs in a primary care population.

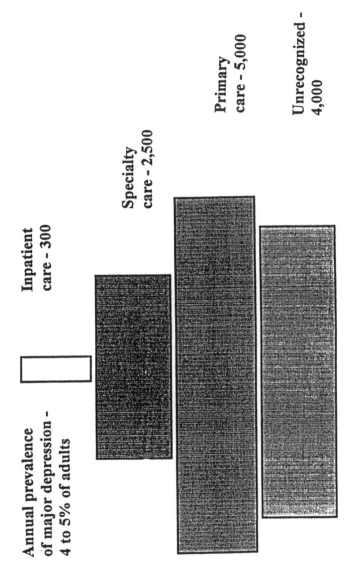

Figure 3.2.   Sources of care for depressed patients in the primary care population.

studies examining the prevalence of mental disorders and psychological distress in primary care patients (Spitzer et al., 1995; VonKorff, Shapiro et al., 1987). Each piece of the "pie" represents a potential programmatic need, ranging from general psychosocial services to more specialized treatment pathways. As can be seen, when one begins to calculate the number of primary care patients with behavioral health service needs, the task of building a comprehensive system of integrated care seems formidable indeed. Figure 3.2 looks at population-based planning as a function of the source of service, with a hypothetical population of 300,000 primary care patients, of whom 4 to 5% will have diagnosable major depression at any given time, again based upon available research data (Simon, VonKorff, & Barlow, 1995). Note that behavioral health services delivered in mental health clinics constitute a relatively small proportion of the total service volume. The obvious planning conclusion is that for integrated care to succeed, service capacity in primary care (and associated staffing patterns) may need to double for specialty mental health delivery sites.

As we shall discuss later, this capacity demand can be met either by shifting more mental health staff into primary care and/or developing a model of care that can address a larger number of service needs, without a dramatic increase in personnel.

HORIZONTAL AND VERTICAL INTEGRATION: TWO TEMPLATES FOR INTEGRATIVE PRIMARY CARE

The population-based care framework also suggests that there are two different, complementary approaches to addressing the behavioral health needs of the primary care population. As can be seen in Figure 3.3, horizontal integration is the platform upon which all other forms of integrated behavioral health care reside, because most members of the primary care population can benefit from a behavioral health services delivered from a generalist service delivery model. A distinguishing feature of horizontal integration is that it "casts a wide net" in terms of

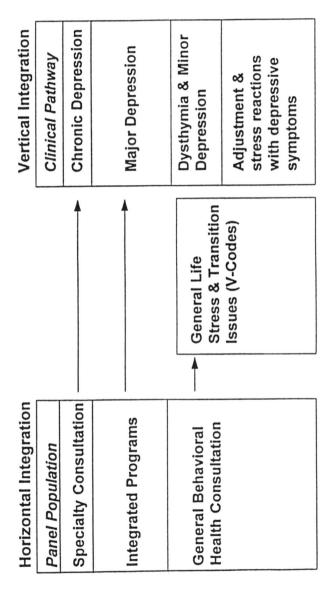

Figure 3.3. Two models of population-based care.

who is eligible. From a population-based care perspective, the goal is to enroll as many patients as possible into brief, general psychosocial services. Traditional primary care medicine is largely based upon the horizontal integration approach. The goal is to "tend the flock" by providing a large volume of general health care services, none of which is highly specialized. Patients who truly require specialized expertise are usually referred to medical specialties. Similarly, patients with behavioral health needs can be exposed to nonspecialized services; those that truly require specialty care are referred into the specialty mental health system.

Vertical integration involves providing targeted, more specialized behavioral health services to a well-defined, circumscribed group of primary care patients, such as patients with major depression. This is a major contemporary development in primary care medicine, i.e., the use of a "critical pathway," "clinical roadmap," or "best practices" approach. Targets for vertical integration are usually high frequency and/or high cost patient populations such as depression, panic disorder, chemical dependency, and certain groups of high medical utilizers. With respect to frequency, a complaint that is usually represented in the population (like depression) is a good candidate for a special process of care. With respect to cost, some rare conditions are so costly that they require a special system of care, for example, patients with chronic behavioral health problems. A good example of this type of problem involves patients with Acquired Immune Deficiency Syndrome (AIDS). In the behavioral health arena, high utilizers of medical care, by definition, are a small but costly group that often are the targets of vertical integration programs (Strosahl & Sobel, 1996).

Primary Mental Health Care: A Model of Integrated Care

Elsewhere, a *primary mental health care* model of integrative primary health care has been described (Quirk et al., 1995;

Strosahl, 1994b, 1996a, 1996b). This model of behavioral health care is consistent with the philosophy, service goals, and health care strategies of primary care medicine. It is also capable of addressing the increased service demands likely to be encountered in a fully integrated behavioral health system. This approach involves providing direct consultative services to primary care providers and engaging in temporary comanagement (with the primary care provider) of patients who require more concentrated services, but nevertheless can be managed in primary care. Both consultative and condensed specialty treatment services are delivered as a "first line" intervention for primary care patients who have behavioral health needs. If a patient fails to respond to this level of intervention, or obviously needs specialized treatment, the patient is referred on to the specialty mental health system (Strosahl, 1994b). Consistent with the service philosophy of primary care, the goal of primary mental health is to detect and address the broad spectrum of behavioral health needs among the primary care cohort, with the aims of early identification, quick resolution, long-term prevention, and "wellness." Most importantly, primary mental health is designed to support the ongoing behavioral health interventions of the primary care provider. There is no attempt to take charge of the patient's care, as is true in specialty mental health care. The goal of primary mental health is to resolve problems within the primary care service context.

LEVELS OF PRIMARY MENTAL HEALTH CARE

Primary mental health services also exist on a "levels of care" continuum, that correspond to (1) the level of complexity of the problem and (2) the proportion of the primary care population that will "penetrate" the service. Most patients who receive such care will participate in behavioral health consultation which is based in the horizontal integration approach. Patients with more complicated behavioral health needs will receive services in "critical pathways," based in the vertical integration approach. Both approaches are required

to fully enable an integrated delivery system. Patients who do
not respond to either service approach are then referred on for
specialty mental health care. Clinical experience and program
research suggest that this percentage is low, between 10 and
20%.

The foundation of an integrated delivery system is the *general behavioral health,* which has a "see all comers" program
philosophy. Primary care providers are encouraged to refer any
patient for any reason to on-site behavioral health consultants,
who have a set consultation schedule that is utilized only by
the primary care team. Most patients in a primary care cohort
are best served in the general consultation service delivery
model. These services are brief (15–30 minutes) and time limited (1–3 visits). Many patients who ordinarily would be eligible
for critical pathway services (i.e., depression, panic disorder)
can still benefit from consultative intervention. A secondary
goal of the consultation model is to raise the skill level of the
referring providers so that, over time, "routine" problems are
handled more effectively within the forum of the routine medical visit. Eventually, primary care providers may be able to handle routine behavioral health and medication needs with very
little consultative assistance.

The *specialty consultation* level of primary mental health
care is for patients with chronic psychosocial and/or physical
problems who need longer term management by the primary
care team, in consultation with the behavioral health specialist.
Commonly, this service is needed by patients with personality
disorders, chronic pain–disability issues, or adjustment–compliance issues involving a chronic medical illness. The program is
delivered in the consultative service model, but visits with the
behavioral health consultant are less frequent and spread out
over time. The goal of this service is to help the primary care
team efficiently manage the patient's health and behavioral
health care needs.

This *integrated program* service level is designed for high
frequency primary care populations such as major depression.
It involves using highly condensed, specialized medication
and/or behavioral treatment packages that are tailored for the

fast work pace of primary care. The intent is to treat the condition in a temporary comanagement partnership with the primary care provider. To achieve this end, the consultant and primary care provider comanage the patient using a structured program of care. More behavioral health visits may occur in integrated services than is true in general consultation (4–6 visits of 30 minutes), although the emphasis is the same: patient education, self-management skills, compliance with medication, and intervention feedback for the primary care provider. An excellent example of this service is the Integrated Care Program for Depression, in which a primary care provider and behavioral health consultant work together in a structured program which uses medication and/or cognitive behavioral treatment for patients with syndrome depressions or depressive symptoms secondary to life stresses/transitions (Robinson, 1996; Robinson, Wischman, & Del Vento, 1996). Research indicates that, when applied to depressed primary care patients, the integrated care approach produces superior clinical outcomes, better medication compliance, better management of side effects, more satisfied patients and more satisfied primary health care providers (Katon et al., 1996; Robinson et al., under review).

MILEPOSTS IN DEVELOPING AND EVALUATING INTEGRATED CARE PRODUCTS

While the opportunities involved in integrative care are endless, there are many potential barriers to achieving the best system architecture in this rapidly growing area. As has been discussed, the most important obstacle is the lack of a widely accepted framework that would propel the development of industry standards regarding integration products. Currently, programs as diverse as off-site classes for high utilizers of health care, conducting conjoint therapy visits with physicians in training, or offering health improvement programs to any interested patient, are viewed as examples of integrated care products. The point here is not to belittle these efforts or the individual creativity which breeds them, but rather to suggest that there is currently no established method for determining whether an integrated service program meets even minimal product standards. Purchasers and consumers of integrated behavioral health services need a set of standards upon which to evaluate whether a system of care is integrated or not. Table 3.1 presents a sample "report card" listing key criteria for optimally integrated behavioral health primary care systems. In general, the main "mileposts" revolve around three core issues: Colocation of services, building services that address the full spectrum of need, and consistency with the mission of primary care. Almost any integration product can be analyzed and evaluated using these three parameters.

On-site services are a critical component of a desirable integrated care system. In this author's opinion, the most effective integrated services involve having a behavioral health specialist on site, practicing in the medical cluster as a part of the primary care team. Unfortunately, this design requirement is frequently ignored or overlooked, as both behavioral health and primary care executives are put off by the potential costs of providing on-site staff. Many behavioral health "carve-out" and "carve-in" companies may have to go to a mixed model and have a staff component that provides integrated services in primary care. This will not be popular, but it should be an industry requirement.

Many behavioral health companies now offer phone consultation on demand to primary care providers. While this is a nice gesture, emergency consultative services have little impact on overall integration of routine behavioral health and primary care services and do little to raise the skill level of primary care health providers with respect to the thousands of routine psychosocial interventions that are employed in the daily practice of primary health care. The most effective vehicle for touching the lives of thousands of primary care patients remains the on-site consultant, who is a member of the primary care team and has a weekly presence in the medical practice area. Enough consultation time is needed to guarantee acceptable access for newly referred patients, generally within 5 days

TABLE 3.1

Sample "Report Card" for Integrated Primary Care Behavioral Health Programs

Dimension	Inadequate Grade	Passing Grade	Superior Grade
1. Program planning approach	No research or public health basis, little connection to health care delivery system objectives, no assessment of priority behavioral health needs in resource planning	Uses some research and public health concepts; system design only partially addresses priority population needs; resources support some low impact programs	Population-based care planning framework based in epidemiological assessments, priority behavioral health needs addressed first in resource allocations
2. Integration models employed	Isolated programmatic effort; no critical pathways or general behavioral health services models used	Systems uses either at least one critical pathway or general behavioral health services approach	System employs both at least one critical pathway and general behavioral health services
3. Predicted population impact	Low impact on both health costs and behavioral health of the primary care population; services in free standing program for small segment of population, cost returns small relative to total health care budget	Some population impact possible; however, it is limited to a specific segment of primary care population or service density is too light to address existing needs in a particular area; only modest cost returns possible	High population impact; services target high areas of behavioral health need; service density great enough to service a variety of behavioral health needs; large cost returns possible because of multiple population targets
4. Service locations	Off-site services or programs for physician referred patients; phone consultation available with off-site behavioral care	On-site service delivered in a space separate from medical practice area, often a "mental health wing"	On-site services delivered within medical practice area as part of general health care process

TABLE 3.1 (continued)

Dimension	Inadequate Grade	Passing Grade	Superior Grade
5. Service philosophy	Behavioral health constructed as a specialty service; service goal is to treat patient by delivering mental health specialty services; physicians kept informed at "arm's length"	Behavioral health viewed as a special to service, practiced in collaboration with physician; goal is to resolve patient problems via delivery of specialty mental health treatment	Behavioral health part of primary medical practice; both services integrated in primary care team; goals consistent with primary mental health care model
6. Service characteristics	Behavioral health delivered in "50 minute hour" model; behavioral health providers responsible for care; perceived by provider and patient as separate specialty service; service length varies dependent on diagnosis; mental health access standard used	Behavioral health offered in "collaborative care" model; may involve physician as part of specialty care; behavioral provider responsible for care; seen as "specialist" by the physician and patient; 50 minute hour is still dominate approach; service length varies depending on diagnosis; mental health access standard used	Behavioral health delivered in consultation model; physician remains in charge; visit pattern designed to integrate activities of both providers; behavioral health providers seen by patient as adjunct to primary care team; service length is short by program design; primary care access standard used
7. Service penetration	6% or less due to small target population; time intensive delivery model	15% of entire primary care population; program capacity improved but limited by lack of pathways or general services	20% or more; program capacity great due to consultative services and multiple critical pathways
8. Referral and case finding impacts	Program has no appreciable impact (less than 10% reduction) on overall rate of physician referrals for specialty mental health; 25% or more patients enrolled in program referred on to specialty care	Program reduces physician referrals for specialty mental health by at least 25%; 20% or fewer patients enrolled in programs referred on to specialty care	Program reduces physician referrals for specialty mental health by at least 50%; 20% or fewer patients enrolled in program referred on to specialty care

of referral. This requires between 2 to 4 hours weekly consultation time for every 1,000 primary care patients, depending upon the characteristics of the population. A final caveat is that colocation of services does not in itself guarantee an integrative service philosophy, but it is a critical first step.

A second critical parameter is that the integrated service program show evidence of both evaluating and addressing the full spectrum of behavioral health needs within the primary care population. This requires the development of both horizontal and vertical integration programs, that are systematically interlaced. When resources are limited, it is possible to use the population-based planning framework to determine which vertical programs (critical pathways) are likely to have the largest impact on the population. Similarly, adopting a horizontal integration strategy in the form of a widely available general consultation program makes sense when the goal is to offer limited behavioral health services to a large proportion of the primary care population.

The main point here is that "integrated" behavioral health programs that tackle a small segment of the primary care population, no matter how appealing the social philosophy, simply do not "make the grade" in the larger picture of integrative system planning. Often, the marketing for such programs provides cost offset data (we saved $81,000) or patient enrollment data (3,200 patients have completed this lifestyle class) as a way of promoting the product. However, the background context is missing in terms of the percent of the total primary care population that is being served or the total primary care budget for that system. Without these comparison points, there is no way to really evaluate whether the program meets the population-based care standards already described.

In terms of developing industry standards, fully integrated systems should show evidence of delivering behavioral health services to 15% or more of the primary care population annually, using a combination of critical pathways and general behavioral health consultation services. While this figure seems high by specialty mental health standards, where annual penetration rates hover between 3 and 7%, it is important to remember that the annual penetration of primary care medical services is between 70 and 80%. Further, since the estimated behavioral health need in the primary care population is 70%, a 30% standard means that only 25% of the patients with probable need are entered into services. As integrative primary care systems mature, it is highly likely that this standard will be increased in a way that parallels our service expectations regarding childhood immunizations, breast cancer screening, and so forth. Similarly, the rate of patients referred by physicians directly into specialty mental health should decline. From the integrated service end, the percentage of patients referred out of primary mental health programs should be low, no more than 20%.

The degree to which behavioral health services are consistent with the philosophies, goals, and strategies of primary care is a subtle but powerful determinant of successful integration. For example, many systems have placed psychotherapists on site in primary care clinics, to provide specialty mental health care to physician referred patients. Physicians may receive intake reports, copies of session notes and may even participate in a conjoint session, when the occasion demands it. All parties will readily agree that collaboration between mental health and primary care providers is good, but is this an example of a model of care that is consistent with the primary care mission? In reality, this type of approach does little more than open a mental health specialty service in a primary care clinic. Responsibility for care shifts to the mental health provider, who fundamentally is seen as a treating specialist by the primary care team. Because of decades long segregation of mental health and primary care services, it is tempting to see such attributes as colocation or collaboration as sure signs that integrated care is occurring. If we use the philosophies, goals, and strategies of primary care as the yardstick, colocation and collaboration are necessary, but not sufficient to yield integrative care.

In fully integrated systems, behavioral health is not a specialty service, but is a routine component of medical care. A patient is just as likely to see a behavioral health consultant as he or she is to see a registered nurse during an appointment. The behavioral health provider is part of the primary care team, not part of a specialty mental health group located in the same professional office complex. The cost of primary mental health care is absorbed as a part of the patient's medical benefit. Accordingly, it is billed as a medical service, similar to laboratory, pharmacy, or nursing support services. At the level of medical service provision, behavioral health occupies a leading role in evidence-based practice algorithms. The patient with recurrent tachycardia is never referred to a cardiologist without first being evaluated for panic disorder. The patient who experiences a major life stress such as divorce, death of a parent, or recently diagnosed chronic illness is sent to the behavioral health consultant for prophylactic stress management and coping skills planning. Goals generated in consultation become part of the patient's general medical record and strategies are reinforced during all routine health care visits. The patient with recurrent major depression who recovers in response to integrated care provided by the behavioral health consultant and health care provider forms a relapse prevention plan that involves participation by the nurse, physician, and consultant. It is discussed during the primary care team meeting and becomes a part of the patient's priority health care objectives. There are many other examples of how the missions of primary care and behavioral health can be "seamlessly" integrated. Most importantly, the behavioral health provider functions as part of a system of medical care, and takes on the goals and strategies of primary health care. The advantages of such a system are obvious: better coordination of care, better clinical outcomes, reduced medical practice costs, and increased customer satisfaction. Perhaps most important, such a system would give primary care and behavioral health providers the opportunity to learn from each other so that the mind–body schism is forever sealed.

SUMMARY

In this chapter, the reader has been exposed to both a horizon and a compass. The horizon is a vision of integrated behavioral health primary care services that is based upon systematic population-based planning and a set of theoretically complementary approaches to integration. The vision ultimately involves melding primary health and mental health into a "seamless" system, that shares basic philosophies of care. The compass is designed to help us stay on track, at a time when the path to success is not clear. As we develop the first generation of integrated primary care behavioral health services, it is important to have mileposts to tell us whether we are journeying in the right direction. As a foil to the Chinese saying used earlier, we want to pick where we're headed, so that when we reach there, there is where we want to be.

PART II

Models of Integration

4.

Integration of Behavioral Health and Primary Care Services: The Group Health Cooperative Model

**Kirk Strosahl, Ph.D., Neil J. Baker, M.D.,
Mick Braddick, M.B., Ch.B.,
Michael E. Stuart, M.D., Matthew R. Handley, M.D.**

As the era of health care reform continues toward its second decade, there has been a steadily increasing interest in the integration of primary care and behavioral health services. The rationale for integration has been well described in the introductory chapters of this book. Suffice it to say that there are significant cost, clinical outcome, and customer satisfaction influences which are driving the integration initiative. What is still lacking at this point, however, are convincing demonstrations of full delivery system integration. While there are many

Acknowledgments. The development of the Group Health primary care behavioral health programs described in this chapter would not have been possible without the pioneering program development efforts of many Group Health Mental Health Department staff over the years. These pioneers include Dave Kanofsky, Ph.D., Patricia Robinson, Ph.D. and Greg Simon, M.D. Visionary leadership was provided by Dave Brubakken, Ph.D., who assembled the first primary care integration work group. Without the staunch, ongoing support of Mike Quirk, Ph.D. in his role as Mental Health Director, full implementation of integrated behavioral health services at Group Health would not have been possible. To all these courageous professionals, we are deeply indebted.

creative and praiseworthy programs that emphasize integration, few encompass the full spectrum of behavioral health needs known to exist in primary care populations. Many could be characterized as first generation pilot programs; in other cases, the program has matured and is oriented toward a single segment of the primary care population. These efforts have been both natural and necessary to help the development of the generally favorable view of integration that now exists in both the primary care and behavioral health sectors. What is needed to move into generation 2 is the development of specific delivery system models that are both effective and have the potential for widespread application in the behavioral health industry.

As was spelled out in the previous chapter, fully integrated behavioral health primary care systems must be able to have a wide spectrum impact on the health and mental health of the primary care population. They must essentially be "cost neutral" due to current trends toward shrinking behavioral health and primary care resources. They must be consistent with the mission of primary care and must have a workable service delivery model that allows behavioral health providers to practice in the same style as primary care providers. This type of integration can only be achieved through extended planning and effort over time. Such has been the case at Group Health Cooperative of Puget Sound, where the task integrating behavioral health and primary care services has been underway for nearly a decade. The purpose of this chapter is to describe the integrative primary care system at Group Health, using as a template the horizontal and vertical integration models described in chapter 3. First, we shall briefly review the primary mental health care service philosophy and how it supports both horizontal and vertical models of integration. Second, key attributes of our primary care behavioral health consultation service will be described. This, the Group Health Depression Clinical Roadmap will be discussed to highlight organization, systemic, and service philosophy issues that must be addressed to have a successful integration program. Finally, we will describe a program for disseminating a consistent set of primary mental health products throughout the Group Health delivery system, via the development of content and skill based training systems.

PRIMARY MENTAL HEALTH CARE: THE GROUP HEALTH MODEL OF INTEGRATED CARE

Delivering integrated behavioral health services within a specialty mental health model, even in an organizational context where brief therapy is a dominant approach, introduces a myriad of philosophical and logistical problems. These problems include inadvertently reinforcing the stereotypic separation of health and mental health, resistance by primary care patients, lack of capacity, and creating unmanageable demands on scarce mental health resources. As a cost and quality oriented alternative, we developed a primary mental health care service model which is conceptually similar to other consultation services that exist within most primary care clinics (Quirk et al., 1995; Strosahl, 1994a, 1994b, 1996a, 1996b). There are a variety of conceptual and related practice style issues that make this form of service dramatically different from traditional specialty mental health care. Undoubtedly the most important difference is the primary mental health care service philosophy, which emphasizes resolving behavioral health problems within the primary care service structure, as well as engaging in health promotion, relapse prevention, and preventive care for at-risk patients. In general, the defining strategy of the primary mental health care model is to position the behavioral health provider in a front line position, on a par with other primary care team members. Like other members of the team, the behavioral health specialist brings specialized knowledge to bear on problems that require additional expertise. Consistent with the primary care team philosophy, the physician or primary health care provider remains in charge of the patient's care. The activities of the behavioral health provider are always designed to support the interventions of the primary care provider. To summarize, the primary mental health model is tailored to and integrated within the process of routine primary health care

services. Referrals for behavioral health support can come from
any member of the primary care team. Depending upon the
practice settings, referrals may predominantly come from physicians, midlevel providers or nursing staff.

Addressing the needs of the primary care population from
using a consultation paradigm has dramatic implications for
both the mission and goals of integrative services as well as the
clinical practice of the behavioral health provider. Some of the
defining differences between this model of care and traditional

TABLE 4.1
**Distinguishing Characteristics of Primary and Specialty
Mental Health Care Models**

Dimension	Specialty M.H. Care	Primary M.H. Care
1. Mission	Provide specialty mental health care as adjunctive service to primary care	Provide primary care service focused on behavioral health issues
2. Location	In separate location or colocated in "mental health wing"	In medical practice area
3. Provider	Therapist	Health care provider
4. Service Modality	Psychotherapy session (individual, group, family), usually 50 minutes; length of treatment highly variable	Consultation session, 15 to 30 minutes long, usually 1 to 3 sessions
5. Team Membership	Specialty mental health peer review team	Primary care team
6. Primary Customer	Client, then other providers	Physician or referring provider, then client
7. Primary Service Goal	Resolve client's mental health issues as primary provider	Help physician and team to be more effective in treating client's mental health problem
8. Philosophy of Care	Behavioral health is a specialty service done outside the context of routine health care	Behavioral health is part of the process of general health care
9. Patient's Perception	Work with a specialist apart from primary health care context, a separate service	Looks like, feels like a routine aspect of health care

specialty mental health care are summarized in Table 4.1. In general, the behavioral health consultation model does not involve providing any extended mental health care to the patient. Most consultations involve a single visit with the patient, followed by immediate feedback about medication and/or psychological intervention strategies to the referring primary care provider (i.e., physician, physician's assistant, clinical nurse specialist, etc.). Any intervention strategies recommended to patients are simple, bite sized, and compatible with the types of interventions that can be provided in a 15-minute health care visit. It is also clear to the patient that the consultant is being used to help the health care provider and patient come up with an effective "plan of attack" to target the patient's concerns. Follow-up consultations (when appropriate and requested by the referring provider) are choreographed to reinforce and build upon the health care provider's interventions. The goal is to maximize the impact of a small number of visits to the consultant and health care provider. An important goal is to identify and monitor patients who show some type of behavioral health risk, in a manner which is very consistent with how primary care providers manage their at-risk patients. At all times, care is coordinated by the referring provider, who is still responsible for choosing and monitoring the results of interventions. The behavioral health consultant is also responsible for triage and referral to specialty mental health, in cases where the patient has failed to benefit from primary care-based services or obviously requires extended specialty care.

One advantage of the primary mental health model is that our consultants can deliver a wide array of clinical services, all within the consultation framework. Table 4.2 summarizes the core consultation services that we have found are frequently requested and valued by the primary care team.

Frequently requested services may involve providing assistance with treatment planning and monitoring, addressing community resource needs of patients (including specialty mental health referrals), follow-up consultation services as part of either a chronic or acute care treatment plan as well as services directed toward the staff itself to address team building or personnel issues.

TABLE 4.2
Frequently Requested Services In Primary Mental Health Care

Requested Service	Key Attributes
1. Behavioral Health Consultation	Initial 15- to 30-minute consultation visit for evaluation by prescribing or nonprescribing consultant; focus on diagnostic and functional evaluation, recommendations for medication and psychological treatment strategies for use by referring health care provider
2. Behavioral Health Follow-Up	Follow-up visit to review progress with a behavior change plan or treatment started by a primary care provider
3. Triage/Community Resource Visit	Visit designed to determine appropriate mental health specialty or community referral outside the care setting; usually a single visit
4. Treatment Compliance	Visit designed to help patient comply with medication initiated by provider; focus on education, addressing negative beliefs, or strategies for coping with side effects
5. Relapse Prevention	Visit designed to help patient who has responded to treatment to prevent recurrence
6. Integrated Care	Visit as part of "clinical pathway" patient education package conducted by consultant, usually in tandem with primary care provider, for high frequency conditions (depression, anxiety, somatization)
7. Case Management	Visit designed to support functioning in multiproblem patient; visits infrequent but continue over time; often part of a visit package that is designed to reduce unnecessary medical utilization
8. Behavioral Medicine	Visit designed to help patient cope with a chronic medical condition or those who are "at risk," emphasis on life-style issues/health risk factors
9. Patient-Physician Consultation	Visit with provider and patient designed to address working relationship

TABLE 4.2 (continued)

Requested Service	Key Attributes
10. Provider Consultation	Face-to-face visit with physician to discuss treatment planning issues; often involves "curbside" consultation; can include formal case conference with provider and health care team
11. Team Building	Meeting with members of the health care team to address peer relationships, job stress, or process of care issues
12. On Demand Consultation	Phone or face-to-face contact with provider, usually occurs with emergencies; focus on immediate care planning

Well conceived consultative services will eventually raise the skill level of the referring providers so that, over time, "routine" problems are handled effectively within the context of the routine medical visit. With consultative feedback regarding hundreds of patients with behavioral health issues, primary care providers begin to see the same themes recur in their panel of patients, and also gain first-hand experience using effective intervention strategies, while being supported by the primary mental health provider. Clinical experience as well as research suggest that integrated services improve the process of care for behavioral health issues including both medication practices and the more frequent and appropriate use of psychosocial intervention strategies.

HORIZONTAL SERVICE INTEGRATION

As was discussed in the previous chapter, integration models can be divided into those that attempt to provide a general response to the diverse needs of the primary care population (horizontal programs) and those that focus on a specific segment of the primary care population (vertical programs). Our experience at Group Health is that both types of programs are needed to accomplish the full integration of behavioral health and primary care services. In this section, we will describe the Primary Care Consultation Service, an example of a horizontally integrated system of care.

General Consultation Services

The platform of the Group Health Integrated Services Model is the general consultation service. In general, this service is available to any primary care patient that a physician or primary care provider is concerned about. The "see all comers" access philosophy both reduces the pressure on the health care provider to prescreen referrals and makes it clear that addressing behavioral health issues is a routine part of primary care service. The goal of the 30-minute consultation visit is to help the referring provider and patient work more effectively to target any behavioral health problems that have surfaced. The consultation model is very flexible in that it may involve the consultant, patient and primary care provider in any combination. Normally, the behavioral health specialist will see the patient and, less frequently, the patient and primary care provider together. The main service goal is to increase the impact of the provider's medication and psychosocial interventions. In order to achieve this objective, the consultant must develop intervention strategies that fit the "15-minute hour." In reality, the behavioral health intervention, whether it involves medications and/or behavioral strategies, must not consume more than 2 to 3 minutes of the health care visit, or it will not be seen as useful by the primary care provider. Typical consultative interventions are limited behavioral activation, psychoeducational readings, or initiating a medication and working briefly with the patient concerning compliance and side effects. If one to two follow-up consultations will help increase the chances of success, the consultant may see the patient again. In all such cases, it is clear that the consultant is not engaging in psychotherapy, and the primary care provider will remain responsible for all decisions concerning the patient's health and behavioral health care. In general, the average number of consultative visits per referred patient is two, with a range of one to three visits.

In the Group Health model, the general consultation service is the platform for all other integrated services. The limited visit span and compressed session length result in greatly expanded impact in the primary care population. For example, a consultant can see six to eight patients in a half day of practice, and still have time to provide face-to-face and written feedback to referring physicians. This capacity is amplified by a current service staffing ratio that calls for 2 hours of weekly consultation service for every 1,000 panel lives. A primary care group practice responsible for 10,000 patients would have 20 hours of scheduled consultation service weekly. The capacity of this service is 40 patients per week, meaning that between 15 and 20% of the entire primary care population could receive consultative behavioral health services on an annual basis. In order to further impact the behavioral health needs of primary care patients, current strategic planning calls for a doubling of this staffing ratio during 1997.

Eventually, we will begin to offer the consultative service option to patients who self-refer for specialty mental health services. This is being done because consumer focus groups at Group Health have suggested that approximately 70% of all consumers would actually prefer to receive behavioral health services at their primary care center. Shifting interested consumers to a primary care based consultation service not only carries promise of increasing consumer satisfaction, but may also allow patients who truly require specialized mental health services to access them more immediately. The long-term vision of the primary care and behavioral health leadership is to shift the locus of care for patients with routine mental health needs into primary care, while providing specialized services using a core group of more expensive, highly trained mental health providers in a multi-specialty mental health clinic.

One potential drawback of the consultation model is that it could become a gigantic "case finding" service, resulting in a deluge of referrals to specialty mental health. In fact, this has not been the case. Approximately 15 to 20% of all patients seen for behavioral health consultation are eventually referred for specialty mental health care. In view of the fact that these patients have already been clinically evaluated by the consultant, further efficiency is obtained by directly placing the patient with the "correct" specialty mental health provider based upon the consultant's recommendation.

Specialty Consultation

The specialty consultation level of primary mental health care
is for patients with chronic, multiple behavioral health and/
or medical illness that will require longer term management.
There are many groups of patients like this in primary care.
Some of the most common include patients with chronic, progressive diseases, personality disorders, long-term evolving
stress factors (i.e., caregiving for a parent with Alzheimer's disease), or high utilizers of medical services. In order to successfully manage these patients, consultative support is often
required over longer periods of time. For example, many patients with personality disorders also have serious medical problems that result from the condition itself (i.e., diabetes) and a
failure to comply with self-management programs. Many of
these patients are unwilling to accept a referral to specialty
mental health. They feel most comfortable working on their
many issues with the primary care team. The life circumstances
of this type of patient can change dramatically over time and
each change brings with it a challenge to the medical and behavioral health management team. Consequently, maintaining
a consultative presence over time increases the patient's sense
of continuity and helps primary care providers follow a consistent longer term approach. While more consultation visits may
occur over time, the service delivery structure is less concentrated (i.e., once quarterly) and may be continued over months
or years. Consultative interventions focus on care management
or community resource networking, managing unnecessary
medical utilization and working with the patient to improve
functional outcomes. At all times, the activities of the consultant are designed to help the primary care team efficiently
manage the patient's routine and emergent health and behavioral health care needs.

VERTICAL INTEGRATION AT GROUP HEALTH: THE
DEPRESSION ROADMAP

The hallmark of the vertical integration approach is that a
population with a specific disorder (e.g., depression) becomes

the focus of an organized process of care. The aim is to restructure the delivery of care throughout an entire health care system so that health care outcomes in four areas (health status, patient satisfaction, provider satisfaction, and cost/utilization) are improved (Handley & Stuart, 1994; Handley, Stuart, & Kirz, 1994; Stuart, Handley, Chamberlain et al., 1991; Stuart, Handley, Thompson et al., 1992). In prior years, Group Health has selected such clinical issues as diabetes management, heart disease prevention, use of lipid lowering agents, and smoking cessation as the focus of "clinical roadmap" projects. In approaching depression, the guideline is intended for the *entire* population in need, not just those patients presenting to mental health. Therefore, mental health and primary care must jointly assess and plan the delivery system changes which need to be made.

The Group Health model involves developing clinical guidelines to close gaps between current and optimal practice by bringing about changes in provider behavior (Handley & Stuart, 1994; Handley, Stuart, & Kirz, 1994; Stuart, Handley, Chamberlain, et al., 1991; Stuart, Handley, Thompson, et al., 1992). Guidelines are systematically developed statements to assist practitioners and patients in choosing appropriate health care for specific conditions. *Assist* is a key word—clinicians must have the latitude to make judgments about what is best in an individual situation. A guideline cannot be written to apply to every patient. There are very few circumstances in which "rules" or "standards" are appropriate.

Organizational, Systemic, and Service Planning Considerations

It is through guideline development and implementation that the information and tools necessary to treat depression in primary care are brought to the decision-making frontline. An integrated care system for depression is not possible without a comprehensive, systematic approach involving multiple layers and components of the delivery system. In the process of developing a comprehensive process of care for depression, or any

disorder, organizational, systemic, and service philosophy issues inevitably surface that need to be addressed and resolved.
In this section, the critical elements for success of such systemwide organizational change will be identified. Emphasis will be
on the types of issues that must be addressed, rather than an in-
depth review of what the evidence is that supports a particular
conclusion to a clinical process question.

Topic Selection—Suitability for Delivery Systemwide Efforts. Suitability is a critical question because we have limited resources
for improvement efforts and we want to know that there is a
likelihood of significant improvement in the four outcome areas. We must know that we can measure a proposed change,
that internal data establish a gap between current and optimal
practice, and that an initial overview of the literature provides
evidence on which a guideline can be based. The suitability of
depression as a roadmap condition was based upon epidemiological research done within Group Health by the Center for
Health Studies. Various studies suggested that approximately
14% of enrollees in a primary care system suffer either major
or minor depression, while 6 to 8% of patients presenting for
care have major and minor depressions. Of these, 80% initiate
treatment in primary care. Primary care providers recognize
80% of patients with major depression as "cases" of psychological disorder while identifying 50% of cases involving minor
depression (Simon & VonKorff, 1995a). Most patients (65%)
with major depression will not only be recognized, but will elect
to initiate treatment with their primary care provider. Other
studies have shown that patients with depression have a 40%
relapse rate and 7 to 10 disability days per month as opposed to
8 days per year for asymptomatic patients. In addition, patients
identified with some form of depression are 4 times more likely
than the rest of the population to have coronary artery disease
and two times more likely to have diabetes. Depressed patients
are also more likely to smoke.

Randomized controlled studies involving more than 900
Group Health patients (Katon, VonKorff, et al., 1995; Katon,
Robinson, et al., 1996; Simon et al., 1996) clearly demonstrated
a gap between current and optimal outcomes; only 40% of

patients starting on antidepressants achieve 50% or more reduction in symptoms by 4 months of treatment compared to 70% achieving this level of reduction in structured research programs. These studies also demonstrated the potential capacity to measure changes which might be implemented delivery systemwide. In addition, the studies were unique in measuring not just health status outcomes but also improvements in patient satisfaction.

Focus groups of patients who had received treatment for depression at Group Health also suggested that care processes were highly variable and this had a direct effect on consumer satisfaction. These enrollees perceived that Group Health had no unified program of treatment even though they had a high level of confidence in their individual providers.

Finally, organizational costs were a major force in the development of the depression roadmap. The introduction of SSRI drugs, combined with a growing awareness of recognizing and treating depression, resulted in more and more primary care physicians prescribing antidepressants, to the point that SSRI drug costs accounted for $1/7$ of the entire pharmacy budget for the GHC population (500,000 enrollees). The costs generated a controversy within and between medical clinics concerning the appropriate use of new antidepressants. Not only were costs an issue, but research within the GHC delivery system suggested that fully half of all patients started on antidepressants actually might have minor depression, i.e., patients who in structured interviewing did not meet criteria for major depression (Katon, VonKorff, et al., 1995; Katon, Robinson, et al., 1996). Should these patients with mild depression be started on antidepressants? Should all of them receive a behavioral health consultation prior to prescription of medication?

Buy-in of Medical and Administrative Leaders. Creating systemwide change inevitably involves so many parts of the organization that it is absolutely critical for senior medical and administrative leaders to "buy into" the need for complete organizational change. These leaders must "own" the guideline and accept accountability for its success. This is best accomplished through consistent involvement of senior leadership at key stages of development and implementation. The determination of which topics are suitable for an evidence-based improvement process and final selection for a roadmap is made through structures which involve these medical and administrative leaders. By the time implementation occurs, the leaders have been exposed to the key delivery systems questions and solutions many times. It is truly their roadmap.

Assembling the Teams. To achieve significant organizational change, guidance is required from steering committees and senior decision-making bodies. Ultimately, however, the guideline team is the single most important entity in developing a set of coherent recommendations regarding the treatment of depression. At Group Health, the guideline team is responsible for defining the problem, posing questions to the medical literature, retrieving and evaluating the literature, creating evidence tables, synthesizing the evidence, reviewing organizational data, and drafting the guideline. In addition, they develop a program implementation and evaluation plan as the roadmap is "rolled out" into the delivery system.

Assembling an effective guideline team is a critical step toward implementation. The guideline development process should involve key clinical opinion leaders both in the health and behavioral health systems. Maintaining integrity in distinguishing conclusions based on expert opinion versus conclusions based on systematic grading of evidence is a core value of our process. Credibility of the guideline is at stake. Opinion leaders play an important role in promoting acceptance of the guideline, even in the numerous controversial areas that exist in the depression literature.

The depression guideline team involved two primary care physicians and a pharmacist, in addition to several mental health representatives. Several nationally known researchers from the University of Washington and from the Group Health Center for Health Studies also served as consultants to the guideline team. As might be expected, the team represented a wide range of viewpoints. The ability to generate conclusions based on consistent criteria and values have contributed strongly to the initial positive reaction we have received to the guideline.

Group Health has chosen an explicit evidence-based process for evaluating the medical literature rather than reviewing and revising outside guidelines. All of the evidence in a topic area is reviewed systematically through a careful grading of the study by design (i.e. randomized controlled study vs. historical cohort vs. case series) and external validity, which is a by-product of general methodological rigor (Handley & Stuart, 1994).

As Eddy (1993, 1994) has discussed, guidelines developed by consensus of experts inevitably contain significant biases. It is simply not possible for individuals to consider an entire body of literature that they have not systematically analyzed. An anticipated change in outcomes is more likely to occur when based on multiple randomized controlled studies than when based on such "gestalt" of the evidence. This scientific way of looking at the evidence impacts on one of the most crucial aspects of the decision-making environment. Providers want to believe that there is evidence for what they do, that the benefits and risks have been adequately studied. Yet, few providers have the time or expertise for completing a critical review of the literature. Instead, we have been acculturated into a system which emphasizes personal experience, reasoning based on pathophysiology or expert opinion. These methods can lead to overestimating benefits and underestimating harms or costs.

Our emphasis on randomized controlled clinical trials is not without its difficulties. Controlled trials may not yield similar results or may not even be feasible to answer certain key clinical questions. Ultimately, the quality of the guideline depends on the quality of the team which meshes expert opinions with graded evidence. This is particularly true in the area of depression, where there are many controversies about which type of treatment works the best, what types of patients are best suited for a treatment, and which treatments produce the best long-term benefits.

Develop a Cost Model. Ideally, cost modeling incorporates scientific evidence and organizational data to provide a summary of the benefits, harms, and costs of different practices. The guideline team projects what changes in health outcomes would occur with the recommended practice changes. Looking at the current cost of treating depression, we were unable to construct a specific balance sheet because neither mental health nor primary care providers made reliable diagnoses of major or minor depression. Patients received treatment under more general diagnostic categories (e.g., Depression NOS, V-codes, etc.). This simply reflected the very reason for engaging in a roadmap project in the first place. As a result, the first year of guideline implementation will allow us to collect baseline data on the costs of treating depression in both the specialty mental health and primary care populations. For the present, research within Group Health can inform us regarding such population indicators as the prevalence and ratios of major to minor depression diagnoses. These benchmarks can be used to detect any pattern of over- or underdiagnosis within our system, pending the time when more formalized assessment data allow us to create more precise expectations. Further benchmarks involve the percentage of patients with major or minor depression who receive either tricyclic antidepressant (TCA) or serotonin-specific reuptake inhibitor (SSRI) medication. Employing readily available initial indicators will help us make early determinations about the impact of the depression guideline, especially in primary care practice settings, where the majority of diagnosis and medication treatment occurs.

CLINICAL CONTROVERSIES: AN EVIDENCE-BASED APPROACH TO RESOLUTION

As might be expected, the development of a clinical practice guideline for depression will raise many controversial issues. Some of these issues can be answered by the literature, some can only be approached by melding slim or nonexistent research with expert opinion. To establish a firm base of evidence for these sometimes difficult discussions, the guideline team assembled over 7,000 abstracts, reviewed over 500 articles, and constructed approximately 150 evidence tables. To highlight the importance of this process to conflict resolution and acceptance of the guideline by both primary care and behavioral health practitioners, it will be useful to examine some key controversies that were addressed.

Should Patients with Minor Depression Receive Drugs or Therapy?

We could not find evidence to support the routine use of medications or psychotherapy in minor depression (in our guideline this includes DSM-IV dysthymia and depression NOS). There was considerable sentiment among some experts to separate dysthymia and recommend the use of antidepressants for this disorder. Unfortunately, studies looking at treatments for dysthymia are quite limited and are generally small in size, with varying diagnostic criteria, widely varying minimum severity criteria, and methodological flaws (Baker, Stuart, & Braddick, submitted a).

While the evidence did not provide guidance in the treatment of minor depression (including dysthymia), both the mental health and primary care providers on the team were quite concerned that these patients "receive something." Such patients can be quite distressed and can demand expensive treatments (e.g., with antidepressants, particularly SSRIs). Also, the diagnostic criteria for major depression are not precise and patients with prodromal symptoms, patients who have not fully recovered from a previous episode, or patients with recurrent illness who are decompensating might be missed. The team was in agreement that all patients should first receive help with a program of self-care with physician support and careful follow-up. Further, if patients with minor depression did not improve with active support/self-care over 1 to 4 weeks, a general behavioral health consultation should be considered to assist in further care planning which then might include an antidepressant or further psychotherapy. Thus, the primary care consultation service is a crucial component of the process of evaluation and treatment of patients with minor depression.

Can Major Depression Be Treated In Primary Care?

For major depression, there was strong evidence that medications or psychotherapy provide significantly better outcomes than no treatment or control interventions. In particular, several studies demonstrated that structured clinical protocols used by primary care providers and supporting behavioral health specialists resulted in significantly better outcomes than usual care alone (Katon, Robinson, et al., 1996; Katon, Von-Korff, et al., 1995). Effective primary care based treatment programs for depression typically incorporate a cognitive behavioral approach that emphasizes patient education, depression management strategies, personal problem solving skills, compliance with medication and strategies for managing side effects (Robinson, 1996). This is combined with on-site behavioral health consultation available to treating primary care providers and to assist patients in their self-management efforts (Robinson, Wischman, & Del Vento, 1996).

SSRIs vs. TCAs

The most controversial topic in the guideline concerned the class of antidepressant medications which should be used as the "frontline" treatment of depression. The evidence reviewed suggested that SSRIs and TCAs are equally effective but SSRIs have a lower discontinuation rate due to side effects (I. Anderson & Tomenson, 1995; Baker, Stuart, Braddick, & Simon, submitted b; Simon, VonKorff, Barlow, Pabiniak, & Wagner, 1996). The only prospective review of cost differential between classes of medications was done within our own clinics and demonstrated significantly greater drug costs for SSRIs (Simon et al., 1996). We concluded that, in the absence of medical contraindications, TCAs should be considered first for initial antidepressant treatment based on cost considerations.

ROADMAP IMPLEMENTATION

Roadmap implementation begins with a systematic consideration of the nature of current practice and how the roadmap process can change current practices (Handley, Stuart, & Kirz,

1994; Stuart et al., 1991). At multiple levels (organization, systemic, individual practice) there are always influences promoting use of the guideline by providers and restraining forces which impede adoption of practice changes. For example, the forces promoting change in current practice include feedback from patients who want consistent educational materials and more supportive care, strong evidence that structured primary care based treatment improves outcomes for major depression, the cost implications on a clinic basis of using SSRIs when less expensive, equally effective drugs exist. Restraining forces include strong advertising influences on patients who in turn pressure physicians for SSRIs, expert opinion preferences for SSRIs, expert opinion advocating medication treatment of minor depression and dysthymia, the need for additional education and training programs for physicians in the algorithm and evidence, the use of new diagnostic tools, and active support of patients in a program of care that might require additional medical visits.

To maximize the influence of "prochange forces," the depression roadmap includes components which are made available to all providers at Group Health. Many of these components are designed to make change "easy," and to remove unnecessary obstacles to adhering to the guideline.

Clinical Decision Support for Providers

All providers have a computer which gives them the algorithm, explanatory notes, and evidence tables. The decision support modules address all stages of care, from accurate diagnosis of depression, to treatment indications, to data addressing the cost implications of different treatment options, to recommendations regarding follow-up care and strategies for preventing relapse. The system also contains computer generated patient education handouts. Most importantly, the system is designed to insure easy access to primary care providers, so that it can be incorporated into the 4- to 5-minute time frame available during a typical medical visit. Behavioral health consultants working in primary care practice teams also have access to the same system, so they can support primary care providers in decision making under the guideline.

Continuing Education Programs

Grand rounds and other large continuing medical education (CME) offerings have been and will be used to generate awareness and bring providers together for informal discussions. On a clinic by clinic basis, there is a CME offering in which providers role-play use of the diagnostic tool as well as active support for patients within a program of self-care. As a stimulus for the role-playing, they will observe both an experienced primary care physician and psychiatrist using these tools. Behavioral health consultants in each clinic also attend a related course which teaches them how to provide consultation with physician referred depressed patients, thus enhancing use of the guideline and supporting materials.

Academic Detailing

This procedure involves one-to-one conversations between an "expert" local opinion leader who is chosen to champion the roadmap and another primary care provider in the same practice group. The goal is to both teach the provider to use new clinical strategies through the use of information and evidence and to counteract various influences that may impede the provider's willingness to change.

Opinion Leaders

Multiple studies have shown that individuals who are respected as clinicians and advisors may frequently assist in clinical practice change implementation. As described, opinion leaders were selected to be part of the guideline team. The physician leading this project will be present on a regular basis at the pilot site for support and consultation. Local opinion leaders are also identified, to "champion" the use of the guideline at the level of daily practice.

Systematic Feedback

Provider specific and peer comparison feedback is absolutely crucial to influencing practice change. Initially, primary care providers receive information about numbers of patients diagnosed with major or minor depression, the ratio of major to minor depressives diagnosed within a practice, as well as the ratio of SSRI to TCA prescriptions. This allows comparisons to be made within a medical practice group as well as among clinics. While there is no "gold standard" implied in these data, the effect is to pull practitioners and clinics closer together so that between-practice and among-clinic variation in the treatment of depression is reduced.

Clinical Process Redesign

At the system level, clinical process redesign incorporates many of the changes in provider expectations previously discussed and, at the same time, builds a system that can sustain this change through the provision of equipment, facilities, and structural aids to practice. For example, the guideline recommendation to detect major depression requires the availability of a primary care "friendly" diagnostic tool, a way of establishing severity, readily available patient education materials, to name only a few. Many attempts to change systems of care fail because the "tools of the new trade" are simply not thought through at the applied level. A primary component of the Group Health depression roadmap is the infrastructure necessary to support changes in primary care practice.

Patient Tracking System

Diagnostic and treatment information will be provided on individual patients through use of a patient tracking system which is computer based. Both primary care and behavioral health providers are expected to document a diagnosis of major and minor depression which will eventually become part of a computerized "depression registry" as a routine part of visit information. Along with computerized records of visits and pharmacy information, primary care providers will receive information about whether the patient obtained refills and if medication dosages are within the recommended ranges. Patients who have not had visits within the time frames recommended by the guideline will be highlighted for providers.

Consumer Education

This component involves an active outreach program to Group Health consumers, with the intent of educating them regarding the philosophies and decision-making basis of the guideline and how it is implemented by the primary care provider. For example, one of the most popular recent outreach efforts was a public lecture on a new depression guideline which was advertised to patients through our information lines.

Outcomes and Process of Care Measurement

There are two fundamental outcomes that are being sought in the depression roadmap. First, we hope to close the gap between current and optimal practice in the treatment of depression in primary care. Second, we assume this improved process of care will result in more favorable clinical outcomes. However, to verify that these goals have been attained, as well as to engage in a cycle of continuous improvement, the roadmap must be informed by an ongoing process of outcome and process of care information. Our initial systemwide plan involves the establishment of baseline diagnoses and treatment with medications. Subsequently, we will be able to measure outcomes through use of changes within each patient using the depression severity tool. Ongoing consumer satisfaction surveys will tell us whether Group Health consumers feel they are receiving quality care from their primary care and behavioral health providers.

The Group Health depression roadmap represents a fundamentally different approach to integrating the primary care and behavioral health treatment of depression. In a sense, it brings together two different "players" who have much to say about the quality of depression treatment in primary medical care. Capitalizing on an organizational commitment to a fully integrated delivery system, and a specific model of care to guide us, success in improving the clinical and functional outcomes of depressed primary care patients seems highly likely.

TECHNOLOGY TRANSFER: THE KEY TO PRODUCT FIDELITY

Developing methods for disseminating the primary health care service philosophy and "product line" throughout the Group Health delivery system has been a major focus of both senior leadership and program developers. Two key issues have emerged which have guided development of the Group Health technology transfer package. First, we needed to develop consistent service definitions, associated service policies, and core administrative mechanisms. Second, we needed to address the fact that line clinicians consistently expressed a need for training in behavioral health consultation practices.

The Consultation Service Product Manual

A product manual approach was taken to address the issues associated with building consistent service philosophies, definitions, policies, and core administrative processes. For example, the manual spells out the core ingredients of effective consultation with primary care providers and lists a series of steps clinicians should take to start up and maintain effective practices within the primary care team. The manual details what consultative services are to be offered and describes the role of different disciplines within the consultation service. Service policies are also articulated. For example, there is a consistent stance all consultants are to take when a primary care provider asks them to provide psychotherapy, instead of consultation, to a patient. Core administrative processes are also listed. For example, the product manual details how a consultation visit is to be counted against the patient's mental health benefit and how any copayment is to be calculated and collected.

Taken as a whole, the product manual serves as an "end users" manual for clinicians, managers, primary care support staff, and system administrators. It creates a consistent set of service expectations and administrative procedures specific to the behavioral health consultation service. Most importantly, the product manual approach allows the general consultation "product" to be implemented in different practice settings with a high degree of fidelity.

Clinical Training Package

The clinical training package developed for Group Health mental health providers is both cost effective and results in increased provider competence in the delivery of general consultation to primary care providers. The training package emphasizes both content and the development of clinical skills using a mentoring system. The content requirements are to know the basic features of the primary mental health care philosophy, how it differs from specialty mental health, how to work with patients and providers in highly abbreviated time frames, how to write a good consultation report, to name only a few. This information is delivered in a workshop format, replete with both written examples and videotaped demonstrations of real consultation sessions. The goal of the workshop is to give mental health providers the basic information needed to be effective in delivering the various primary mental health-care products.

The only way to assure that basic knowledge is being converted into effective clinical practice is to provide in vivo training using a supervised practice model. The mentoring model used at Group Health involves pairing an "expert" consultant with a "novice" trainee. The expert first demonstrates appropriate consultative practices in a normal daily practice environment. This allows the trainee to see a variety of patients and different consultative issues emerging in routine clinical practice, along with the expert consultant's way of handling various practice demands. After an appropriate period of time (usually four half-day sessions), the roles are reversed. The expert observes the practice of the trainee and offers supervisory input, again for perhaps four half-day sessions. Throughout the process, expert and trainee discuss a wide range of clinical, policy, and administrative process issues, as they surface in the context of providing patient care. These content issues are also reinforced in the product manual described earlier, which serves as a reference during the training process. Before a trainee can "graduate," he or she must be evaluated by the expert as meeting competence criteria on a number of different clinical practice dimensions. Throughout the training process, the expert and novice are discussing these competency parameters and identifying areas of strength and weakness in the trainee's performance.

Because Group Health has a geographically and structurally diverse delivery system, the training package was developed to "train trainers." Graduates of the mentoring program are also taught mentoring skills that they will be expected to apply when they train other "novices." In this way, the panel of consultation experts widens throughout the delivery system. Local clinics and group practices always have access to a consultation expert, who not only provides the same type of training, but also acts as a local "champion" for the consultation service and keeps other providers abreast of new products, policies and administrative processes.

SUMMARY

In this chapter, we have attempted to highlight the key features of the primary mental health care model at Group Health Cooperative of Puget Sound. It should be noted that this approach has evolved over the years and, in many respects, is a living process. We fully expect that as our experience with integrated primary care behavioral health services grows, new service philosophies will appear, new products will be developed, and we will continue on toward our goal of building a seamless interface between health and behavioral health services. While this would be a crowning achievement for many of us professionally, the real beneficiaries are the consumers of health services, who no longer would be confronted by the artificial division of services and stigmatization that is still apparent today.

5.

The Emergence of New Possibilities for Medical Practice, and the Relation to Environmental Change

Matthew A. Budd, M.D.

A nation's armies can repel an invader from its borders, but no force can resist an idea whose time has come.

Voltaire

Behavioral medicine, characterized as it is by its holistic and integrative focus toward patients, is historically well positioned not only to deliver much needed care to our society, but also to serve as a catalyst for the next stage of development of our health care organizations.

Kuhn (1962) in his now classic work, *Structure of Scientific Revolutions,* points out several patterns of change in human practice. First, there is incremental change of practice to meet new needs, demands, and adjustments. This is sometimes referred to as first order change. Then there is another kind of change in which basic philosophic assumptions are supplanted by new structures of understanding which organize the activity around ongoing human concerns to a higher level of effectiveness and satisfaction. These changes threaten contemporary

power structures, and force structural change in the very culture that generates the shift. The new ways of thinking may be
theoretical, but the social practices that they generate become
anchored with recurrent use. A new "common sense" emerges
with secondary reformulation of the professional and social
structures that are involved in supporting the behavior.

These underlying structures are thought of as "invisible
fabrics" of assumption that guide action. We are at a moment
in medical history when the social and economic pressures being exerted on the health care industry are revealing basic
limitations in our way of thinking about health and illness and
these forces are encouraging the development of new understandings about health and illness, really about human beings
themselves, that will reshape care delivery in the future. These
changes are part of a larger revolution in the thinking about
human nature itself that has roots in biologic (Maturana,
1972), philosophic (Heidegger, 1962), physical (Zohar, 1990;
Bohm, 1992), educational, and organizational (Greenleaf,
1977) thinking.

This chapter will outline some of the basic assumptions of
the traditional thinking about human nature and illness and
will propose a new model for thinking about people. Then it
will describe a learning program that has been designed in the
new paradigm. While this new program was being developed
and tested, it was implemented within an organizational setting
that was governed by "rules" that supported the old paradigm.
A new program is sensed as "foreign" by a traditional organization much as a foreign protein will be sensed as foreign by the
body. An "institutional stress" results that can be addressed
either by denial or resistance, or by the development of new
and compatible organizations. This chapter will conclude by
outlining some of the organizational principles that can support a new kind of health care and demonstrate a striking similarity between the new organization and the new view of health
care that generated the program itself.

THE OLD PARADIGM: BASIC ASSUMPTIONS

The paradigm in which medical care is delivered, in which
physicians and other health professionals are trained, and in

which patients themselves build their expectations has come to be known as the Cartesian paradigm. In the 16th century the medieval notion of an organic, spiritual universe was supplanted by a mechanistic or mechanical view of the world whose new deity was rational analysis. This was embodied in the following quotation:

> I . . . am a thinking thing. And although . . . I have a body with which I am closely *conjoined* I have, on the one hand a clear and distinct idea of myself as a thinking non-extended thing, and on the other hand a distinct idea of my body as an extended, non-thinking thing; it is therefore certain that I am truly distinct from my body, and can exist without it. (René Descartes, *Passions of the Soul*)

Translated to medical care, this worldview leads to three basic assumptions:

The Mind–Body Dichotomy

In this understanding, the mind and the body are separate, in fact governed by different rules, and made of different substance. The body can be understood by mechanical (later chemical and biochemical) principles. The mind is governed by spiritual and other principles, which are nonmechanistic. The sense of this point of view is that mind matters and body matters are separate, and not connected.

Understanding of Parts

In this set of assumptions, the behavior of whole organisms can be understood fully by understanding the function of their parts. This set of assumptions has been the underpinning of the "reductionistic" approach which reduces the understanding of wholes to the understanding of its parts. The parts are best understood in scientific terms: anatomic, physiologic, chemical, biochemical, and biophysical.

The Professional Corollary

Since professionals are trained in the language and distinctions of the parts, and understand the mechanisms involved in the function of organs, their knowledge and actions are likely to affect health outcomes powerfully. Whereas the patient understands only the function of the whole, his or her self-knowledge is less powerful and peripheral.

The introduction of this chapter emphasized that paradigmatic shift and the making of new and valuable offers go hand in hand. In fact, the vast array of effective treatments that mechanistic medicine has developed are staggering. We can prevent, cure, transplant, and control many of the historic scourges of mankind. It should be recalled also from the introduction that as contextual demands shift, paradigmatic weakness is revealed, and the need for a thought shift develops. Managed care has been a major provocateur in the development of a new way of thinking about health, wellness, and illness.

Managed care, for the sake of this conversation, can be seen as a commitment to deliver health care to a population of people, not to a population of patients (here defined as people with disease). Moreover, the commitment includes an obligation to do so with resource conservation. Thus prevention and self-care become central to the mission of managed care, alongside the appropriate application of technology.

Many formal studies (Kroenke, 1989) have shown beyond doubt that a considerable portion of a managed care population that seeks care does so for symptoms that cannot be diagnosed as body diseases. In these cases, the lesion is a dysfunction of wholes, not a diagnosable problem with parts. Additionally, it is well-documented that emotions such as anger, depression, and anxiety actually can result in real disease. For example, anger is a major cardiac risk factor (Williams & Williams, 1995), and depression interferes with immunity. These mood states are examples of predispositions of wholes, affecting health in a negative way, and if ignored increasing both human suffering and medical care costs.

Reductionistic thinking also has little to add in the preventive domain in which a behavior or ontological shift of whole people is the desired objective. Smoking, alcoholism and drug addiction are problems of whole organisms, not isolated parts, and cannot be effectively treated by our reductionistic-based treatments. Drawing from the work of others (Edelman, 1992; Maturana, 1987; Wingrod, 1986), there can be brought to health care a notion of human life that includes the possibility for reductionistic intervention, but also provides a basis for holistic interventions. The next section will describe the basic assumptions behind this new way of thinking, then further describe a program that has been developed to allow people to engage in deep behavioral change.

A NEW WAY OF THINKING: BASIC ASSUMPTIONS

There are three basic pillars that support our work as manifest in the Personal Health Improvement Program (PHIP) which will be described subsequently. In contrast to the Cartesian mind–body duality, our notion is that a human is a "self-generating biologic system of knowing." The three foundational constructs are the following:

People Are Biologic Beings

The great Chilean biologist Humberto Maturana (1987) put forth the thesis that biologic systems, including human beings, are "closed systems of knowing." His investigations of color perception led to his discovery that the nervous system operates as a closed network of interactions in which every change of relationships among certain components always results in a change of the interactive relationships among the same or other components.

In plain talk, the nervous system (the entire body, for that matter) does not take information from the outside in, but is available for coupling to the environment according to the universe of reactions possible for the particular structure at the moment in time. The activities of nerve cells do not reflect an environment independent of the living organism and hence do not allow for the construction of a separate external reality. What is known is a function of what can be known given a particular moment in one's life, not what it is possible to know, or what someone else knows.

People Are Historic Beings

If we call the inherited structure that we are born with our "first nature," then our "second nature" is a reflection of all of the learning, or structural modifications that our structure undergoes in the course of living. This is what the philosopher and physician Medard Boss calls our "biohistory." People act in particular ways structurally supported by an amalgamation of their first and second natures. These two natures generate how we take care of concerns like career, education, shelter, transportation, etc. But in another sense these structurally-based actions can be a trap; people's perceptions can be damaging to their self-esteem, corroding to their relationships, and crippling to their self-efficacy. The work of Edelman (1992) and others gives a plausible biologic model for the structural modifications in the nervous system that occur with learning. External events "trigger" the altered structural elements in the nervous system which are then manifested in different thoughts, emotions, actions, and perceptions.

People Live in Language

Heidegger (1962) said that human beings live in a "house of language." He meant by this that people are immersed and created by linguistic acts. In language people bring forth a social space of living where they dwell together. When we make a "request," we potentially build a piece of life together with another human being. When we make a promise, we build a future cocommitment with another and we open the possibility of betrayal, anger, and resentment. The declaration, "I am incompetent and will not attain much," does not describe something external, but rather brings forth an array of actions consistent with the declaration that constitutes an external manifestation of "self." There is another fascinating consequence of "living in language," i.e., self reflection and awareness. As described by Capra (1996), our linguistic distinctions are not isolated but exist in the network of structural couplings that we continually weave through language. Meaning arises as a pattern of relationships among these linguistic distinctions and thus we exist in a semantic domain created by our language. Finally, self-awareness arises when we use the notion of an object and the associated abstract concepts to describe ourselves. Thus the linguistic domain of human beings expands further to include reflection and consciousness. These, then, are the three pillars of the PHIP program. They provide a non-dualistic (in the Cartesian sense) framework for observation of behavior and change. These concepts are consistent with certain philosophical and psychological principles, but they have the exquisite advantage that they are grounded and validated by the best of current neurobiologic research, thus returning to firm biological footing the initial concern to relieve human suffering.

The Personal Health Improvement Program (PHIP)

The PHIP program is an improved version of the Ways to Wellness program which was developed at the Harvard Community Health Plan (now HPHC) 13 years ago. More than 3,000 people have gone through the program. Five evaluations have been performed (Colasante, in press; Glick, in press; Hellman, Budd, Borysenko, McClelland, & Benson, 1990; McClelland, in press; McLeod, in press) which describe patient results in this program.

The program is a 6-session learning experience. The classes are led by facilitators specifically trained for this and come from a variety of professional backgrounds: physicians, physician assistants, social workers, psychologists, nurses, and health educators. There is a detailed "facilitators guide."

Instruction is given in meditation, and at every session the participants are encouraged to practice it daily. It is represented as a cornerstone activity facilitating learning. In the classroom at least six kinds of activities occur: (1) New distinctions regarding how the mind works and how moods arise are presented in video "master teacher" format. (2) Patients interact with the material by listening, questioning, and reflecting on their behavior and their thoughts in light of these distinctions. (3) Patients perform classroom exercises, allowing them to experience some of the distinctions in actions. (4) They listen to the reports of others engaging in the same learning, and learn from this. (5) They are given elaborate daily homework assignments, thus allowing them to practice the work of the course. (6) They begin each session with an open sharing of the questions and experiences that arose as they did their homework.

At the HPHC setting, most patients are referred by their primary care physician because together they suspect that "stress" or emotional upset is playing a role in generating their symptoms, or altering the course of their chronic disease. Many patients are referred for unique circumstances which have resulted in upset such as job loss or change, divorce, recent diagnosis of chronic illness, recent heart attack, winning the lottery, workplace conflicts, accident prone-ness, addiction recovery, living with cancer and AIDS, etc.

HOW PEOPLE INTERACT WITH THE PHIP PROGRAM

It is useful to indicate from experience with this program some of the ways that people interact with this learning experience. The following are some of the observed patterns:

Failure to Be Referred, or Failure to Accept Referral to the Course

By best estimates, a tiny fraction of patients in a managed care population who could benefit from the course are actually referred. A state of "cognitive blindness" to mind–body issues or unwillingness to raise "personal" matters on the part of clinicians is certainly one factor. Remember that "all" currently practicing physicians have been trained in a rigidly Cartesian paradigm, and only "marginal" individuals think in a holistic paradigm. Additionally, resistance of the patient to a nonphysical solution, or fear of being labeled "crazy" is sometimes present. Clinician skill in addressing and allaying these fears and in building trusting partnership relationships with patients helps to mitigate these barriers.

Engagement with a Learning Program

The serious learning challenge presented by the program brings to the surface three kinds of resistances:

(1) "I can't learn." Many people have the assumption that we have fixed personalities and can't change. (2) "I don't see how this learning can help my problem anyhow. How can a mental program help my physical problem?" As we teach the course, we must remember that patients live in the same Cartesian paradigm as all of us. This program challenges this "common sense" as well as the tendency of people to want a quick fix medical solution. (3) "The problem isn't me, it's my former spouse." We all live under the illusion that if we could have the world be just right, then we could be happy and satisfied. But it never is. The challenge of mature living is to produce satisfaction in our lives by expanding the limits of our possibilities, and building trusting networks of people around us. Role modeling by the course leaders, which includes engaging stories about themselves, helps the students to gradually suspend doubt and begin to learn.

Assuming "Beginner's Mind"

In Eastern cultures the state of acknowledgment of "not know mind" is a state of high attainment. We sometimes call this being "open" to learning. To us in our culture this looks like revealing incompetence publicly rather than seeing it as an opportunity. In the course, this issue is addressed repeatedly and the leaders strive to have "inquiry not answers" be the mantra. A mood of inquiry and dialogue facilitates learning, in contrast to the conversation-collapsing tendency of a search for answers.

Learning with Dignity

A major issue for learners in any domain is that as one starts to learn one is uncertain, makes mistakes, and even (in one's own eyes) looks foolish. In fact, this is not a property of a particular learner, but of all learners. As one begins to learn and to build a new structure (vide supra) there is a long period of transition going from beginner, to competent, to expert. Along the way one stumbles. It is emphasized over and over that this sequence is natural and expected, and reflects the learner's commitment rather than incompetence. The course further emphasizes commitment, not an absence of mistakes.

Learning to Learn

The distinction is made in the course between representational learning, and true learning. The ability to recite a menu, for example, is not equivalent to competence in cooking a meal. Yet the Cartesian view restricts one's ability to see this aspect of learning in its fullest dimension. In the course it is emphasized that learning occurs in new practices, when practiced recurrently over time with self-reflection, and more importantly with coaching. The course talks about how to find teachers, and when to build the trust necessary for learning.

It is the deep conviction of the author that the act of becoming a learner in areas of certainty and rigidity is more important to behavioral change than even the material of the course. In the course room one experiences this shift from rigidity to openness as an almost physical experience, the creation of a human environment, in which intimacy, sharing, and a thirst for inquiry flourish.

Results of the PHIP Course

The course has been studied in groups of patients referred with varied complaints (Edelman, 1992; McClelland, in press; McLeod, in press), patients with irritable bowel syndrome (Glick, in press), patients with temperomandibular joint syndrome (Colasante, in press), patients with panic disorder, and patients with bronchial asthma (Catherine O'Brien, Personal Communication, 1997). The following summarizes the results of these studies:

1. Patients referred who were tested prior to the course scored higher in measures of anxiety, depression, and somatization than "healthy" people.
2. After the course there is improvement in these indices of uneasy mood.
3. There is a measurable decrease in physical symptoms after the course. In the case of disease or condition specific groups (e.g., irritable bowel, temperomandibular joint syndrome) the improvement is seen in these conditions.
4. The utilization of medical care decreases from 30 to 50% in the period following the course. These results have been followed for up to one year.
5. Psychological testing for "affiliative trust" and "self-efficacy" has shown that improvement in these scores is highly correlated with clinical improvement.
6. Functional status measures after the course show striking improvements in the important areas of living, such as mental health, relationships, and general vitality.

7. Patients like the course. They report a sense of fulfillment in the course, are very satisfied with the opportunity to have this kind of learning, and believe this learning is important to their well-being and health care.
8. Prior to the course patients show a high incidence of alexithymia. This decreases after the course and is in fact a strong predictor of patient improvement.

It continues to amaze the clinicians involved in this project that patients are as willing as they are to become responsible partners in their health care by seriously engaging in learning. If this is true, and the evidence strongly suggests that it is, why is it that even in managed care settings in which one would expect rapid adoption of such a new treatment its acceptance has been so slow? Here is an intervention that helps to appropriately address the distress of a population for which managed care is responsible, and to do so in an efficient, acceptable, and cost effective way.

Unfortunately, the organizational environments in which programs are developed are also dominated by the same Cartesian assumptions as the health care professions themselves. Unless new organizational practices and awarenesses are developed, the introduction of behavioral medicine programs will continue to be a struggle.

ORGANIZATIONAL EMBODIMENT OF THE CARTESIAN PARADIGM

It is to be expected that organizations of people will reflect the "invisible fabric" of the assumptions of the culture. This is certainly true of our medical care organizations. Returning to the three cornerstones of the Cartesian paradigm, it is seen how they are imbedded even in our managed care organizations.

The Mind–Body Dichotomy

The training of physicians is highly Cartesian. Until recently only lip service was given to the psychosocial aspects of health and illness in most medical school curricula. Moreover, medical student admissions and postgraduate training have emphasized technical rather than human competence. The skill set of most physicians to recognize, discuss, coach, or treat common behavioral problems is woefully underdeveloped.

The mind–body dichotomy has been institutionalized in the existence of separate mental health and physical health departments. This is patently dysfunctional when it is recognized that 60% of problems that present for primary care attention are neither body nor mind problems, but mind–body problems. There is a remarkable by-product of the "cognitive blindness" that results from this divided view of human nature. Sobel (1995a) has pointed to dozens of solidly grounded interventions in health care that assume a mind–body unity. These interventions are effective, not costly, and mostly unknown or not implemented in daily practice.

As medical care moves into a cost and result conscious future, continued ignorance of the considerable number of practices that suggest a new theoretical framework is no longer tolerable from a patient or payor point of view.

Understanding of Parts

The understanding of organ systems, organ functions, and even subsets of organ systems (e.g., white cells), has been the focus of modern medicine. Moreover, communities of concern with the function of parts have developed. These are called departments. Around these departments power structures, traditions of funding, competition for staffing, training programs, and other struggles have developed. Yet patients are whole people with unified concerns. A program such as PHIP clashes with the traditional "Balkanization" of medical practice in that it is holistic, not reductionistic. The concerns of patients and payors, traditionally, have had little political or economic clout so the silolike departmentalization has continued. This is changing as customers and payors become the major industry stakeholders rather than the professionals. This will be discussed subsequently.

The Professional Corollary

In the old paradigm, the physician-scientist had knowledge and experience with the patient's disease that was "senior" in value to that of the patient. The professional has voluminous answers to "why" and "how," but all of the answers are in the mechanistic domain. The patient (customer) is equally interested in the "what" questions. What is it to have a myocardial infarction? This is the question that the patient lives in even as the clinician asks questions in a different domain.

Moreover, the importance of addressing the "what" question is being shown as a major determinant of the outcome of the disease. For example, depression is a major determinant of the subsequent course of a myocardial infarction. The "meaning" or "what" is being shown to be as relevant as the "how and why." In the "what," the patient is the expert. This is even more so for psychosomatic complaints, health habits, prevention, and chronic disease management. What is being called for is a new kind of partnership between professionals and patients, a partnership which honors the point of view of each in a nonhierarchical way, and maximizes the resources of each in arriving at a shared plan. For medical practice this represents a social revolution of Copernican proportions.

THE ARRIVAL ON THE SCENE OF THE PAYOR AND THE PATIENT

Before the oil crisis, Japanese engineers found little interest in innovations for automotive production systems. By using the oil crisis they created an opportunity through which a revolution in attitudes and systems occurred, and the rest is history: the Japanese automakers quickly became the most successful in the world. In medical care today, especially managed health care, the marketplace has entered as an increasing force. This is seen in terms of demands for cost containment, results assurance, and patient satisfaction. The old system was sheltered from the marketplace, but it is being forced to reexamine its values, processes, and assumptions as well as the skills of its workers.

Patient loyalty, once assumed, is now showing up as a major economic success factor: consumers look for the "best" health plan. In some markets, Medicare patients change health plans every 3 years, hardly a sign of loyalty. But what determines patient loyalty? Certainly technical competence is one cornerstone, but it is not enough. Study after study is showing that patient loyalty is correlated with patient trust, and this is grounded in the patient's assessment that the clinician is interested in the "what's" of life, not just the "how and the why."

But what will make the clinician interested in the living context of the patient, the "what," a matter of equal concern to technology? This is a complex issue, but certainly the norms, the traditions, the mood of the managed care organization itself are major determinants. A clear commitment to "deep" patient service is key. The Samaritan tradition of empathy and caring is one of the pillars of medical tradition, which recently has been eclipsed by technologic excellence. Even more important is how the entire staff is treated. Are the "what's of the staff" as important as their technical proficiency? Are their person vision and values honored, their intelligence and passion aligned with the company, or are they at war with the company? These are central questions for the leaders of managed care companies.

Behavioral medicine can be a major resource to the emergence of managed care, not only in the succor and relief that it brings to patients, but in its proficiency in asking "what" questions, in its respect for the dignity and knowing of the other, and in the inclusion of the knowing of the other in the learning process. Our organizations need this as much as do our patients.

If what we know and do in our behavioral practices, like PHIP, can be brought to the thinking and the organization of the entire system, then our visions for health care will be closer to our grasp, and our thinking will mature to the next level. Behavioral medicine, by virtue of the assumptions that it embodies, can contribute to our managed care organizations becoming healing communities.

6.

Integration: A Case For Putting Humpty Dumpty Together Again

Jaylene Kent, Ph.D., Malcolm Gordon, M.D.

Health care is in the midst of a reengineering revolution and integration is crystallizing as a prerequisite for achieving the benchmark standard in the industry. The arguments for integration are numerous, compelling, and inescapable. They include: (1) reducing cost through "appropriate staff mix" with roles assigned to the most appropriate and cost effective health care providers; (2) shifting away from a Hippocratic approach (the traditional one-on-one, physician to patient, paradigm) to a population-based approach in which care is delivered by health care teams utilizing best practices guidelines; (3) assigning broader responsibilities to primary care physicians who are themselves leveraged by collaborating with other less costly or more appropriate providers; (4) moving from hospital-based to outpatient-based care which creates a need for a continuum of services embracing both health and illness in the outpatient setting; (5) shifting clinical care demands to encompass both acute and chronic needs; (6) designing health care delivery systems that are customer and service (management of demand) driven rather than physician driven; and (7) employing clinical interventions with demonstrated optimal health outcomes.

A CASE FOR PUTTING BIOLOGY BACK IN PSYCHOLOGY

The current hierarchical, fragmented health care delivery system artificially separates psychology from biology. There has been limited application of Engel's (1993) biopsychosocial model in the practice of mainstream medicine and even less focus on creating the infrastructure within organized systems of health care to deliver such a model.

Much research has suggested that thoughts, feelings, coping style, mood, and life-style choices can have a significant effect on health status (Bandura, 1991; Kobasa, Maddi, & Kahn, 1982; Wiggins, 1994) and that the traditional "biological" or "medical" evaluation and treatment which focuses on organicity alone may not be enough to achieve optimal health care outcomes. For instance, research has demonstrated that more than 60% of all chief complaints presenting in primary care have a behavioral or psychological basis (Wiggins, 1994). Even more startling is the finding by Kroenke and Mangelsdorff (1989) that a biological basis for "new" complaints in primary care was found only 16% of the time. Lyn Payor (1988) writes:

> . . . it is still the case that only 15% of all contemporary clinical interventions are supported by objective scientific evidence that they do more good than harm. On the other hand, between 40% and 60% of all therapeutic benefits can be attributed to a combination of the placebo and Hawthorne effects, two code words for caring and concern, or what most people call an individual's personal responsibility for their health status. (p. 9)

In general, the current health care system and medical culture reduces an individual's personal responsibility for their health status. This philosophy runs counter to the evidence which suggests people provide a large percentage of their own health care and new evidence which suggests they want to be involved in their health outcomes. We live in an increasingly health conscious society with an explosion in the availability of information on health and disease in the media and the Internet. Patients want to be involved in the decision-making process regarding health and disease and be partners with the health care team (Vickery, Kalmer, & Lowry, 1983).

Another interesting perspective which has been studied for over two decades and is gaining increased prominence is that psychological events themselves, such as emotions, beliefs, coping styles, and learning, may have a direct impact on physiological systems, most likely by interacting with the central nervous system, endocrine system, and the immune system, thereby influencing the onset and course of disease (Bandura, 1991; Kent, Coates, Pelletier, & O'Regan, 1989; Sobel, 1995b; Solomon, 1985). This line of research further supports the health benefits which may accrue from adding the patient to the health care team.

It is especially the burgeoning clinical needs and financial costs of the chronically ill that currently challenge the system. Chronic disease accounts for 90% of all morbidity, 80% of all mortality, and 80% of all health care dollars (Scott & Robertson, 1996). An appreciation of these numbers explains how a system designed for acute, defined episodes of care is challenged. In summary, we are in the midst of a revolution which challenges not only our fundamental assumptions in evaluating and treating illness, but also the very paradigm utilized to deliver that care.

KAISER SAN JOSE EXPERIENCE: INTEGRATION BEFORE IT WAS "COOL"

This chapter tells the story of the evolution of integration at one medical center, Kaiser San Jose, in primary care. In 1989, the physician-in-charge at Kaiser San Jose Medical Center made a decision to develop specialized services for patients with chronic benign pain syndrome. To this end, resources were allocated for the Skills Not Pills program, staffed by a health psychologist, clinical social worker, and a physician. Although a programmatic, multidisciplinary team approach in traditional primary care managing a chronically ill population may have been considered a novel approach, the idea was accorded support. Why?

The pioneering work of Dr. David Fordyce, a psychologist, and Dr. James Bonica, a physician, both at the University

of Washington in Seattle, had clearly demonstrated the need
for an integrated, multidisciplinary team approach to manage
this very difficult, refractory population. Additionally, a similar, pioneering, multidisciplinary approach at another Kaiser
facility had demonstrated success. Consequently, the integrated team concept was nearly undisputed in the prevailing
medical culture at Kaiser San Jose. A health psychologist was
given an administrative title and the responsibility for further
development of services. This gesture was a harbinger of the
recognition that would come 8 years later from the highest
levels within the medical group for integration in all of
primary care. So began the Department of Behavioral Medicine and Health Psychology.

Behavioral medicine, by definition, is a multidisciplinary
approach to clinical care. True to this model, the arrangement at the San Jose Medical Center has a multidisciplinary
staff directed by a health psychologist. Health psychology is
a specialty area within psychology characterized by skills and
knowledge in prevention of medical illness, behavioral and
nonpharmacologic treatment of existing medical illnesses,
recovery from, or adjustment to ongoing medical illness,
compliance with medical regimens, and maintenance of good
health. Health psychologists are most often trained as clinical
psychologists and then obtained the requisite specialty training in health psychology, most often at medical schools.

This department has extensive collaborative relationships
with the departments of psychiatry, nutritional services, health
education, adult primary care (of which behavioral medicine
is a division) and specialties of oncology, neurology, cardiology,
pulmonology, rheumatology, endocrinology, nephrology, and
specialty clinics such as the pain clinic and spine unit. In fact,
staffing for nearly all clinical programs and services are provided through "chargebacks" from sponsoring or "mother"
departments. The psychiatry department, in particular, has
been especially generous with resources and support.

As it came to pass, the administrative and clinical culture
designed to support a multidisciplinary approach to meet the
needs of one chronic, clinical population, that with chronic

benign pain syndrome, proved to be a natural one for organizing services to meet the needs of other populations with chronic needs. But, in the beginning there was and continues to be the Skills Not Pills program.

SKILLS NOT PILLS: A BREAK FROM THE MOLD

This is a 10-week, multidisciplinary, cognitive/behavioral outpatient program which provides medication tapers, medication adjustments, psychological interventions, education, and physical reconditioning for Kaiser members with chronic benign pain syndrome. Patients eligible for this program include those who have completed all appropriate medical and surgical evaluations and interventions. The focus of the treatment program is on skill building and restoration to the highest possible level of functioning. The program structure relies very heavily on learning theory with close attention to reinforcers of pain behavior. In addition to behavior modification, skill building (which includes pacing, assertiveness, psychosocial strategies, and stress management) and reconditioning are also emphasized.

The clinical treatment consists of a health psychologist, nurse, physician, and clinical social worker. Together with their spouse or support person, the patient meets with the entire treatment team prior to entering the program. This preliminary team meeting is held for a variety of reasons: (1) to establish a clinical alliance between the participants and the providers; (2) to answer questions; (3) to review the participants' commitment to the program; (4) to clarify that the staff will not "cure" their pain; but support them as they learn to manage it more effectively; and most importantly (5) to communicate that the treatment team recognizes that their chronic problem affects all areas of their life: social, psychological, and biological, and the team has the expertise and commitment to function as their consultants in all these areas during the program.

A new program begins every 5 weeks. This structure allows new members to join "veteran" members who can encourage and support new member participation. "Lay leadership" or "peer support" is a powerful ingredient in the program. The professional staff repeatedly stress their "consultant role only," emphasizing that program participants are "in charge" of their pain, not "the doctors." When joining the program, the members have agreed to forego seeing any other health care professionals during the 10 weeks, limiting their contacts with their health plan to the Skills Not Pills treatment team only. It is stressed neither the physician, nor any other team member, is available to hear complaints about their pain problem once the program starts.

Patients come to the clinic on Mondays and Thursdays for $3^1/_2$ hours on each day for 10 weeks. On Monday evenings, program participants meet first with the team nurse who oversees the reconditioning exercise portion of the program. Subsequently, they meet with a team health psychologist and social worker who teach a variety of skills including relaxation, cognitive techniques, and stress management. On Thursday nights, support partners attend the program with the core group member participating in a didactic presentation by a member of the professional staff. Since chronic pain affects the entire family system, participation in the program by a support person is mandatory. On nonclinic days, program participants are expected to complete and chart daily homework, which includes twice daily stretching and strengthening exercises, a walking program, and relaxation. Once the 10-week, intensive portion of the program is completed, there is a 10-month follow-up program. In this phase, graduates of the intensive portion of the program attend a monthly group meeting with the program health psychologist. Upon completion of the program, participants return to their original primary care providers.

ONE SIZE DOES NOT FILL ALL

As more and more referrals for pain management came into the department, it became clear demand outstripped supply. A waiting list for evaluations by the psychologists developed, and access to services became problematic. The physicians in the Spine Unit especially needed better access to pain services. In an effort to better meet the need, a health psychologist spent 2 hours a week in the Spine Clinic and a pain management program that did not require a psychological evaluation was developed. Physicians could refer directly to the program, called the Pain Education Group (PEG).

The Pain Education Group (PEG) is a lower intensity 8-week, multidisciplinary intervention for patients with chronic benign pain syndrome. Staffed by a primary care physician and a health psychologist, this program captures the best aspects of a psychoeducational approach and combines it with the advantages of group therapy and support. This program also allows for medication management and when appropriate, drug tapers, in the nonaddicted patient by the PEG physician. This occurs in a group setting rather than in the traditional, one-on-one, patient to doctor paradigm.

A more limited version of the Pain Education Program is also offered in Spanish under the direction of a Spanish-speaking psychologist.

The Chronic Daily Headache Program was conceived because of our ongoing desire to meet the needs of our medical colleagues. Following a collaborative meeting with the San Jose Neurology Department and an invited guest neurologist from Hayward Kaiser, the behavioral medicine staff set as its goal the identification of a subpopulation of patients who could benefit from a collaborative relationship between neurology and behavioral medicine.

The neurologists identified analgesic rebound headaches as a diagnosis most likely to benefit from such a collaborative approach, and the Chronic Daily Headache Program was created to serve the needs of members with pain problems. This is an 8-week group program that treats analgesic rebound headache through appropriate drug tapering, group support, and relaxation. The program structure is similar to the Skills Not Pills program in that new members have the benefit of "experienced" group members to encourage and support them. This particular population invariably must experience more head pain before a lessening of head pain occurs and it requires a leap of faith to believe that program participation will eventually lead to increased comfort. The professional staff consists of a psychiatric social worker and a primary care physician.

CHRONIC IS CHRONIC

As referrals of patients with other chronic medical conditions, e.g., diabetes or hypertension or members placing excessive demands on the primary care physician, began coming into the department, we knew we would need again to broaden our services in a cost efficient way. Efforts to work with these members in a one-on-one paradigm was too labor intensive and perhaps not the treatment of choice.

ONE GOOD THING LEADS TO ANOTHER

One day, an innovative approach to meeting the multiplicity of clinic needs-demands of both our referring colleagues and our heterogeneous patient population began to take shape. It was clear that many of the services required for good pain control were useful in the management of other chronic conditions. For instance, they include learning skills for self-management of common symptoms, achieving a sense of control over one's health, support, exercise, stress management, relaxation training, and caregiver support. Although some diagnoses require unique knowledge and skills specific to their illness, e.g., mastering self monitoring of blood sugars in the case of diabetics, or achieving competency in using a blood pressure cuff for hypertensives, it appeared there were many more common needs than differences in patient populations having heterogeneous chronic medical diagnoses.

Additionally, it also appeared to be an opportunity not only to improve patient care, but also to support physician recommendations. Although most primary care physicians would recommend exercise or stress reduction to many of their patients with chronic problems, there were limited internal programs or resources to support that component of their treatment plan. This approach might also provide a line of service for many of the most vexing patients seen in primary care: somatizers and those presenting with nonspecific medical complaints, such as fatigue, dizziness, or poor sleep, all in the absence of manifest physical disease.

The Health Modules were created as a treatment option which offered a solution to these problems by providing a variety of clinical opportunities for patients to learn self-management techniques which can minimize their symptoms (e.g., good stress management), optimize their sense of control over their health, increase their sense of support from the medical community, and promote healthy life-styles.

HEALTH MODULES: PROGRAMS FOR HEALTH AND ILLNESS

The specific services for self-management offered in the Health Modules are not disease specific and can be mixed and matched according to the needs of the patient, caregivers, and providers. For instance, some individuals may be interested only in the Reconditioning Exercise Program (REP) and not stress management. Some of the modules require a physician referral, some do not. Nearly all of the programs are staffed with a provider from the "world of psychology and behavior" and a provider from "the world of biology and disease" and occur in a group setting.

The Health Modules are as follows:

SLEEP (Sleep Easy Education Program) is an 8-week program with a multidisciplinary staff for members with insomnia. Education materials (on sleep disorders, circadian rhythms, sleep and aging, sleep hygiene, snoring, relaxation techniques, and other sleep-inducing strategies), as well as sleep logs and medication evaluation are used to identify causes of insomnia and to improve sleep.

REP (Reconditioning Exercise Program) is a 9-week program for patients with chronic medical illness who would benefit from reconditioning exercises, aerobic walking, relaxation techniques, and increased participation in activities of daily living.

Meditation for Health trains members in a specific relaxation technique called Mindfulness Meditation. Research has amply demonstrated that relaxation can help individuals regain a sense of control over their minds, their bodies, and their lives. This experience can enhance one's sense of well-being.

Stress Management for Individuals with Chronic Illness (also known as "Caring Not Curing") is an 8-week stress management group program for members with medical illness whose symptoms are exacerbated by stress. It is also useful for individuals who have nonspecific medical complaints which may be exacerbated by stress. The topics covered include assertiveness training, anger management, "making the most of your medical appointment," medication management, relaxation, and communication skills.

Caring for Caregivers is a group program focused upon the intense emotional and psychosocial needs frequently experienced by caregivers (spouse, family member, significant other, domestic partner) of medically ill patients. It is open to referral from primary care and subspecialty providers who find these caregivers to be overwhelmed, psychologically symptomatic, or in need of support in order to effectively continue their caregiving.

The Extra Care Group is an ongoing group program for medical patients who are especially problematic for physicians, e.g., utilizing inappropriately, demanding, argumentative, unrealistic in their expectations, hostile, and time-consuming. The physician coleading this group also utilizes this meeting as a group appointment for delivering medical care to his own patients participating in the group.

Major Medical Illness Program is open to members suffering from any major medical illness who are experiencing psychiatric symptoms or having difficulties coping. Every effort is made to collaborate with the primary care physician in better meeting the psychosocial and emotional needs of these members.

PSYCHIATRIC DIAGNOSTIC SPECIFIC SERVICES

Providing integrated services for the chronically medically ill and empowering members in patient self-care are only two broad areas of service provided by behavioral medicine in primary care. Another fundamental service and need are those for more traditional psychiatric diagnoses. The services for depression and anxiety delivered in primary care demonstrate the interface between mental health and primary care.

The *Depression Program for Primary Care* is a collaborative endeavor between the Departments of Psychiatry and Behavioral Medicine, and with the Anxiety–Panic Program for Primary Care, is one of two new key programs. It is a multidisciplinary, brief, cognitive–behavioral depression treatment program specifically for depressed medical patients being treated by primary care physicians. It is designed for primary care clinicians who want an alternate treatment to antidepressants, or more than just medications, but without the stigma of a psychiatry referral.

The *Anxiety–Panic Program for Primary Care* is a multidisciplinary, brief treatment program using cognitive–behavioral behavioral techniques and appropriate medication management. It is characterized by rapid access and timely feedback to the referring primary care physician. Entry into the anxiety management program is through a triage group intake appointment with a psychiatrist and a social worker. Once a specific diagnosis is established, the appropriate referral is made. This may include services in the Psychiatry Department for anxiety disorders or additional services within behavioral medicine. Options within behavioral medicine include group psychotherapy with a psychologist, medication groups, or relaxation trainings.

The department of Behavioral Medicine also participates in diagnostic specific programs for medical conditions:

The *Multidisciplinary Oncology Program* is a service designed to meet a broad cross-section of psychological, medical, and educational needs for cancer patients, family members, and caregivers in a cost effective manner. This program is a model of multiple disciplines and multiple departments collaborating to deliver integrated care. An oncologist, nutritionist, health educator, and health psychologist all work together in this 8-week time limited program. It couples the best of a health education approach with a psychodynamic group process. It also allows for the nutritionist and oncologist to deliver some care in a group appointment format, rather than a one-on-one format.

The *Chronic Fatigue Syndrome and Fibromyalgia Program* offers emotional support and relevant information regarding these conditions. The focus is on the positive with goals to reduce stress, to cope with depression and anxiety, to improve physical endurance, and to regain a sense of control in one's life.

THE HYPERTENSION MANAGEMENT PROGRAM

This program is a collaborative group appointment project between internal medicine and behavioral medicine. Based on the belief that members want to be involved in their health care and that human behavior influences health and health care outcomes, a pilot project cosponsored by the Departments of Medicine and Behavioral Medicine for managing uncomplicated hypertension was implemented.

Several factors influenced the decision to develop this innovative approach to high blood pressure management. Hypertension is a chronic, usually lifelong medical condition with a high prevalence in the general population and in managed care memberships. Health care resources devoted to this condition are considerable, yet blood pressure control is often not optimal. Life-style modification alone or in combination with pharmacologic agents is the currently accepted treatment regimen for hypertension. Research indicates that nonpharmacologic treatments, e.g., weight loss, dietary sodium restriction, low saturated fat diets, routine aerobic exercise, relaxation techniques, and stress management are effective in lower blood pressure. Educational information describing the disease helps individuals understand the disease process and note life-style changes in controlling their condition (Groth-Marnat & Edkins, 1996; Joint National Committee on Detection, Evaluation, and Treatment of High Blood Pressure, 1993; Neaton, Grimm, & Prineas, 1993; Langford, Davis & Blaufox, 1991).

Extrapolation from other research on chronic disease management suggests that group interaction and support aids in blood pressure control. Developing self-efficacy skills also enables hypertensive patients to take a more active role in treating their own chronic condition and literally become active members of the health care team. This is critical as patient compliance with both behavioral and medical aspects of the treatment regimen is crucial for adequate blood pressure control.

A description of the current hypertension management group program might be helpful. The management team consists of a primary care internist, a health psychologist, and a medical assistant. The group members are invited from the physician's patient panel. Inclusion criteria are: (1) Diagnosis of stable, essential hypertension, with minimal other complicating medical diseases (although hyperlipidemia, mild diabetes mellitus, mild coronary artery disease are acceptable), and (2) a willingness to participate in this new program. Members are invited to participate by letter, phone contact, or a personal invitation from the physician. The target group size was 15 and after experience with 6 groups, the attendance was found to average 12.

There is an introductory series of three sessions, each of $1^1/_2$ hours duration, which meets weekly. These meetings cover group introductions, the completion of forms, the distribution of information/program packets, and educational presentations in the following areas: (1) hypertension diagnosis pathophysiology, and behavioral and pharmacological treatments; (2) dietary considerations including weight control and sodium and fat intake (the importance of regular exercise is also covered); (3) stress management and relaxation techniques. The group members are strongly encouraged to purchase a home blood pressure cuff and demonstrate competency in the group session in its use. All participants are required to keep a home blood pressure log which they bring to the meetings. The work of Pickering (1994) suggests that home pressure readings are better predictors of how well blood pressure is controlled than blood pressure readings taken in the medical settings.

Clinical decisions regarding treatment modification are based on home blood pressure readings at the third session and at the 4-month follow-up sessions. The appropriate treatment regimen is based on input from the patient, the physician, and the psychologist. Telephone follow-up and treatment regimen modification is done by algorithm by the medical assistant after the initial sessions and between follow-up group appointments.

At follow-up meetings which occur every 4 months, didactic information regarding hypertension, health topics, life-style interventions, and routine health maintenance measures are covered. It is also an opportunity for group support and "peer counseling." At all group meetings, participants are encouraged to discuss any health-related issues and make certain any acute health problems are addressed by the staff.

At the time of this writing, six groups comprising a total of 70 members have participated in the program. Recidivism for members who start the program has been negligible. Patient satisfaction scales have shown unanimous delight with this program as a way to manage their hypertension, yielding an average satisfaction score of 4.9 on a scale of five. Blood pressure control in the participants has been excellent with many patients decreasing their medication and several discontinuing their medication altogether. An economic analysis indicates this collaborative group appointment approach will be slightly more costly than the traditional, one-to-one physician to patient paradigm, in the first year of treatment and cost neutral thereafter. The management team's professional satisfaction is higher in this paradigm than the traditional one. The primary care physician feels more comfortable dealing with behavioral aspects of care; the health psychologist is more familiar with the technical aspects of care; and the medical assistant has become an extremely active and valuable team member.

The collaborative group appointment for managing hypertension helps to address aspects of the patient's life, as they interface with their chronic medical condition: the biological, psychological and social preliminary data suggest, as predicted by other chronic disease management research (Groth-Marnat & Edkins, 1996) is associated with (1) improves clinical outcomes; (2) is cost effective; (3) improves patient and professional staff satisfaction; and (4) actively engages these patients in their own care.

THE BEHAVIORAL MEDICINE LIAISON SERVICE

Since putting Humpty Dumpty together requires all the king's horses and all the king's men, psychology has joined the primary health care team in San Jose. This section describes behavioral medicine's role in the most common portal of entry: the primary care practitioner's office. Front line clinicians have become increasingly aware that current demands, ranging from health promotion and prevention to complex clinical problems, requires collaboration with other professionals. No single discipline embraces all of the knowledge and skill required to provide seamless, high quality care (Hinshaw & DeLeon, 1995). As noted above, behavioral and psychological issues drive 60% of primary care visits. It naturally follows that adding a psychologist to the health care team optimizes the skill mix to meet these demands.

A NEW ROLE FOR PSYCHOLOGISTS ON THE PRIMARY CARE TEAM

The responsibilities of the health psychologist on the primary care team fall into two broad categories: clinical–consultative and educational. Each will be discussed separately.

The *clinical–consultative* responsibilities of the team psychologist include the diagnosis, management, and referral when appropriate of:

1. Somatizing patients who are high utilizers of primary care services.
2. Patients whose medical conditions have compromised their daily functioning.
3. Patients with longstanding medical complaints for which there is no clear organic etiology.
4. Patients who comply poorly with needed medications or other prescribed therapies.
5. Dysfunctional patients who are resistant to mental health referrals, whose management requires close collaboration with the physician, or with patients whose behaviors place them at risk for adverse health consequences, e.g., patients who are oppositional in ways that prevent the delivery of adequate healthcare.
6. Consultation on medications for disorders that affect behavior, mood, thinking, and cognitive functioning in patients with an uncomplicated medical status.
7. Patients in early stages of substance abuse.
8. Patients with chronic and life-threatening diseases.
9. Chronic pain patients.

Additionally, the health psychologist will identify patients who can be treated effectively in primary care without referral to psychiatry. Services available from the behavioral medicine staff will include brief (1–3 sessions) crisis intervention and/or cognitive–behavioral therapy, brief evaluation, and triage to appropriate services with health education, psychiatry, behavioral medicine, or the community.

The *educational role* can be conceptualized as providing three broad aspects to the primary care setting: (1) Training primary care physicians to enhance their own skills in diagnosis and management of patients presenting with mental health and behavioral health needs. (2) Education on appropriate utilization of psychotropic medications to enhance clinical outcomes and minimize need for referral. (3) Education regarding which kinds of patients may benefit from referral to other services.

A PARADIGM SHIFT AT THE EDGE OF THE ENVELOPE

Teams of multidisciplinary providers working collaboratively in primary care to meet the needs of empaneled patients are currently being assembled at Kaiser Permanente Medical Center San Jose. It is expected that characteristics of a behavioral medicine approach to medical care will be manifested in this reorganization. In summary, Hinshaw and DeLeon (1995) identify a number of the quintessential aspects and benefits of multidisciplinary collaboration: (1) Merging of expertise—smooth functioning multidisciplinary teams allow for a blending of expertise and seamless utilization of team expertise by members. (2) Shared responsibility and situational leadership—unlike the historical tradition of the physician routinely remaining the "captain of the ship," particularly on clinical care issues, multidisciplinary collaboration is built on shared clinical responsibility and flexibility with primary clinical responsibility driven by patient care needs (*Primary Care Weekly*, 1995). (3) Collegiality—the daily work experience of providing frontline clinical care can be deeply enriched, invigorated, and enhanced when sharing with other colleagues from different disciplines who are similarly invested in a common outcome. (4) Distribution of power—equitable and appropriate distribution of power and influence is fundamental to multidisciplinary, collaborative care. Because it is assumed that expertise from each team member will be needed at various times in the collaborative process, the unique contributions of each team member is valued and respected.

This multidisciplinary approach affirms that primary care is dealing with the whole person and providing appropriate expertise for all aspects of their case.

BARRIERS TO INTEGRATION

The professional and economic climate and culture at the San Jose/Kaiser Permanente Medical Center were right for the undertaking of the first step in integration: The initiation of a specialized integrated service for patients suffering from chronic benign pain. It was also the right climate and culture to allow one good thing to lead to another, until there were a multitude of integrated programs. Nonetheless, throughout the years integration was progressing, a number of potential difficulties could be seen, although fortunately because of professional and management enthusiasm, they never seriously threatened the process. (1) Respect and knowledge regarding each team member's capability and potential contribution to patient care is crucial. Traditional practice has not fostered this level of professional understanding. Instead, patients have simply been referred to another "specialist" rather than another member of a clinical team. (2) Traditional hierarchies have always characterized the practice of medicine. The idea of collaborative clinical care, reliance upon the expertise of a clinician other than a physician, and distribution of power run contrary to an old and powerful medical tradition. (3) "Turf Issues" whether between physicians and nurses, psychiatrists and psychologists, or orthopedic surgeons and podiatrists always have the potential for sabotaging team work.

A secure professional identity, clear assignment of roles, and good understanding of legal issues surrounding scope of practice and open communication may help to diffuse these issues.

CONCLUSION

In the Humpty Dumpty nursery rhyme, "all the king's horses and all the king's men could not put Humpty Dumpty together again." Fortunately, this is only a children's story. In real life, the model of integrated care is empirically and intuitively persuasive. At Kaiser San Jose, we continue to build an integrative, collaborative care model based on our successful, historical experience and guided by the exploding scientific literature in this field.

7.

Evolving an Integration Model: The *HealthCare Partners* Experience

James D. Slay, Jr., Rel.D., Caroline McLeod, Ph.D.

HEALTHCARE PARTNERS

HealthCare Partners is a large multispecialty medical group in Los Angeles County, serving over 250,000 patients at 37 medical sites. Owned and managed by physicians, the organization is committed to designing clinical and operational innovations that fulfill the promise of managed care. In implementing managed care, the consequences and problems resulting from the fragmentation of services became apparent. Collaborative care has been identified as an emerging solution to the problems of service fragmentation.

HealthCare Partners resulted from a recent merger of three groups: Huntington Medical Group, California Primary Physicians, and Bay Shores Medical Group. With the merger came the consolidation of over 25 years of combined managed care experience, along with expertise in programs applying psychosocial interventions to medical care. From the combined experience has come a vision of a collaborative health delivery system that bridges the traditional fragmentation between psychosocial and biomedical services. This chapter will review guiding principles of managed care and the problems presented by a fragmented delivery system, and then will discuss the processes developed within HealthCare Partners to integrate behavioral and biomedical services into a collaborative system of care.

The Vision of Managed Care

The original vision of managed care involved the reduction of health care costs through maintenance of good health and the prevention of health crises by means of early and appropriate intervention in illness and illness-producing behaviors. Paid a fixed sum (capitation) to maintain the health of a given population, managed care providers have the incentive to develop programs that produce good long-term clinical outcomes, decrease costs, and increase efficiency of care. Recognizing that a health care delivery system has to be financially viable in order to provide access to a large number of people, managed care in its ideal form represents a solution to limited resources while providing improvements in the quality of care.

Managed Care in the Three Worlds of Health Care

In order to realize the vision of managed care, it must operate well within what Peek and Heinrich (1995) call "the three worlds of health care." These authors propose that the clinical, the operational, and the financial worlds are really different dimensional views of the same underlying reality. Systems cannot be financially viable in the long run if clinical effectiveness is compromised. Similarly, if a system is hampered by poor operational structures, appropriate care ends up being delayed and financially unsupportable. If a process fails in any of the three worlds, it will ultimately fail in all three.

The Promise of Managed Care

Capitation represents a large innovation in the reimbursement structures of the financial world. To be effective, managed care must evolve corresponding innovations in the clinical and operational worlds. To the degree that its focus remains on reducing expenditures while ignoring the other two worlds of health care, managed care is untenable. The promise of managed care lies in the redesign of a fragmented health delivery system that was left over from a fee-for-service health care system.

Fragmented care involves financial, clinical, and operational structures that support different disciples conducting their business independently. In order to capitalize on the vision of managed care, systems must be redesigned to overcome this fragmentation. Such innovation requires the active, coordinated participation of clinicians involved in the day-to-day care of patients. Berwick (1996) offers important guidance for the redesign process:

> Without a clear focus on the needs and experiences of individual patients, much of the financial and structural reorganization now rampant in health care will be unlikely to yield improvements that matter to the patients we serve. As we change the system of care, five principles can help guide our investment of energy: (1) Focus on integrating experiences, not just structures; (2) learn to use measurement for improvement, not for judgment; (3) develop better ways to learn from each other, not just to discover best practices; (4) reduce total costs, not just local costs; and (5) compete against disease, not against each other. (p. 839)

This chapter will describe problems presented by fragmented care, and the experience of HealthCare Partners as it developed programs to solve these problems.

FRAGMENTED CLINICAL CARE

Understanding the importance of integrating clinical services became clear to clinicians at HealthCare Partners as the organization moved from a fee-for-service setting toward managed care. The problems of fragmentation of care became more apparent as centralized organizational structures became available to track patient outcome.

Fee-for-Service and Fragmentation

In our experience, under a fee-for-service system, treatment is highly specialized and technologically sophisticated. Patients are referred and often self-refer to practitioners having expertise in the particular body system seen to be problematic. If multiple body systems are involved, the patient bears much of the responsibility of integrating the different pieces of advice rendered by multiple providers. Since provision of care is oriented toward the method of reimbursement, treatment in a fee for service structure is likely to involve face-to-face meetings and procedures that are billable. Less emphasis is placed on education, healing aspects of a relationship, and continuity of care outside of office visits.

While there are probably many inefficiencies in this fragmented system, this chapter will focus on fragmentation between psychosocial and biomedical aspects of care.

Understanding Mind–Body Fragmentation

The traditional split between mind and body is reflected in the separate systems of training and caregiving that have predominated in this country over the last century. The current system of fragmented care involves clear clinical, financial, and operational divisions between biomedical and psychosocial treatment. Patients are treated as if they have discrete medical or psychiatric illnesses. Expertise developed to treat biomedical crises such as cancer and systemic infection have required the mastery of considerable technological knowledge. In the face of immediate, life-threatening illness, psychosocial aspects of care are frequently considered to be secondary. Thus, the training focus for biomedical providers has been technological intervention.

Psychosocial providers, on the other hand, have focused on diagnosable mental illness with treatment plans independent of the medical condition. Behavioral health treatment is thus seen as a parallel specialty, with minimal interaction with medical treatment. Its focus has traditionally been on persons with major mental illness, with serious disorders of thought and mood.

Though both biomedical and psychosocial disciplines have made tremendous progress in treating the most severe forms of physical and mental illness such as cancer and schizophrenia, in separation they are inadequate to the task of treating the more predominant illnesses of today, which are stress and behaviorally related (Wickramasekera, 1989).

Illness Has Biomedical and Psychosocial Components

Illness has both biomedical and psychosocial aspects that need to be addressed to provide effective care (Kleinman, 1988). We have discovered that four problems are poorly addressed in a fragmented system. Three of them are well documented in the literature. The first involves the problem of somatization. Between 50 and 80% of visits made to primary care are made for symptoms that are shown to have no organic or psychiatric basis (Cummings & VandenBos, 1981; Kroenke & Mangelsdorff, 1989; VandenBos & DeLeon, 1984). Commonly known as "somatizers," these patients experience psychosocial stress primarily through bodily sensation (Barsky, Goodson, Lane, & Cleary, 1988). These patients tend to overutilize medical resources (Anderson, Francis, Lion, & Daughety, 1977; Mumford, Schlesinger, & Glass, 1982), returning in distress again and again to medical providers who may lack the time, skills, and treatment orientation necessary to be of help. Indeed, these patients are at risk for iatrogenic complications, as repeated testing introduces unnecessary medical procedures and reinforces the patient's perception that something terrible is wrong and has not been identified (Katon & Sullivan, 1990).

Prompt identification and treatment of somatization would greatly improve the health of the population we serve.

The second problem is the fact that behavioral issues have a profound impact on outcome in situations where medical conditions are present. Studies have shown that a high proportion of patients are noncompliant with physician recommendation (Pomerleau, 1979). Increased morbidity, mortality, and dysfunction has been associated with depression and negative affect in patients with various diseases (Carney et al., 1988; H. S. Friedman & Booth-Kewley, 1987; Lustman, Griffith, & Clouse, 1986; Wells, Golding, & Burnham, 1988). Thus, psychosocial intervention is needed in conjunction with medical treatment in order to enhance the possibility of improved clinical outcomes.

The third problem is that disorders of mood are prevalent and disabling to patients in primary care. Estimates of clinical depression range from 5 to 13% (Blacker & Clare, 1987; Neilson & Williams, 1980); the addition of persons with subclinical depressive symptoms raises the incidence to around 20% (Zung, Broadhead, & Roth, 1993). Primary care doctors are frequently slow to diagnose and treat depression (Gonzales, Magruder, & Keith, 1994; Magruder-Habib & Zung, 1990). Furthermore, depression should be of major concern because the functional status of patients with depression is as low as that in patients with chronic disease (Wells et al., 1989). Effective health care must address this issue.

The fourth problem involves a lack of communication between biomedical and psychosocial providers, with the traditional understanding of patient confidentiality a major barrier. Our experience is that this gap seriously compromised effective care, particularly in cases of addiction where medical detoxification and behavioral intervention must be coordinated, in psychopharmacological intervention which requires monitoring of physical side effects, and in somatization and chronic pain where aggressive medical–surgical intervention without attention to psychosocial issues can do harm to the patient. Thus, the operational and clinical divisions between behavioral health providers and physicians result in poor coordination of care and poor outcome.

Financial Consequences of Fragmentation

Because behavioral health has been seen to be a discipline so specialized and because behavioral health has been situated in offices usually separate from medical offices, it has been vulnerable to "carve-out," where a portion of the health care capitation is given to a specialized managed care organization responsible for providing behavioral health services. For several reasons, this arrangement is disastrous for a multispecialty medical group which is paid on a capitated basis. First, communication between biomedical and psychosocial providers is virtually nonexistent, compromising the quality of patient care, which in turn threatens the desirability of the product and the profit margins dependent on maintaining the health of its capitated population. Second, the provider of medical care bears the costs of poor access and inadequate behavioral health treatment when dissatisfied, distressed patients with psychosocial issues return again and again to the primary care physician. Because the carve-out company does not directly bear the consequences of its poor service, it is relatively impervious to financial incentives for quality care. Finally, revenue given to the carve-out company is lost to the multispecialty group, which can capitalize on the efficiencies of integrated care.

THE PROMISE OF INTEGRATED CARE

Clinical and Operational Advantages

An integrated care delivery system has several advantages within the clinical world. First, it provides for the diagnosis and treatment of "somatizers," individuals with mood related physical distress who access primary care. Second, it attends to behavioral aspects of health care, increasing continuity of care and addressing issues of mood, compliance, and education that profoundly impact clinical outcome. Third, it establishes good communication between behavioral health and medical providers as a standard for good clinical care. Fourth, it makes available early and appropriate behavioral intervention at time of crisis, resulting in more positive outcomes and appropriate sub-sequent utilization of medical services. Fifth, it provides sup-port to family members in time of medical crisis, with resultant mobilization of family resources for the improved health of the entire family system.

Financial Advantages

Because integrated care involves better, more effective treat-ment, it can produce financial savings. Cummings and Follette (1968), Glazer (1993), Mumford, Schlesinger, Glass, Patrick, and Cuerdon (1984), and others have reported that even within a fragmented care system, treatment of psychological distress leads to decreases in medical costs. They have dubbed this "the medical cost offset."

Cost offset occurs with the appropriate and timely treat-ment of psychological distress, resulting in decreases in overall health costs for the individual, the family, the payor, and the medical group. It is important to note that in an integrated system of care, as biomedical and psychosocial costs are com-bined into total costs, traditional cost offsets might become difficult to detect. Berwick (1996) calls for a refocusing of atten-tion, from the reduction of local costs within a fragmented system to the reduction of total costs. He notes, however, that such a shift will require new financial understandings. "Inte-grated delivery systems may have a better chance at unifying views of cost, but that unifying will require many departures from classic, fragmenting assumptions about how budgets are made and monitored" (p. 842).

Thus, in understanding the costs and benefits of integrated care, we must develop ways of valuing elements that are im-portant in the clinical and operational worlds. What is the cost of a dissatisfied patient, of limited access, of poor quality of life, and of days lost from work? What are the benefits of patients' positive relationships with their providers, of families that de-velop resilience to stress, and of a system that provides a seamless continuity of care? As innovations in the clinical and operational worlds evolve, systems in the financial world must be developed to accurately measure the impact of these innovations.

DEVELOPMENT OF INTEGRATED PROGRAMS AT HCP: WHAT WE HAVE LEARNED

The development of integrated programs at HealthCare Partners occurred simultaneously within different parts of the organization as providers gained experience with managed care. Innovations were developed spontaneously in the day-to-day process of the delivery of care. The innovations presented below illustrate the processes involved and the improvements that are afforded by implementation of collaborative care at a program level.

Providing a Forum for Discussion

In order to develop integrated programs, it is necessary to bring together the appropriate experts. One important group that provided a forum for discussions among key leaders was the Health Care Integration Task Force. It was established as a team of interdependent, transdisciplinary, cross-functional experts who worked to redesign and rethink the delivery system. Members of the task force included administrators, medical directors, psychologists, primary care physicians, a physical therapist, nurse practitioners, and addictionologists. These individuals were highly respected within the organization, and had the unique ability to think and work outside of the boundaries that traditionally defined their professions. They helped to develop and operationalize pilot programs, and provided advice as the pilot programs expanded to the larger organization. Because of their standing within their professions, these individuals provided the means for internal marketing, communication, and education within HealthCare Partners.

Team Vision

HealthCare Partners began to develop the vision of collaborative care teams, with caregivers having general expertise in biopsychosocial aspects of health as well as in their area of specialty. In other words, providers would develop a basic understanding of how psychosocial issues and pathophysiology can interact and influence one another, and would become familiar enough with the expertise of other people on the team to be able to speak a common language. Providers therefore become managers and integrators of care, working together to support the long-term health of patients and their families.

Team-Based Culture and Accountability

The development of good collaborative care requires an environment that fosters commitment to personal learning and to patient care as well as a sense of personal accountability. A good example of collaborative care development comes from a site chosen as a pilot for a biopsychosocial model of care. Five physicians and one behavioral health specialist were selected as the professional staff along with appropriate accompanying supportive staff. Two physicians, Matthew Budd, M.D. and Andrew Epstein, M.D., of HSC Associates, who specialize in organizational and clinical team development, were employed to help develop a team-based culture. The full staff met intermittently with the consultants over several months in order to establish an interdisciplinary team that is directly accountable for the care of patients in their geographic area.

The site team developed several innovations including expanded hours of service and a new program of outreach to the bilingual population. In addition, the team developed regular case discussions which involved all members of the staff. Since collaboration is not a skill taught to most providers under the current training system, time must be set aside for providers to work out the interface between the biomedical and psychosocial cultures.

The results have been significant in terms of the satisfaction of both patients and providers. Significant also is the sense of pride and ownership claimed by all members of the staff. This kind of environment is optimal for the fostering of clinical and operational innovation necessary for good collaborative care.

Behavioral Health Providers at Primary Care Sites

Based on experience within the organization and this pilot site, behavioral health providers have been moved from separate mental health buildings into primary care sites throughout HealthCare Partners. The proximity of behavioral health to primary care greatly improved access for distressed patients. As biomedical providers recognize the need for psychosocial intervention, they walk the patient down the hall to introduce him or her to the behavioral health provider. We call this the "hallway handoff." The following example is typical of many cases which are difficult to treat under a fragmented system of care.

Lydia is a 73-year-old woman who was known to the staff of the medical site as a frequent visitor for a variety of physical complaints, including back pain, insomnia, dyspnea, heart palpitations, and anxiety. She had previously refused to see a behavioral health specialist at a nearby behavioral health site. She made an appointment to see her physician because of several attacks of anxiety, and in the doctor's office she experienced an extremely unpleasant panic attack.

The physician arranged for the patient to meet with the behavioral specialist on the spot, the specialist's office being right down the hall. The counselor's discussions with the patient and her husband revealed major family and grief issues contributing significantly to her anxiety and general sense of "dis-ease." Having recently lost a number of her friends through death, the patient was also socially isolated. After meeting with a counselor for several sessions, the patient's experiences of panic and anxiety diminished. If so desired by the patient, she will be able to attend a group setting to ease her social isolation and to provide ongoing stabilization.

In a brief survey, 21 providers who practiced in collaborative sites estimated that 70% of their patients who needed behavioral health services actually accessed the system under collaborative care. The same providers estimated that only 45% of their patients followed through on the referral when behavioral health was off-site. One provider remarked that when behavioral health is off-site, it may take as many as four or five visits before a patient will agree to be seen there. The provider reported that the "hallway handoff" was immediately successful in helping the patient make the transition to behavioral health.

Collaborative Communication

Collaborative skills are developed through informal discussions in offices and the lunch room, along with regular presentations of more formal cases. Emphasis is placed on teamwork, with the patient belonging to the group of people working together, rather than to providers working independently. The next case is an example of how team case management provided timely care of high quality, supporting family systems and avoiding hospitalization.

Sally is a 14-year-old white female who was brought to her pediatrician by her mother who was concerned about the child's lack of appetite and weight loss. Despite being evaluated by the pediatrician, a behavioral health specialist, and an endocrinologist, no immediate clear clinical picture emerged. As the providers worked to understand the complex nature of her problem, Sally's weight approached critically low levels. Family members as well as the health providers became alarmed. Working together with a psychiatrist and an eating disorders specialist who were on staff, the providers quickly developed a plan of action which successfully contained the anxiety of the family as well as safeguarding the health of the child.

This complex case is memorable because of the family's immediate need for coordinated, expert care in multiple specialties. This kind of rapid response would be extremely difficult to organize and implement in an outpatient setting under fragmented care.

Operational and clinical innovations are necessary to support the kind of teamwork described above. Communication among providers is greatly enhanced through the accessibility of medical information via an electronic medical record. The information can be entered or reviewed from different locations within a building or within the region. Because information is shared among providers, ongoing consent for the sharing of information is obtained from the patient and documented in the medical record. Contrary to the expectations of some behavioral health specialists, when psychosocial needs are presented as a part of their overall health care, most patients have few qualms about allowing relevant information to be shared.

Family Psychosocial Intervention at the Time of Medical Crisis

Collaborative care can be particularly important and effective at times when a family member has been diagnosed with a major medical illness. Early support and education of the patient and family members can forestall major psychosocial crises and improve the quality of life for the family.

John is a 14-year-old Caucasian male who sought help from the pediatrician for hearing loss. John's mother had died of a chronic disease which had produced increasing disfigurement, disability, and pain over a period of 20 years. John had witnessed his mother's progressing disease with horror, and had confided to his father that he would shoot himself if he ever were to be diagnosed with it.

Results from testing revealed that John was, in fact, in the early stages of the disease. The physician determined that intervention was necessary in order to prevent deterioration of John's hearing. At the same time, this pediatrician recognized the sensitivity of the issue to the father, who was just coping with the loss of his wife and who now would have to mobilize to support the child. Inviting the father to her office to discuss the results of the test while John was visiting relatives, the physician introduced a behavioral health specialist, and the three of them discussed the ramifications of the test for the father and the son. Plans were made over how to discuss this with John. When John was told about his illness and the recommended treatment, he was supported by his father, his physician, and a counselor. He is now doing well and the father and son are prepared to meet the challenges posed by a potentially crippling disease.

Collaboration among Providers Treating Different Family Members

Sometimes the source of recurrent illnesses in children can be linked to stresses within the family system. Under collaborative care, family dysfunction can be more readily identified and treated, resulting in a better quality of life and a lower medical utilization by family members.

> An 8-year-old boy was brought to the pediatrician for recurrent colds and reported behavioral problems. The pediatrician walked the boy and his mother to the behavioral health specialist on site. With discussion, the counselor found that the father had unrealistic expectations about appropriate behavior for a child of that age. Furthermore, the mother seemed overwhelmed and depressed, and was receiving counseling for this. She denied substance abuse issues.
>
> Discussion of the case on the health care team revealed that the father had been diagnosed several years before with an alcohol problem, but had refused treatment at that time. The issue had not been linked to the fact that the rest of the family had been high utilizers of medical treatment for colds and flu, with the mother in counseling for depression.
>
> As a result of the collaborative discussion identifying the larger family issues, a treatment plan for the family was developed involving multiple caregivers. Al-anon was recommended for the mother and a treatment plan addressing the substance abuse was formulated for the father.

Treating Somatizers

Patients presenting with somatization in primary care present two kinds of problems. First, they are often not open to psychological intervention. Second, providing individual therapy for so many is not operationally or economically practical. Fortunately, a good solution exists: Many individuals who will not accept counseling will accept a psychoeducational course to treat stress-related physical disorders. One such course is the Personal Health Improvement Program. The principles it teaches about self-reflection, dignity, requests, and promises are useful and practical for everyone, although individuals in distress are likely to find knowledge in these areas particularly relevant to their life situation.

The Personal Health Improvement Program (PHIP) is a 6-week course developed to address the needs of patients with stress-related illness. Patients meet in a class format once a week for 2 hours; the class consists of in-class activities, video presentations, educational lectures, awareness and imagery exercises, as well as supplemental readings and homework.

PHIP has proven to be an excellent intervention for individuals who are overwhelmed and in distress. In two published controlled studies, the precursor to PHIP, Ways to Wellness, was shown to significantly reduce somatization, anxiety, and depression in those who attended the course. An evaluation of PHIP at Harvard Pilgrim Health Plan revealed similar findings as well as a 45% reduction in health care visits among 110 patients receiving treatment in eight different health care sites. An evaluation of the program in our system confirmed these findings.

PHIP is particularly useful in an integrated setting because it provides an extremely effective front-line intervention at low cost, and it is easily accessible to patients because it is an educational "course for effective living" rather than a psychotherapy group.

Relationship-Centered Care

Collaborative care is centered on the patient's experience and is designed to optimize the effects of healing relationships. The relationship between providers and the patient is central. This important shift in health care orientation is beautifully explained by Trussolini and the Pew-Fetzer Task Force (1994). Relationship-centered care recognizes that:

In order to be therapeutic, the relationship between healer and patient should have as its foundations a shared understanding of the meaning of the illness. This requires the healer to respond to the experience of the patient. In some cases, the healer also must be able to understand the meaning of the illness to and through a person who is close to the patient, such as a parent, a caregiver, or a spouse. . . . The capacity in a healer to sense the meaning is not in the first instance a discrete competency to be learned, but rather a different way of seeing or an awakening to a different way of being a healer. Only when this has occurred can competencies be learned and applied. (pp. 22–23)

As an example, the application of this orientation is the recognition that the identity of the primary contact between the patient and the health care team will depend on the patient's problem, not on an arbitrary role within the health care system. For most patients, this will be the primary care provider; but for other patients with severe illnesses, a specialist may be more appropriate for this role. For example, a person with chronic obstructive pulmonary disease may rely most on a pulmunologist for care. Similarly, a psychiatrist may be the primary contact for a person with major mental illness.

HealthCare Partners has designed other patient-centered programs to meet special needs both in and outside of the primary care setting. These programs implement a biopsychosocial team approach.

Chemical dependency intervention in primary care has been one of our most successful innovations. The medical provider, addictionologist, behavioral health clinician, and often the urgent care provider collaborate in detoxification, rehabilitation, and outpatient treatment. For example, the clinician specializing in chemical dependency who works in family practice is able to meet, in a shared session with both the family practice physician, the addictionologist, and the patient needing medical detoxification. The combined intervention increases the likelihood that the patient will return for chemical dependency treatment, as no time elapses between the visit to the physician and the initial visit with the chemical dependency clinician.

The Touch Program is a return to home-based visits. It involves outreach and behavioral health treatment of patients who are at risk due to (1) family or patient inability to adjust to chronic illness; (2) being homebound with mental health problems; and (3) patient/family/caregiver dysfunction or noncompliance. Most Touch Program patients are over 65 years of age.

Primary care providers typically contact the program because of problems with a particular patient. A provider with dual licenses in nursing and behavioral health then meets with the patient and family members at the patient's home to assess his or her needs. The provider then collaborates with the primary care provider, with social workers, with home health, and with psychiatric consultants in order to determine the best treatment for the individual involved. Treatment is provided at home for the patient and the family. After the situation has been stabilized, the patient is followed by telephone on an ongoing basis. Additional home visits are scheduled if needed.

A study of 45 seniors in the program showed that 87% of the patients moved from high intensity crisis care to less intense levels of care. A large number of the patients had visited emergency and immediate care centers prior to being contacted by the Touch Program. Patients reported extremely high satisfaction with the program, and the total cost savings was $7,019 per patient per year.

The Transplant Program supports patients and their families who are waiting for or going through organ transplants. The biopsychosocial team to care for these patients is composed of the medical–surgical team plus the psychiatrist, a psychologist, and a social worker. These team members work collaboratively to support both patient and family as their needs arise.

The "Options" Program addresses the medical, psychosocial, and legal needs of terminally ill patients and their loved ones. The program was developed according to the belief that involvement in end of life decisions enhances the patient's feeling of self worth and the quality of life. Additionally, family members' involvement reduces the stress of making these difficult decisions and ensures that the patient's wishes are carried out. The collaborative care service is offered to all HCP patients.

Lessons Learned

This section has described a number of programs that involve collaboration between psychosocial and biomedical providers, and has demonstrated several advantages to the integration of care. It is important to have a forum for discussion for biomedical and psychosocial providers, in order that they may teach and learn from one another. A collaborative system is more sensitive to the whole range of patient and family needs, which increases compliance with medical treatment. Underscored is the effectiveness of short-term interventions at time of acute need with people who would not have accessed a separate behavioral health site. It was observed how interventions that include family members decrease distress and physician visits by all members of that family. It was found that relationship-centered care increases patient satisfaction and trust in providers, which seems to optimize the effects of the healing relationship. Finally, providers report greatly increased satisfaction with their roles. These lessons learned from various integrated programs are now being consolidated and applied to the health delivery system as a whole at HealthCare Partners.

NEXT STEPS: SYSTEMWIDE IMPLEMENTATION OF COLLABORATIVE CARE

As a result of the successes with collaborative care in various parts of the organization, HCP has launched a project known as the Collaborative Care Project to further develop the biopsychosocial model as a clinical innovation to be used throughout the organization. The project's goal is to improve the quality of health care by integrating the clinical delivery system. This is to be accomplished through the creation of service units in which all or most health care needs are met by a biopsychosocial treatment team. The development of collaborative clinical care throughout the organization will involve the consolidation of collaborative skills as a core competency within the company, as well as the redesign of operational and financial systems to evaluate, optimize, and support this method of delivery.

In moving toward a companywide implementation of collaborative care, several issues to be addressed have been identified.

Behavioral Health in Primary Care and Regional Centers

It is estimated that up to one behavioral health provider is needed to provide services for the caseload of every four primary care physicians on site. Intervention for patients in primary care tends to be family based and solution focused, and will usually consist of one or two sessions. Behavioral health appointments on site are scheduled with gaps so that "same day" appointments are available.

When possible and appropriate, psychosocial treatment is provided through groups of either a psychoeducational or psychotherapeutic nature. Longer term therapy and group therapy will tend to take place at a regional behavioral health center rather than a primary care site to meet the increased space required for specialized groups and to accommodate patients with major mental illness.

Development of a Team-Based Culture

Site-sharing by psychosocial and biomedical providers does not in itself promote collaboration. Education, empowerment, and commitment at a site level are required for providers to develop a common language and orientation to meet the biopsychosocial needs of their patients.

Consistent System to Identify Psychosocial Distress

There is considerable variation in primary care providers' ability to identify psychosocial needs. Therefore, HCP is developing a patient questionnaire system to consistently identify persons with these needs. Results from the questionnaires are given to the providers to assist them in evaluating and treating their patients at the time of the visit.

A Forum for Discussion

Collaborative care involves the development of new clinical skills. Therefore, a forum is needed for systematic study of cases and situations which exemplify best and worst care. This forum will eventually lead to the development of treatment guidelines.

Modifications in Operational and Financial Systems

Crucial to innovation in health care is the involvement of all three worlds in the redesign process. As clinical guidelines are developed, individuals with financial and operational expertise must be involved to consider implementation.

Ongoing Assessment

Ongoing assessment of clinical effectiveness, operational efficiency, and financial viability is necessary in order to ensure that collaborative care is useful and supports the concerns of the organization.

SUMMARY

HealthCare Partners has made a philosophical and organizational commitment to the biopsychosocial model of care for its patients. With the development of collaborative teams, HCP is able to attend to the major medical and mental conditions of its patients as well as deliver care to the 50 to 80% of patients who present to primary care with nonorganic and subsyndromal distress. In addition, the system is well positioned to offer patients health education, enrichment, and enhancement.

There is a tremendous need and opportunity for provider education in this integrated system. As providers are placed in proximity to each other, new learning and new ways of caring are a natural consequence. The move from independence to interdependence produces an environment in which appropriate and timely care can be delivered.

HCP providers have responded enthusiastically to all its collaborative care initiatives. The patients have responded with equal enthusiasm. As an integrated multispecialty provider group utilizing the collaborative care model, it is uniquely positioned to reclaim the original vision of managed care.

PART III

Research and Training

8.

Is the Integration of Behavioral Health Into Primary Care Worth the Effort? A Review of the Evidence

Gregory E. Simon, M.D., M.P.H.,
Michael VonKorff, Sc.D.

Over the last decade, clinicians, insurers, and professional societies in the United States have directed increasing attention to the management of mental disorders presenting in primary care. A major stimulus for this shift in focus has been the growing body of research on the epidemiology and management of mental disorders in primary care. Early epidemiologic studies (Regier, Goldberg, & Taube, 1978) clearly demonstrated that traditional specialty mental health services reached only a small portion of those in need of care. This epidemiologic evidence prompted a generation of research focused on the reintegration of mental health services into primary health care. After approximately 20 years of research, a substantial research database is now available to guide the development of integrated general medical and mental health care. This chapter will review that research database with specific focus on the following questions:

- How prevalent are anxiety, depressive, and substance use disorders in primary care?

• What is the impact of mental disorders in primary care on individual patients, the health care system, and the larger society?
• Are primary care patients with mental disorders currently recognized and treated?
• Are those recognized and treated receiving appropriate and effective care?
• Will integration of mental health services into primary care reduce the prevalence and impact of mental disorders in the population?
• Will more effective treatment of mental disorders in primary care lead to cost savings or cost offsets?
• What are the implications of research findings for program design?

The complete body of research on mental disorders in primary care is too broad to be covered in detail here. This selective review presents key studies and highlights work over the last decade at Group Health Cooperative of Puget Sound.

EPIDEMIOLOGY OF MENTAL DISORDERS IN PRIMARY CARE

Research over the last 20 years has demonstrated that mental health problems are common among primary care patients. Data from the Group Health Cooperative (GHC), site of the World Health Organization multicenter primary care survey, estimated prevalence rates of 8% for current major depression, 10% for current anxiety disorder, and 8% for current alcohol use disorder (Simon & VonKorff, 1995b). These findings are generally similar to other primary care surveys which have found prevalence rates of 6 to 14% for current depressive disorders, 6 to 12% for current anxiety disorders, and 5 to 8% for alcohol use disorders (Nielsen & Williams, 1980; Philbrick, Connelly, & Wofford, 1996; Spitzer et al., 1994; VonKorff, Shapiro, et al., 1987). These surveys have included a wide range of patient populations (urban and rural, higher and lower socioeconomic status) and practice settings (prepaid, fee-for-service, academic, community). Prevalence rates for anxiety and depressive disorders among primary care patients are typically twice as high as seen in community samples, reflecting the association between psychological distress and use of primary care services (Kessler et al., 1987).

Among community residents with mental disorders, approximately half are treated exclusively in primary care. Data from both waves of the Epidemiologic Catchment Area survey indicated that approximately 28% of community residents satisfied criteria for any mental or substance use disorder over a 12-month period (Regier et al., 1993). Of that group, approximately 45% received some treatment in the general medical sector while 43% received some specialty mental health services (Narrow et al., 1993). These proportions did not include those seen in primary care or other medical settings but not recognized or treated.

A variety of sociodemographic factors are associated with decreased use of specialty mental. health services. Data from Group Health Cooperative suggest that primary care patients less likely to use specialty mental health services include men, the elderly, and those with fewer years of education (Simon, VonKorff, & Durham, 1994). Data from community surveys also suggest that whites are more likely to use traditional specialty mental health services than members of other ethnic groups (Olfson & Klerman, 1992; Padgett et al., 1994).

Characteristics of the health care delivery system may also affect relative use of primary care or specialty services for mental health needs. Data from the 1970s and 1980s indicated significant differences in patterns of specialty mental health service use between pre-paid and fee-for-service health plans. Members of prepaid plans were more likely to use any specialty services but less likely to be treated intensively (Diehr, Williams, Martin & Price, 1984; Manning, Wells, & Benjamin, 1987; Norquist & Wells, 1991). These studies did not clearly indicate whether higher rates of service used in prepaid plans resulted from the method of payment or the system of care (organized system with clear referral pathways). Use of specialty mental health services is clearly affected by out-of-pocket costs (Hankin, Steinwachs, & Eldes, 1980; Manning, Wells, Duan, Newhouse, & Ware, 1986; Simon, Grothaus, Durham, VonKorff, &

Pabiniak, 1996). Modest increases in copayments or coinsurance appear to reduce likelihood of mental health service use without respect to level of need. The common policy of higher cost-sharing for mental health than for general medical visits will increase the proportion of patients with mental disorder managed exclusively in primary care where out-of-pocket costs are lower.

IMPACT OF MENTAL DISORDERS

Mental disorders among primary care patients have a major impact on daily functioning and quality of life. Epidemiologic surveys of primary care patients consistently demonstrate that anxiety and depressive disorders are associated with significant impairment of work and social functioning and health-related quality of life (Ormel, VonKorff, Ustun, Pini, Korten, & Oldehinkel, 1994; Spitzer et al., 1995; VonKorff, Ormel, Katon, & Lin, 1992; Wells et al., 1989). The impairment associated with mental disorders appears as great as or greater than that due to chronic medical conditions such as diabetes or arthritis (Ormel et al., 1994; Wells et al., 1989). Longitudinal studies demonstrate synchrony of change in depression and functional disability. Improvement in depression is associated with improved daily functioning (VonKorff et al., 1992; Ormel, Von-Korff, VanDenBrink, Katon, Brilman, & Oldehinkel, 1993) while onset of depression is associated with onset of functional disability (Bruce, Seeman, Merrill, & Blazer, 1994).

Lost productivity attributable to the mental disorders commonly seen in primary care has a major economic impact. Epidemiologic surveys estimate that anxiety and depressive disorders are associated with 4 to 5 days of lost productivity per month above that due to comorbid medical conditions (Ormel et al., 1994; Spitzer et al., 1995). Improvement in depression is associated with reduced disability and improved work productivity (Ormel et al., 1993; Mintz, Mintz, Arruda, & Hwang, 1992). From the perspective of an employer (or society as a whole) the economic value of 4 days of lost productivity by an hourly worker is often greater than $400. This monthly "cost" of depression far exceeds the typical costs of depression treatment in primary care (Simon, VonKorff, & Barlow, 1995).

A growing body of evidence demonstrates that anxiety and depressive disorders among primary care patients are associated with large increases in use of general medical services. An early study of "high utilizers" of general medical services at GHC found high prevalence rates of current and lifetime anxiety and depressive disorders (Katon et al., 1990). In a similar sample of "high utilizers" from the DeanCare HMO in Wisconsin, depression was associated with an approximately $1,500 increase in overall costs (Henk, Katzelnick, Kobak, Greist, & Jefferson, 1996). Data from the GHC site of the WHO primary care survey indicated that primary care patients with current depressive or anxiety disorder had overall health care costs 50 to 75% higher than comparable patients without mental disorder (Simon, Ormel, VonKorff, & Barlow, 1995). Improvement in anxiety and depression was associated with reduced cost, but this relationship did not reach statistical significance (probably reflecting the modest sample size and the large variability in costs). In a larger sample of GHC patients with depression identified through administrative data systems, current depression was associated with a similar 50 to 75% increase in overall utilization after adjustment for comorbid medical illness (Simon, VonKorff, & Barlow, 1995). Less than 25% of these excess costs were attributable to mental health treatment. In a sample of GHC Medicare enrollees, level of depression (as measured by CES-D score) was strongly associated with use of general medical services (Unutzer, Patrick, Simon, Grembowski, Walker, & Katon, 1996). In this sample, improvement in depression was associated with significant decreases in overall health services cost.

ARE THOSE IN NEED RECOGNIZED AND TREATED?

Epidemiologic studies demonstrate that a substantial number of patients with anxiety and depressive disorders are not recognized by primary care physicians. While reported "nonrecognition" rates range as high as 80 to 90%, studies with highest rates of nonrecognition have often relied on screening scales or other self-report measures to assign diagnoses. Studies using structured diagnostic assessments and formal diagnostic criteria have typically reported recognition rates of 45 to 60% (Gerber et al., 1989; Nielsen & Williams, 1980; Schulberg, Saul, McClelland, Ganguli, Christy, & Frank, 1985; VonKorff et al., 1987). Among GHC patients in the WHO primary care survey, primary care physicians recognized approximately 55% of those with current major depression, 50% of those with current anxiety disorder, and 50% of those with current alcohol dependence (Simon & VonKorff, 1995a, 1995b).

More detailed study of patients with "unrecognized" disorders, however, yields a somewhat more reassuring picture. In the GHC sample described above, patients with unrecognized depression were less severely ill and less disabled than those with recognized depression (Simon & VonKorff, 1995a). A similar result has been reported in a sample of Michigan family practice patients (Coyne et al., 1995) and the Dutch site of the WHO primary care study (Tiemens, Ormel, & Simon, 1996). Across all sites of the WHO collaborative study, recognition of anxiety and depressive disorders by primary care physicians was strongly related to symptom severity (Simon, Ustun, & VonKorff, 1996). When the sample of cases was limited to those with disability attributed to mental disorder, rate of recognition by the treating primary care physician was considerably higher. These data suggest that primary care physicians' likelihood of recognizing anxiety and depressive disorders is related to severity of illness and need for treatment.

Available data do not clearly indicate that screening to improve recognition of mental disorders in primary care will improve outcomes. At the GHC site of the WHO study, patients with major depression who were not recognized by the primary care physician improved over the next 3 months at a rate comparable to recognized cases (Simon & VonKorff, 1995a). A longitudinal study of recent onset psychological disorders among Dutch general practice patients found an association between recognition and more rapid recovery among patients with anxiety disorders, but found no effect of recognition for depressive disorders (Ormel, Koeter, VanDenBrink, & VandeWillige, 1991). More recent data from the Dutch site of the WHO study show no association between recognition and outcomes for patients with anxiety or depressive disorders (Tiemens et al., 1996). A similar finding was reported in a smaller sample of depressed primary care patients reported by Schulberg, McClelland, and Gooding (1987). While these data suggest that increasing recognition might not improve outcomes, experimental studies yield stronger evidence. In a randomized trial conducted among psychologically distressed "high utilizers" in the GHC population, increasing physicians' awareness of psychiatric diagnosis did not improve patient outcomes (Katon, VonKorff, Lin, Bush, Lipscomb, & Russo, 1992). Dowrick and Buchan (1995) recently reported a randomized trial of depression screening in primary care with feedback of screening results to treating physicians. Such feedback of screening results did not improve clinical outcomes. Mathias, Fifer, Mazonson, Lubeck, Buesching, and Patrick (1994) described a randomized trial of anxiety disorder screening and feedback among primary care patients and physicians in a Colorado health plan. Increasing recognition rates through screening had no effect on patients' clinical or functional outcomes.

The absence of a clear association between recognition and outcomes suggests two explanations. Some patients may experience good short-term outcomes with or without recognition by the primary care physician. A substantial number of patients with unrecognized anxiety or depressive disorders appear to have less severe conditions with little associated disability. Spontaneous improvement without specific treatment is highly likely. For some primary care patients with more severe conditions, recognition alone may be insufficient. Diagnosis by the primary care physician will have little impact unless it is followed by initiation of effective treatment and adequate follow-up care. This argument is supported by the studies of primary care treatment programs (both effective and ineffective) described below.

EFFECTIVENESS OF CURRENT TREATMENTS IN PRIMARY CARE

Prescription of psychotropic medication is the most common treatment provided for mental disorders presenting in primary care. Epidemiologic surveys of primary care patients suggest that one-third to one-half of patients with current depressive disorder receive antidepressant drugs (Simon & VonKorff, 1995a; Wells, Katon, Rogers, & Camp, 1994). Of patients with recognized anxiety or depressive disorder, approximately 60% receive some psychotropic medication (Simon & VonKorff, 1995a). Primary care physicians account for the majority of treatment with both antidepressant drugs (Beardsley, Gardocki, Larson, & Hidalgo, 1988; Simon, VonKorff, Wagner, & Barlow, 1993) and benzodiazepines (Simon, VonKorff, Barlow, et al., 1996).

Prescribing of psychotropic medications by primary care physicians often fails to conform to expert recommendations and practice guidelines. Research in this area has focused primarily on antidepressant drugs because recommended levels of antidepressant treatment (dose and duration) are well established. In several samples of GHC primary care patients initiating antidepressant treatment for depression (Katon, VonKorff, Lin, Bush, & Ormel, 1992; Simon et al., 1993; Simon, Lin, Katon, et al., 1995; Simon, VonKorff, Heiligenstein, et al., 1996), only 40 to 50% received recommended levels of acute-phase treatment (i.e., at least 3 months of treatment at minimally adequate doses). In these samples, at least one-third of patients beginning antidepressant treatment discontinued medication early. Of those continuing treatment, a substantial number never received doses within the range recommended by expert guidelines. Analyses of data from the Medical Outcomes Study sample (Wells et al., 1994) and several earlier primary care samples found even lower rates of "adequate" antidepressant treatment. Observational data from GHC samples suggests that premature discontinuation of antidepressant treatment is associated with less frequent follow-up visits (Simon et al., 1993) and poorer patient education (Lin et al., 1995). In contrast with previously described data on recognition of depression, receipt of appropriate pharmacotherapy is not significantly related to severity of depression and patients receiving recommended levels of pharmacotherapy are somewhat more likely to improve during acute-phase treatment (Simon, Lin, et al., 1995).

Few primary care patients presenting with anxiety or depressive disorders receive specific psychotherapies of proven efficacy. Among GHC primary care patients with current depression, only one-third receive any specialty mental health services (Simon & VonKorff, 1995a) and only half of those referred make more than three visits (Simon, VonKorff, & Durham, 1994). While primary care physicians may provide brief counseling (Meredith, Wells, Kaplan, & Mazel, 1996; Robinson et al., 1995), this treatment does not approach the intensity of psychological treatments whose effectiveness has been proven in randomized controlled trials. Nonspecific brief counseling also is unlikely to incorporate therapeutic techniques of proven efficacy in the treatment of depression.

RESEARCH ON EFFECTIVENESS OF INTEGRATED CARE MODELS

Several recent studies have demonstrated the benefits of mental health programs integrated with primary health care. The benefits of integrated programs have been evaluated across a range of practice settings, patient populations, and clinical modalities. These successful programs, however, have several common elements: a specific focus on depression, integration of mental health services (and mental health specialists) into the primary care clinic, a structured program of treatment, and an emphasis on follow-up care to assure appropriate treatment.

Katon et al. (1995) developed and tested a program of integrated care for primary care patients initiating depression treatment. This "collaborative care" program included training for primary care physicians, educational materials for patients, and on-site consultation with a liaison psychiatrist. The primary care physician and psychiatrist shared responsibility for acute-phase treatment, alternating visits over the first 6 to 10 weeks. The program also included active monitoring of patient adherence with feedback to the psychiatrist and primary care physician. When compared to patients receiving usual depression treatment, patients with major depression in the collaborative care program were more likely to receive recommended levels of treatment, reported higher satisfaction, and had significantly better clinical outcomes. Among patients with minor depression, the program was not significantly more effective than usual care.

A second study at Group Health Cooperative found equally favorable results with an integrated program provided by a liaison psychologist (Katon et al., 1996). This program included the same components of patient education and active monitoring. Psychiatric consultation was available, but only used as needed. All patients in the intervention group received a brief psychotherapeutic intervention delivered in the primary care clinic. This program incorporated elements of behavioral activation, self-monitoring, and cognitive restructuring. Outcomes were similar to those of the psychiatrist collaborative care model. There were significantly better patient satisfaction and clinical outcomes among patients with major depression.

Schulberg et al. (1996) recently reported the integrated delivery of either antidepressant pharmacotherapy or interpersonal psychotherapy were both significantly superior to usual primary care. Patients were enrolled by a two-stage screening process intended to identify those with untreated depression of at least moderate severity. This sample of urban primary care patients was generally more severely depressed and socioeconomically deprived than the GHC collaborative care samples. The interventions provided were also substantially more intensive. The interpersonal therapy group received weekly treatment in the primary care clinic for up to 16 weeks. The pharmacotherapy group also received frequent visits with monitoring of antidepressant blood levels. When compared to patients receiving usual care, those in both intervention groups had significantly better clinical outcomes. While the pharmacotherapy group experienced somewhat more rapid improvement than the psychotherapy group, the two groups showed equivalent results by 4 to 6 months.

Mynors-Wallis, Gath, Lloyd-Thomas, & Tomlinson (1995) demonstrated the efficacy of a brief problem-solving psychotherapy for depression among British general practice patients. Patients with major depression were randomly assigned to a brief problem-solving psychotherapy (6 or 7 sessions over 12 weeks), pharmacotherapy with amitriptyline, or placebo treatment. All treatments were delivered in the general practice clinic or the patient's home. Problem-solving therapy was provided by either a psychiatrist or one of two general practitioners trained in the method. Outcomes for the problem-solving group were significantly better than those of the placebo group. The amitriptyline group had somewhat better outcomes than placebo treatment, but this difference was not statistically significant (probably reflecting the small sample size and insufficient statistical power).

The successful intervention studies described are best put into perspective by comparison with a series of negative reports. In the GHC study of "high utilizers" discussed earlier, distressed "high utilizers" of outpatient medical services were randomly assigned to usual care or a psychiatric consultation intervention (Katon, VonKorff, Lin, Bush, Lipscomb, & Russo, 1992). The intervention treatment program included on-site psychiatric consultation with feedback to the primary care physician, but no structured treatment program or active follow-up were provided. Patient outcomes were no different in the intervention and usual care groups. Callahan, Hendrie, Dittus, Brater, Hui, and Tierney (1994) tested an integrated clinical program to improve depression treatment among elderly primary care patients. The intervention program included training of primary care physicians, screening for depression, and feedback of screening results and treatment recommendations to the treating primary care physician. No specific treatment program or monitoring of follow-up care were included. Outcomes for patients in the intervention group were not better than those for patients receiving usual care. In a follow-up evaluation of the two GHC randomized trials described above, Lin et al. (in press) found that improvements in practice during the intervention period did not persist after withdrawal of the research program. Once on-site consultation and treatment monitoring were discontinued, practice patterns and patient outcomes were no different from a "control" clinic receiving no intervention services.

COST OFFSET AND COST-EFFECTIVENESS

A number of quasi-experimental studies have examined the cost-effectiveness of conventional specialty mental health services. Of studies using nonrandomized comparison groups, Follette and Cummings (1967) as well as Goldensohn and Fink (1979) found reductions in general medical utilization associated with initiation of psychotherapeutic treatment. Similar findings were reported by Hankin, Kessler, Goldberg, Steinwachs, and Starfield (1983), Mumford, Schlesinger, Glass, Patrick, and Cuerdon (1984), and Goldberg, Allen, Kessler, Carey, Locke, and Cook (1981): reduced medical utilization associated with use of traditional mental health specialty services. Studies using a before–after design (Goldberg et al., 1970; Jameson, Shuman, & Young, 1978) have consistently found reductions in medical utilization following mental health treatment. While these studies all suggest the potential for cost savings due to effective mental health treatment, none can exclude the potential biases in nonexperimental designs. For example, decreased utilization seen in before–after designs may reflect either treatment effects or regression toward previous utilization levels after a period of unusually high utilization associated with distress. A similar bias can occur in comparisons of treated patients with an untreated (but nonrandomized) comparison group.

Hellman et al. (1990) at Harvard Community Health used an experimental design to evaluate the effectiveness of group behavioral medicine interventions for patients with psychosomatic complaints. When compared to patients in a "control" treatment (stress management information) patients in the behavioral medicine programs experienced greater symptom relief and greater reductions in outpatient medical utilization. These interventions were specifically focused on coping with distressing somatic symptoms and were not general-purpose programs for management of psychological distress.

The strongest evidence for the economic benefits of integrated mental health care comes from studies of medical and surgical inpatients. These studies have typically examined the impact of psychoeducational or brief psychotherapeutic interventions for patients with specific medical conditions. As reviews by Mumford et al. (1984) and Strain, Hammer & Fulop (1994) have pointed out, these studies indicate that effective mental health services can reduce medical utilization (especially inpatient utilization). They also illustrate two important principles for achieving cost-offset effects: focus on patients with high baseline utilization and integration of mental health services into general medical care.

As discussed above, anxiety and depressive disorders among primary care patients are associated with significant increases in use of general medical services. This "excess" utilization occurs across all categories of service (inpatient, outpatient, primary care, medical specialty, etc) and is not accounted for by greater medical comobidity among depressed patients (Simon, Ormel, VonKorff, & Barlow, 1995; Simon, VonKorff, & Barlow, 1995; Unutzer et al., 1996). Greater medical utilization does not simply reflect somatization and excess utilization by the worried well. Depression is associated with even greater increases in utilization among those with serious chronic illnesses than among those without (Simon, VonKorff, & Barlow, 1995; Henk, et al., 1996). It seems plausible that psychological illness impairs ability to cope with either chronic medical illness or nonspecific somatic symptoms.

Research data on the economic value of integrated outpatient programs remains incomplete. The observational data described above indicate the potential for significant cost savings, but only true experiments can determine whether improved mental health treatment in primary care will produce cost savings. While several recent experimental studies have demonstrated the clinical benefits of integrated care programs, none have had sufficient sample size to detect differences in general medical utilization. Given the variability in health care costs, a sample of 400 or more patients would be necessary for such a study. An ongoing collaborative study at DeanCare, GHC, and Harvard-Pilgrim Health Care will examine the cost-effectiveness of systematic depression treatment among "high utilizers" of outpatient medical services. The sample size (over 400 patients) should be sufficient to examine effects on clinical outcomes, direct health care costs, and indirect costs (daily functioning and work productivity).

Available research, however, is sufficient to demonstrate that the cost of proven integrated care programs is small compared to the potential economic benefit. In the two "collaborative care" studies described above, treatment costs for patients receiving the integrated intervention program were only $250 to $400 higher than those for patients receiving usual care (VonKorff et al., 1994). This modest additional expenditure increased the proportion of patients with major depression responding to treatment from approximately 45% among those receiving usual care to approximately 75% among those receiving collaborative care. While this sample was not large enough to rule in or rule out any associated decreases in general medical costs, the increased costs of more effective treatment ($250 to $400) were only 20 to 25% of the excess general medical utilization associated with depression in primary care. This comparison does not consider the potential indirect savings due to improved daily functioning and productivity.

IMPLICATIONS OF RESEARCH FOR PROGRAM DESIGN

Existing research suggests several guiding principles for development of mental health programs in primary care. First, programs based on physician education or simple screening are unlikely to improve patient outcomes. Second, treatments developed and proven in specialty populations appear to be quite effective for depressed primary care patients. Third, structured treatment programs which include patient education, structured care programs, systematic monitoring, and adequate follow-up care are critical to improving patient outcomes.

A review of the research described above also suggests significant gaps. Most intervention research to date has focused on depression. Epidemiologic evidence suggests that anxiety and alcohol use disorders are also prevalent among primary care patients. Research to date has not considered the effect of insurance coverage arrangements and financial incentives. Some financial arrangements may reduce the potential for collaboration between primary care and mental health providers. Consultation models developed under capitated arrangements (Katon et al, 1995; Mynors-Wallis et al., 1995) may prove difficult to implement or maintain in systems which pay providers per unit of service delivered. Copayments and coinsurance arrangements typically imposed on mental health services may significantly affect patient participation and clinical effectiveness. Finally, most studies have focused on acute treatment. Because anxiety and depressive disorders are often chronic or recurrent (Katon et al., 1995; Simon, Ustun, & VonKorff, 1996), programs to prevent relapse may have a greater impact on overall prevalence than programs to improve acute treatment.

Comprehensive mental health programs must balance the proven benefits of condition-specific treatments against the need to meet a wide variety of "real world" clinical demands. As noted above, most intervention studies have focused on specific, well-defined conditions (typically depression). The research advantages of this focused approach are clear (Katon et al., 1995). One is most likely to demonstrate the benefit of an intervention program by focusing on more severe cases of a well-defined disorder in which the efficacy of specific treatments has been well established. Clinical program development, however, has somewhat different priorities. Clinical practice is much more heterogeneous than research samples. Satisfying primary care "customers" (both patients and referring physicians) requires that a clinical program accept and manage the wide range of problems presenting in primary care: anxiety disorders, depressive disorders, somatoform disorders, situational crises, substance use disorders, and family–marital problems. Referrals from primary care providers are likely to span the full range of symptomatic severity. Primary care providers will not be satisfied with a program which accepts only specific groups of patients or which asks referring providers to "sort" patients into narrow referral pathways. Matching patients with the most appropriate type and level of care must be the responsibility of the mental health consultant(s), not the referring provider. The specific treatment models proven effective in clinical trials must be adapted to a more generic system of evaluation and treatment.

SUMMARY

The data reviewed here make a strong clinical and economic case for the integration of mental health services into primary care. Epidemiologic data clearly demonstrate that depressive, anxiety, and alcohol use disorders are common among primary care patients. Mental disorders in primary care account for a large burden of functional impairment, lost productivity, and "excess" use of general medical services. The economic impact of the disability and medical utilization associated with depressive and anxiety disorders far exceeds the potential cost of providing appropriate treatment. While a significant proportion of anxiety and depressive disorders in primary care may go unrecognized, current research does not clearly demonstrate that increased recognition alone will improve patient outcomes. For patients with less severe illness, recognition and treatment may not be necessary to achieve good short-term outcomes. For those with more severe conditions, recognition alone is not sufficient. Given the available evidence, increasing the rates of recognition and treatment is probably not the most important goal of primary care-based mental health programs. In contrast, there is now strong evidence for the value of integrated programs which deliver more appropriate and organized treatment to those already identified. Among primary care patients recognized as depressed, few receive treatment consistent with current practice guidelines. Structured, primary care-based treatment programs can deliver more appropriate treatment and significantly improve patient outcomes. Key elements of effective primary care-based treatment programs include: educating and reactivating patients, integration of mental health clinicians into the primary care practice, structured follow-up care, and systematic monitoring of treatment adherence and clinical outcomes. Future research and development should address a broader range of clinical problems (e.g., anxiety disorders, substance use disorders) and should include efforts to prevent relapse and chronicity.

9.

Training the Primary Care Physician for the Integrated Behavioral Health/Primary Care System of the Future

**Steven Cole, M.D., James H. Gordon, M.D.,
Stephen M. Saravay, M.D.,
Maurice D. Steinberg, M.D.,
Steven Walerstein, M.D.**

OVERVIEW: PROBLEMS, BARRIERS AND SOLUTIONS

The concept of integrating behavioral health care into primary, general medical practice runs counter to the prevailing "biomedical" approach of Western medicine learned and ingrained over the past two centuries (G. E. Engel, 1993). It is little wonder then that the medical profession has been reluctant to adopt such a fundamental reversal in philosophy. To do so now, however, has become a matter of urgency.

Preceding chapters have lucidly articulated the rationale, and indeed the imperative, for incorporating all aspects of well-being into our care of patients. At this juncture in the evolution of our health care system, it has become clear that an integrated approach to health care delivery is no longer a matter of choice

163

or preference, but rather a necessity. The extraordinary, highly competitive demands for efficient delivery and quality outcomes already confronting us mean that we cannot wait for the natural assimilation of knowledge and ideas to run its course, culminating in the eventual adoption of a biopsychosocial model of primary care. We must act now to facilitate moving the process of change more rapidly (Epstein, Budd, & Cole, 1995).

Our objective in this chapter is to outline concrete ways in which the upcoming generation of physicians and those already practicing in the community can be trained in the concepts of integrated and collaborative behavioral care and provided with the tools for efficiently delivering it. Before describing such programs, it is worth briefly reviewing three cardinal barriers to the adoption of an integrated health care model. Overcoming these barriers, therefore, logically becomes the core objective of training or "retooling" initiatives. These key barriers may be conceptualized as attitudinal (mindset), informational (knowledge), and aptitudinal (skills) (Bird & Cohen-Cole, 1983).

Physicians naturally inherit the attitude and cultural mindset of their teachers and mentors. The great tradition of mainstream medicine in the West has been based on the Cartesian belief in the essential independence of physical and mental processes. While physicians may be intellectually aware of the large body of evidence demonstrating the invalidity of this concept, this awareness per se is insufficient to change the notion and related behaviors that biological health is the principal domain of medicine while mental health properly belongs to another, "lesser" branch (Cole & Raju, 1996).

Traditional "biomedical" training does not provide physicians with sufficient knowledge about mental disorders for them to understand, recognize, and diagnose such conditions (Cohen-Cole & Friedman, 1983). By the same token, the implicit irrelevance of the psyche leads clinicians to ignore the humanistic component of the physician–patient relationship and to suppress their own emotional involvement in the process, exactly the opposite of the interaction required to provide effective biopsychosocial care (Epstein et al., 1995).

Even if physicians astutely recognize that a patient may be suffering from a mental disorder, they often lack specific communication skills designed to elicit a concrete diagnosis in an efficient manner as well as the competence to provide effective treatment. Physicians' education and training has omitted or at best has given only lip service to these areas. It is easy to see that these operational barriers powerfully reinforce each other and tend to perpetuate resistance to dealing with behavioral problems in primary care practice.

The question now becomes, can these barriers be broken down and entrenched practice patterns changed? Dozens of training programs intended to educate primary care practitioners in psychiatric aspects of care have been described, but it is apparent that the structure of the training is crucial to its ultimate effectiveness (Cohen-Cole, 1991a). Several studies reported in the literature indicate that the psychiatric training programs evaluated had little educational impact. It has been shown, however, that targeted psychiatric educational programs can improve the level of knowledge among internal medicine and family medicine residents (Cole, Saravey, & Steinberg, 1995). Also, notably, many family practice residencies have for some time integrated practice-based training and supervision in managing psychosocial aspects of care, even though evaluation results are still limited. The following section describes our experience with programs designed for training internal medicine residents for the integrated behavioral health care system of the future.

TRAINING PROGRAMS FOR PRIMARY CARE PHYSICIANS

After 3 years of collaborative effort, a multidisciplinary task force appointed by the Society of General Internal Medicine defined the objectives of a model curriculum for primary care residents aimed at integrating mental disorders and behavioral problems into primary care practice (Cole et al., 1995). The fundamental concept embodied in the curriculum is that primary care providers benefit their patients, as well as themselves, by learning to practice in a biopsychosocial mode, that they can competently manage many uncomplicated mental disorders themselves, while in some cases collaborative management with or referral to a specialist will be appropriate (Cohen-Cole & Levinson, 1994).

In brief, the objectives of this training curriculum include five general areas: (1) the biopsychosocial model of illness; (2) interviewing and formulation skills related to the evaluation of behavioral symptoms; (3) knowledge of the mental disorders that are of central importance in primary care practice; (4) supportive interventions to patients with mental problems; and (5) management of psychiatric emergencies.

Primary Care Residents

While many different training programs could conceivably be utilized to reach these objectives, we propose a systematic curriculum currently being tested at Long Island Jewish Medical Center (LIJMC), which may serve as a model for future efforts. The LIJMC curriculum is unusual in many aspects and readers will be interested in a detailed description of its components, their philosophical rationale, and pragmatic considerations.

Training of medical interns in behavioral aspects of care at LIJMC covers 3 years. In postgraduate year 1 (PGY-1), the course focuses on medical interviewing proficiency, in PGY-2 on acquiring concrete psychiatric knowledge and skills, and in PGY-3 on supervised clinical practice in assessment and management of uncomplicated ambulatory behavioral disorders.

PGY-1. The first year concentrates on medical interviewing, and on incorporating the principles of biopsychosocial medicine. The rotation, entitled "Advanced Clinical Skills" (ACS), is taken by all medical interns at LIJMC (Gordon, Walerstein, & Pollack, in press). The course is given over 4 weeks as a 60-hour, 20-day block curriculum for groups of 4 to 6 interns, who are freed from all but minimal clinical responsibilities for the duration of the rotation.

These parameters are important factors in the success of the ACS program in instilling sound medical interviewing skills. In their first year, interns have not yet solidified problematic techniques or attitudes that have to be unlearned. The intensive block curriculum provides an enculturating immersion in biopsychosocial thinking and uninterrupted processing of complex material that improves learning. A group size of 4 to 6 individuals is optimal for interactive discussions embedded in the course. Limiting other responsibilities reinforces the central importance of the medical interview in medical practice, and it allows the participants to devote all their physical and psychic reserves to what is often an emotionally demanding experience.

The course material is based on the three-function model of the medical interview (Cohen-Cole, 1991b). This model specifically emphasizes the importance of the emotional and behavioral dimensions of the physician–patient interaction, being as consequential as the data-collection process for efficient and effective patient care. In brief, the three functions of the medical interview proposed are: (1) information gathering; (2) establishing a relationship with the patient by responding to his to her emotions; and (3) formulating a joint treatment plan that includes education to change behavior. The ACS course aims to foster and develop the separate skills that are needed by the physician in each of these three areas.

The course is organized and facilitated throughout by a consultation–liaison psychiatrist, namely the second author, who was formerly an internist. The rest of the faculty is made up of five internists who have demonstrated particular facility for the medical interview process and who are comfortable dealing with the emotional content of the course. These five instructors each coteach the course with the psychiatric facilitator on one day per week. The fact that the internists are from the same discipline as the trainees is reassuring and leads to more comfortable role modeling. Having a physician with psychiatric training coordinate the entire course is useful in that skills related to group dynamics and psychodynamic aspects of interviewing can be brought to bear.

From the outset, a supportive, nonjudgmental environment is established by making clear that no grading or formal evaluations will be made, that expression of opinion is encouraged, and that the group decides the direction discussions take.

The first half of the course develops core interviewing skills and includes the use of open-ended questions, facilitation, reflection of emotions, legitimation, respect, and partnering. The second half focuses on "difficult" scenarios, such as obtaining a sexual history, the terminal patient, and substance abuse. Table 9.1 gives the full list of topics.

Most of the 20 sessions are 3 hours in length, and begin with a didactic presentation, sometimes a training video, and a group discussion. The second half of each session is experiential, and usually consists of role-playing to practice skills that have been discussed or feedback on residents' video-taped interviews. Faculty facilitate these interactions, and participants have opportunities to play both the role of the "patient" and the "physician" in each session. After receiving feedback on videotaped interviews, residents also have the opportunity to role-play alternative approaches to difficult situations.

During the ACS program, each trainee is twice videotaped interviewing actual inpatients. The group watches the "live" interview and then reviews the tape, making observations about teaching points that emerge and suggesting alternative tacks the interviewer might have taken. These videotaped interviews and role-playing are consistently mentioned by interns in their evaluation of the course as the most valuable components for effective learning.

For one day of the course, each trainee spends 8 hours as a nursing aide, a feature developed with the Department of Nursing. The purpose is to foster an appreciation of nursing work, and to learn how nursing staff communicate and relate with their patients.

After taking the ACS program, interns experience a degree of personal growth and a reaffirmation of their identity as physicians. One participant, reflecting a feeling expressed by many others, wrote at the end of the course, "I feel I am a complete doctor now." The lessons learned are also evident in practice.

TABLE 9.1
Advanced Clinical Skills Program in Medical Interviewing

Session	Topic
Day 1	Overview, introductions, survey of concerns
Day 2	Initial steps in conducting an interview
Day 3	Gathering data and establishing the chief complaint
Day 4	Emotional and psychological issues
Day 5	Emotional and psychological issues (continued)
Day 6	The meaning of the illness
Day 7	Establishing a treatment plan
Day 8	Mental status exam
Day 9	Personality type and response to illness
Day 10	Transference, countertransference, and the problem patient
Day 11	Informed consent and DNR orders
Day 12	The terminal patient
Day 13	Adopt a Doc—a day with the nurses
Day 14	The HIV patient. Obtaining a sexual history
Day 15	Obtaining the history of abuse: alcohol, drug, physical and sexual
Day 16	Evaluation of depression and panic disorder
Day 17	Therapeutic communication
Day 18	Interns' choice
Day 19	Interns' choice
Day 20	Evaluation and debriefing

Medical and nursing staff often note the difference in interviewing skills and sophistication between ACS-trained interns and interns who have not yet received ACS-instruction. In brief, ACS provides a foundation that serves the participant well during the rest of his or her training and professional life.

PGY-2. In their second year at LIJMC, PGY-2 medical residents learn the cognitive and behavioral skills to assess and manage mental disorders in the primary care setting. These skills are not addressed in depth in PGY-1 in order for trainees to focus on acquiring the more general skills of medical interviewing.

The PGY-2 program on assessment and management of mental disorders consists of nine 2-hour lecture/workshops given once a month. The first session is devoted to teaching the use of PRIME-MD, a 10-minute patient questionnaire and confirmatory follow-up interview designed for primary care diagnosis of mental disorders (Spitzer et al., 1994). Participants also learn to use the Patient Problem Questionnaire (PPQ), a highly structured patient questionnaire which is a modification of PRIME-MD. Patient responses indicate the presence of the following mental disorders: major depression, panic or generalized anxiety disorder, somatoform disorder, eating disorder, or probable alcohol abuse. While this instrument is still under development, it has a high degree of face validity and has become a very useful adjunct to teaching and medical care in our programs.

The rest of the content of the course is based on the principal modules of DSM-IV-PC; that is, a decision-tree approach to the diagnosis and treatment of mood disorders, anxiety disorders, substance abuse, somatoform disorders, cognitive disorders, sleep disorders, sexual disorders, and eating disorders (American Psychiatric Association, 1994).

The primary course coordinator is present at all sessions to provide continuity from month to month. Each session is broken into four 30-minute segments. First, a lecturer gives a highly focused, pragmatic presentation on the assessment and management of the mental disorder itself. That is followed by a demonstration interview, in which an internist plays a patient presenting with the relevant condition and the lecturer conducts the interview. The interview has been scripted to demonstrate several interviewing problems that primary care physicians often face in the assessment and management of common mental disorders. A second facilitator leads a discussion with the audience concerning specific strengths and/or weaknesses of the demonstration interview.

Following this demonstration/workshop, the assemblage breaks into three smaller groups for open discussion of the teaching points made and further role-playing practice of the skills demonstrated. These small groups are facilitated by either the psychiatric lecturer, internist cocoordinator, or senior psychiatric or medical residents. Finally, the separate groups reconvene for a general discussion, to share points that emerged in the breakout segment and to ask specific questions. Specific pharmacological "minicases" are also reviewed in the final plenary segment.

PGY-3. In the next year, PGY-3, medical residents are given on-site clinical training and practice in applying the skills and knowledge they have acquired in their PGY-2 year. (At the present time, due to limited resources, this supervision is limited to the five or six residents on the primary care track. As more resources become available, this training will be extended to all PGY-3s.) Residents are assigned to psychiatrist supervisor for one half-day per week (of their usual medical clinic) and, under carefully monitored circumstances, are given responsibility for treating ambulatory patients with uncomplicated mental disorders.

In most cases, the resident uses the PPQ to identify underlying diagnoses, and employs the communication and cognitive skills learned in the preceding years to formulate a treatment plan in partnership with the patient, under the supervision of the liaison psychiatrist.

This clinical training program is clearly faculty-intensive and is still evolving as experience accumulates. At present, capacity is limited to five residents, one supervised by the attending psychiatrist and four supervised by two psychiatric consultation–liaison fellows.

Evaluation. Anecdotal qualitative evidence validating the effectiveness of the LIJMC curriculum in integrating psychosocial care into general medical practice is plentiful, and some preliminary quantitative (albeit uncontrolled) outcome data based on the first 2 years of the program are now available.

During the PGY-1 ACS course, interns' interviews with medical inpatients were rated by a course instructor using parts I and II of the Brown Interview Checklist (BIC) developed at Rhode Island Hospital (Novack, Dube, & Goldstein, 1992). Precourse and postcourse ratings were compared to provide a measure of educational effect. Statistically significant improvements occurred in 16 of 21 BIC categories. Of the major categories examined, only closing skills did not improve significantly, probably reflecting the artificiality of interviewing a patient who would not be seen again.

In an informal assessment, acquired interview skills seem to be maintained over time. A review of recorded interviews by

PGY-2 primary care residents who took ACS showed that all at least sustained the advances they had made in the previous year and that most had improved further.

COMMUNITY PHYSICIANS

If the integration of behavioral care into primary care residency programs requires effort and dedication, it is a relatively straightforward exercise when compared with the complexities of teaching the biopsychosocial model of behavioral health care to our primary care colleagues already practicing in the community. Nonetheless, the prevalence of behavioral disorders among general medical patients, their widespread misdiagnosis and ineffective treatment, and the focus of managed care organizations on reducing inefficiency and overutilization lead to the inescapable conclusion that primary care physicians must acquire skills in managing mental disorders and related psychosocial problems if they are to survive in practice (Epstein et al., 1995).

Continuing medical education (CME) programs intended to help primary care providers retool for an entirely new style of practice and to provide behavioral health care training must be shaped by the realities of medical practice if they are to be useful (Cole & Raju, 1996). That is to say, training objectives should be concrete, focused, and measurable. Such courses must be physician-friendly rather than physician-critical. That is, they should respect and build upon the skills that primary care physicians have already mastered, and explicitly acknowledge the demands of medical practice. Above all, training programs must be tailored to the everyday pressures experienced by physicians and should therefore set goals that are attainable within severe time constraints.

Roter (1995) has shown that a course structured along these lines, and delivered within a limited timeframe can indeed bring about significant changes in knowledge, skills, and routine behaviors, as well as improving patient outcomes. This model program randomized 69 primary care physicians to one of three groups (to one of two different training programs in communication skills or to a "no training" comparison group) in order to study the impact of training on the process and outcome of care for emotionally distressed patients (Cohen-Cole, Raju, & Barrett, 1993).

The training courses consisted of two 4-hour sessions (separated by 2 weeks) and addressed problem-defining skills or emotion-handling skills. Participants were audiotaped interviewing actual as well as simulated patients both before and after training to evaluate the efficacy of the programs. Audiotape analyses showed that, compared with untrained physicians, trained physicians used significantly more of the skills they were taught and strategies for managing emotional problems, without lengthening the visit. Telephone follow-up of patients 6 months after physician training showed that the emotionally distressed patients of the trained physicians demonstrated significantly less distress than the patients of untrained physicians.

THE MACARTHUR PROGRAM ON DEPRESSION EDUCATION FOR PRIMARY CARE PHYSICIANS

The salient features of the Roter model have been incorporated into a community-based training program funded by the MacArthur Foundation, designed to teach primary care physicians the communication skills and knowledge necessary for the assessment and management of uncomplicated major depression and dysthymia. The course is designed for groups of about a dozen participants and is conducted by a primary care physician cofacilitator and a psychiatrist cofacilitator. The total length of the course is 8 hours, divided into two 4-hour sessions separated by a 2-week interval.

The content of the first session is adjusted to the learning goals of the particular group, identified in a preliminary discussion. Using a slide presentation, participants are instructed on the diagnosis and management of depression as well as the psychosocial aspects of patient care, how to establish emotional rapport with the patient, and how to maximize adherence.

While objectives identified as most important by the participants are emphasized, the paramount importance of communication skills are also stressed. Videotapes are utilized to demonstrate pragmatic communication strategies, and role-playing exercises are employed to practice new skills.

Before the next session in 2 weeks, participants make at least one audiotape recording of a depressed patient in their own practice. Participants bring a 5-minute segment of this tape for review at the second workshop. The second session consists of a review of objectives, discussion of psychopharmacology case studies, and a 2-hour workshop to review audiotapes and to practice new, more effective communication strategies. A manuscript describing this sequence in detail is in preparation.

Formative (qualitative) evaluations of two pilot tests of this program, one with eight internists in New York and one with 12 family physicians in Oregon, demonstrated significant success, judging from participants' systematic evaluations. The robustness of the course material seemed apparent in the uniformly high ratings that all participants gave to the program, despite wide variations in their own level of self-rated knowledge and skills. The internists in New York described themselves as generally lacking in experience in the independent assessment and management of depressive illnesses, while the Oregon family physicians described themselves as already being quite familiar with treating depression in their own practices.

The "learner-centered" nature of the course, along with the flexibility of application of the materials, therefore, seemed able to meet quite diverse learning needs of the primary care physicians. It seemed to the instructors, that the internists in New York reported satisfaction with the course because it gave them the necessary tools to begin assessing and managing some uncomplicated depressions, while the family physicians in Oregon were able to expand upon the knowledge and skills they had already acquired.

A large randomized, controlled clinical trial of the effectiveness of the program for changing physicians' attitudes, knowledge, skill, and routine behavior is now in progress.

TRAINING PROGRAMS FOR PSYCHIATRIC PHYSICIANS
FOR INTEGRATED BEHAVIORAL HEALTH CARE

In the integrated behavioral health care system of the future, many uncomplicated behavioral problems will be managed appropriately by the primary care provider. Clearly, however, severe and complex mental disorders will require the participation of a behavioral specialist, either within the specialty sector itself or within a collaborative specialist/primary care physician approach. In addition, there will be a need for psychiatrists and other behavioral specialists to acquire the educational skills necessary to improve the knowledge and skills of their primary care colleagues, in formal instructional programs as well as in informal consultative relationships.

Psychiatrists of the future can benefit from increased understanding of the context, challenges and opportunities for primary care physicians to practice behavioral health care in the emerging managed care environment. In order for psychiatric trainees to gain this appreciation, each fourth-year psychiatric resident at LIJMC spends 4 hours per week for 6 months in a special rotation on "Primary Care and Psychiatry." The first two months are devoted to a focused "minicourse" on primary care and psychiatry, emphasizing the application of communication skills to primary care psychiatry. The next 4 months place the resident in the primary care attending office, seeing patients along with the internist or family physician.

Finally, the authors have established an innovative consultation–liaison psychiatric fellowship in primary care medicine at LIJCM (Steinberg, Cole, & Saravay, 1996). As part of this training, fellows spend one afternoon per week for one year in a primary care physician's office, observing primary care approaches to behavioral health care as well as offering collaborative psychiatric management; i.e., the fellows observe routine care but are available to assist when invited.

Fellows also learn how to provide supervised one-to-one training of third-year medical residents. Fellows see patients with these residents in medical clinics, assist residents in screening and assessing mental disorders in primary care and then supervise the residents' treatment of uncomplicated behavioral disorders. Fellows receive their own supervision for this complicated clinical–didactic–supervisory work.

SUMMARY AND CONCLUSIONS

In conclusion, the emerging managed care environment presents unusual challenges as well as opportunities for the rapid adoption of an integrated behavioral approach to health care delivery. The diverse training programs developed at LIJMC represent an attempt to meet the varied needs of primary care providers to acquire the cognitive and communication skills required for effective behavioral health care of their patients. The models at LIJMC also focus on the need to develop the knowledge and skills of the psychiatrists of the future to educate and collaborate effectively with their primary care colleagues. The authors hope these new programs and the experience gained so far will be helpful to other centers in developing systematic training initiatives tailored to their particular setting.

10.

Acceptance and Commitment: A Model for Integration

Patricia Robinson, Ph.D., Steven C. Hayes, Ph.D.

This chapter suggests a theoretical model for guiding integration of behavioral health and primary care services. A theoretical model may point the way for educators and providers who develop training programs for professionals and clinical programs for specific patient populations. The proposed model is an extension of the Acceptance and Commitment Therapy (ACT) model (Hayes, 1994; Hayes & Strosahl, 1997). This model evolved from behavior analysis (Hayes, 1987) and places emphasis on contextual variables in understanding and creating behavior change. It appears to be well suited for application to the context of primary health care services. It is hoped that this chapter will inspire development of theoretically based clinical interventions and research designs that further refine theory and practice in this new and growing area.

THE ACCEPTANCE AND COMMITMENT—HEALTH CARE MODEL

In this chapter, the authors refer to the proposed model as the Acceptance and Commitment in Health Care (ACT-HC)

Model. The ACT-HC model suggests that "context" and "control" are important concepts in understanding health care seeking behavior and health care services behavior. Also, the ACT-HC model suggests a distinction between public events (directly observable behaviors) and private events (thoughts, feelings, sensations). The model suggests that all behavior, including that of patients and their health care providers, occurs in a complex context influenced by specific variables. Some of these variables can be manipulated or directly changed while others cannot. Context variables that can be manipulated include patient attendance for medical appointments, patient behaviors regarding management of acute and chronic illness, patient knowledge of health care information, provider prescribing patterns, patient attendance of workplace and primary care health education programs, etc. Context variables that cannot be directly manipulated include the personal histories and current private events of patients and providers. Variables that are less amenable to change need the attention of health care planners, educators, and providers, as these variables tend to be underrecognized and misunderstood.

Health care seeking behavior (or the lack of it) occurs in a complex system involving patient, health care provider, and, often, employer variables. All three players desire control and may participate in experiential avoidance strategies that limit achievement of important health care outcomes. Experiential avoidance is the attempt to escape or avoid certain private experiences, such as particular feelings, memories, behavioral predisposition, or thoughts (Hayes & Wilson, 1993). For example, a chronic pain patient may persist in requesting pain medications rather than learn behavioral management strategies because of an underlying unwillingness to live life with pain. A physician may participate in experiential avoidance by prescribing larger doses of addictive medications rather than experience the discomfort of directly confronting the patient's unwillingness, as well as his or her own sense of powerlessness to offer a remedy for pain. Experiential avoidance is pervasive and often harmful to human functioning (Hayes & Gifford, in press; Hayes, Wilson, Gifford, Follette, & Strosahl, 1996).

Experiential avoidance derives from verbal processes. These include the human ability to associate bi-directionally. In human language, describing an event (e.g., current pelvic pain) can reawaken certain aspects of previous related events (e.g., pain during unwanted intercourse). In ACT-HC, this is referred to as bi-directionality of derived stimulus relations, and it promotes development of experiential avoidance in all verbal human beings.

While bi-directionality of language promotes experiential avoidance, practices within a society may amplify experiential avoidance by promoting verbal rules that directly train experiential avoidance. For example, children learn rules concerning the need to avoid certain feelings, thoughts, etc. Behavior acquired by explicit instruction is often less responsive to changes in the environment than behavior learned by direct experience (Hayes, 1994). Therefore, a person's knowledge that experiential avoidance creates problems is usually not enough to lead the person to modify or abandon the strategy.

People who frequently employ coping strategies aimed at suppressing negative emotions or thoughts tend to have poor health outcomes in numerous areas. The relationship between experiential avoidance and negative outcomes has been shown in depression (DeGenova, Patton, Jurich, & MacDermid, 1994), substance abuse (Cooper, Russel, & George, 1988; Ireland, McMahon, Malow, & Kouzekanani, 1994), and sequela of childhood sexual abuse (Leitenberg, Greenwald, & Cado, 1992). Interventions that disrupt experiential avoidance are often successful and may improve mental and physical outcomes for a large group of patients and for health care providers and employers, as well.

ACT-HC ASSUMPTIONS, TARGETS, PRINCIPLES AND OBJECTIVES

Figure 10.1 provides a process analysis summarizing key basic assumptions in the ACT-HC model. This model demonstrates conditions associated with decisions to use or not use health care services, and patient response when health care services fail to address discomfort and experiential avoidance. In this diagram, ovals represent potential targets for changing patient behavior patterns that are ineffective, including strategies based on misinformation and those that mask discomfort (e.g., alcoholism) and further impair overall functioning. Integration of mental health and medical services will support development of effective therapeutic and educational interventions in these target areas. Further, health care system improvements may be significantly attenuated by workplace programs, as employers may (1) reduce excessive utilization by providing current, effective health education programs to uninformed or misinformed patients, and (2) increase necessary utilization by directing reluctant patients toward needed health care services.

The Diamond-shaped boxes in Figure 10.1 represent change targets within the health care delivery system. Initiatives may promote changes in (1) selection and application of training models used with medical and mental health providers and (2) design and delivery of programs to help patients cope when medical treatments fail to remedy discomforts. Training models deriving from the ACT-HC perspective suggest strategies for improving care seeking among groups who tend to under-utilize health care. These strategies help providers to (1) retain patients who engage in a high rate of experiential avoidance behaviors and (2) design interventions appropriate to the patient's gender, level of motivation, and cultural context. ACT-HC also suggests directions for improving outcomes with patients who tend to over-utilize. These derive from a training model that emphasizes (1) collaboration between medical and mental health providers and (2) availability of mental health services in the primary care setting. All patients may benefit from educational and therapeutic programs that provide skill-development in acceptance strategies, as these may enhance efforts to change public behaviors necessary to improve quality of life when available medical treatments fail to eliminate discomforts.

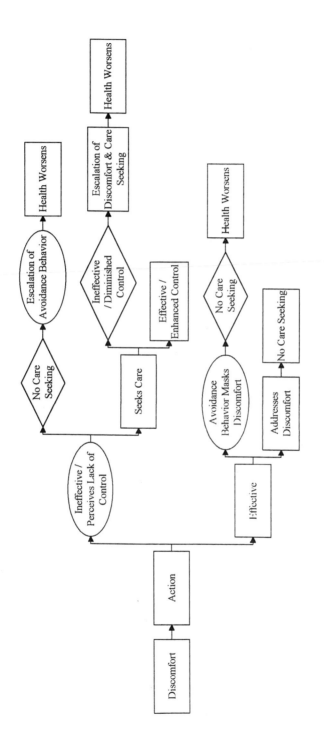

Figure 10.1. ACT-HC paradigm concerning health care seeking behavior.

Principle 1: Health Care Seeking Is Correlated with Discomfort, Distress, Need for Control and Confidence in Health Care Resources.

Discomfort always plays a role in health care seeking behavior. A patient's discomfort may arise from anticipated negative consequences (e.g., "I will contract the flu if I fail to take a flu shot.") or from current discomforts (e.g., "My head hurts."). Patients vary considerably in their level of anticipatory concern with and tolerance for bodily and mental discomforts. Patients also vary in their coping resources, which include health care knowledge, self-management skills, and interpersonal support. Finally, people differ in propensity for using health care services, given wide variation in individual past experiences (i.e., positive or negative) and current access issues (e.g., financial and geographical accessibility).

Patients experience discomfort and employ available resources to address it. Patient-initiated self-management strategies include taking over-the-counter remedies, allowing time for bed rest, talking to a friend about a distressing personal problem, etc. When these strategies fail to provide relief, discomfort continues. The patient perceives a lack of control and may experience increased distress. Patients vary in susceptibility to occurrence of specific physiological components of distress (e.g., increased heart rate, gastrointestinal upset, muscular tension) and beliefs about health care services (e.g., "The doctor knows best"; "Doctors are quacks."). Patients who use experiential avoidance strategies may be at increased risk for poor health outcomes, whether they seek health care or avoid it.

Patients who use experiential avoidance strategies frequently and who also perceive health care services as offering relief may seek care often, even when discomforts are minor. In fact, use of health care services can become a behavior associated with experiential avoidance. The somatizing patient may use contact with the health care system to avoid unwanted thoughts, feelings, and sensations concerning bodily states, illness, helplessness, etc.

When a person who uses experiential avoidance strategies often does not see health care services as a resource, she or he may employ potent self-management strategies when confronted with unwanted feelings, thoughts, or sensations. These may include excessive use of mind-altering, nonprescribed drugs, misuse of food, or workaholism. To the extent that these strategies are overused, they can actually harm rather than protect health. Costs of health care may actually be increased when needed utilization is not sought. For example, a depressed, obese person may avoid seeking care for a chronic cough because she or he is unwilling to be confronted concerning overconsumption of food. Another person might suffer from social phobia and use nicotine to dampen arousal when social interactions are required. In these circumstances, health may decline further, leaving the patient vulnerable to more invasive and costly health care treatments in the future (e.g., removal of a lung instead of participation in a group cognitive–behavioral treatment for eating disorders or a social phobia and telephonic smoking cessation program).

When a person who uses experiential avoidance strategies frequently cannot access health care services, she or he may be more likely to engage in more blatant self-harming behaviors (e.g., uncontrolled alcoholism) or behaviors that harm the individual and society (e.g., violence, property destruction). Unfortunately, health insurance does not guarantee access to primary care, and publicly insured individuals are not accepted by all physicians (Cykert, Kissling, Layson, & Hansen, 1995). Subtle barriers may loom large for economically disadvantaged members of society. Their continued use of experiential avoidance strategies is unlikely to address underlying mental or physical health problems. Further, society at large may fail to understand the context for their behavior and adopt policies that are more costly for the citizenship in the long run. For example, a person with poor control over diabetes may experience depression and use alcohol to avoid unwanted sadness and multiple life problems that complicate life-style changes needed to improve diabetes management. This may lead to job loss, homelessness, and repeated use of emergency services.

Principle 2: Experiential Avoidance Is an Important Control Strategy and Becomes Increasingly Likely as Other Control Strategies Fail.

Patients with continuing discomforts who perceive health care services to offer needed resources will seek out these services. When medical encounters address the discomfort, the patient experiences relief and health care seeking behavior ceases. When medical encounters fail to address the discomfort, the patient continues to experience the discomfort *and* an even greater lack of control. With an increasing sense of being out-of-control, the patient may employ more experiential avoidance strategies. For example, a patient who experiences a panic attack and receives a thorough medical evaluation yielding negative findings may perceive an even greater lack of control ("They cannot find out what's wrong with me, even with the best tests available. I must have a rare and awful condition. I must be more careful than ever before."). The patient may take a medical leave from work, avoid leaving home, or even avoid being left alone.

Patients who use experiential avoidance strategies are vulnerable to mental problems associated with anxiety and depressive disorders. Over one-quarter of primary care patients experience mood disorders and almost 20% present with one or more anxiety disorders (Spitzer et al., 1995). Comorbidity rates are particularly high for major depressive disorder and anxiety disorders, and lowered perceptions of control may account for much of the overlap of symptoms between anxiety and depression (Rapee, Craske, Brown, & Barlow, 1996) and related variability in outcomes among patients with chronic diseases (Kemmer, Bisping, & Steingruber, 1986).

Figure 10.2 provides a schematic of the theoretical relationship among discomfort, perceived lack of control and the common psychological problems of anxiety and depression. Anxiety may be a basic emotional state associated with perceived lack of control over unwanted experiences (Hayes & Strosahl, 1997) and may play a pivotal role in development of other mental disorders. For example, almost 68% of a sample

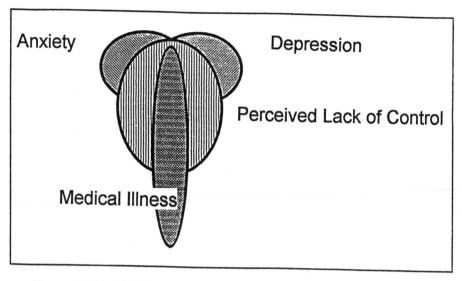

Figure 10.2 ACT-HC paradigm concerning common factors in lack of control

of community-dwelling adults with current major depression reported experience of an anxiety disorder prior to the depression onset (Kessler, Cleary, & Burke, 1985). The "window" of risk between onset of anxiety and development of a major depressive episode appears to be about 18 months. Primary care providers are positioned well for early identification of anxious patients who struggle with accepting a medical diagnosis or implementing behavioral changes needed to successfully manage acute or chronic medical problems. By joining hands with primary care providers, mental health specialists are better prepared to develop cost effective programs that empower patients during the "window" of opportunity between the predisposing state of perceived lack of control and development debilitating mental disorders and patterns of ineffective management of medical problems.

Experiential avoidance appears to be a role in several other disorders that are common in primary care. These include somatoform disorder, alcohol dependence, and eating disorders. All involve an effort to control unpleasant bodily sensations and emotions. Somatoform disorder features significant concerns with control over bodily sensations and may be present in up to 14% of primary care medical patients. Three percent of primary care patients present to their doctors for treatment of eating disorders, where food is used to control uncomfortable emotional states (Spitzer et al., 1995). Patients with potential for development of these types of disorders may become symptomatic when they are confronted with unwanted thoughts, feelings, and sensations associated with illness.

Medical patients with no history of alcohol dependence may resort to problematic use of alcohol when challenged by an unwanted and threatening illness. As many as one in twenty primary care patients suffer from probable alcohol abuse or dependence (Spitzer et al., 1995). Depression is often also co-morbid with drug abuse. Kessler et al. (1996) found that 38.6% of patients with major depressive disorder had some type of substance use disorder. Almost 20% of patients with major depressive disorder report prior substance abuse. One possible explanation for this association is that alcoholism is an attempt to control negative affect through use of a chemically based experiential avoidance strategy.

Principle 3: Emotional Avoidance in Some Contexts Produces Self-Amplifying Behavioral Processes.

Most people feel anxious when they are unable to control mental or physical pain. Most people in America believe that they should be "in control" of their private events (including their thoughts, feelings, and sensations). Current discomforts may provoke current experience of past discomforts associated with lack of control in the past. Providers, like patients, experience a control challenge when they are unable to reduce or alleviate mental or physical pain. Efforts to control discomfort or pain often include rejection of the discomfort through suppression or distraction strategies. These strategies are often promoted by the larger society. For example, common parenting practices include teaching children to conceal their feelings of anger, sadness, and pain ("Don't be sad." "Don't be a baby.") and suppress their thoughts of jealousy and lack of confidence ("You should be thankful for what you've got not mad about what your sister got"; "If you doubt yourself, you'll never get anywhere.").

While many people try to suppress thoughts, this strategy rarely works. Existing studies show, under many conditions, that trying to suppress a thought paradoxically increases the frequency of that thought. This is particularly true for the physical or emotional context in which the suppression took place. This rebound effect has been demonstrated in suppression of somatic and emotional events. For example, research subjects who are instructed to suppress induced pain hurt longer and are more likely to rate subsequent innocuous stimuli as aversive than subjects who are asked to focus on the unpleasant sensations themselves (Cioffi & Holloway, 1993).

Principle 4: Experiential Acceptance Provides an Effective Method of Reducing Self-Amplifying Behavioral Processes Based on Experiential Avoidance

Patients are more likely to have confidence in and respond to treatments planned with health care providers who model or teach an alternative to experiential avoidance. Providers may assist patients in learning alternatives to experiential avoidance in a number of ways. They may help patients to respond to their unwanted thoughts, feelings, and sensations with more openness by modeling such or by providing skill-based learning experiences. Research on general processes of clinical change show that openness to subjective experience is consistently related to positive therapeutic outcomes (Greenberg & Safran, 1989). The most effective treatment for panic disorder serves as an example. This treatment undermines the patient's avoidance of fear and its interoceptive accompaniments (Barlow, Craske, Cerny, & Klosko, 1989).

When providers do not address the patient's struggle with experiential avoidance, patients are likely to be dissatisfied with care and lack confidence in treatment plans. Cancer patients who are more nervous and distressed after diagnosis and have less faith in their physicians are more likely to seek out alternative therapies (Munstedt, Kirsch, Milch, Sachsse, & Vahrson, 1996). In a large study of general medical outpatients in Japan, 23% were classified as "doctor-shopping" patients (Sato, Takeichi, Shiranhama, Fukui, & Gude, 1995). These patients were distinguished by chronicity of illness, difficulties understanding doctors' explanations, and lack of belief in the doctor's diagnosis and treatment.

Patient acceptance of mental and medical problems may derive from an understanding of the context of mental or physical illness or from instruction in skills that empower coping with unwanted, inexplicable, and uncomfortable illness. Mindfulness training is an example of a clinical intervention that promotes experiential acceptance (Kabat-Zinn et al., 1992). Patients with generalized anxiety and panic who attended classes for training in mindfulness maintained reductions in fear over time. Mindfulness training may also help older adults become healthier and live longer (C. N. Alexander, Langer, Newman, Chandler, & Davies, 1989). Patients with HIV/AIDS who learn to practice meditation, which is also an alternative to experiential avoidance, have demonstrated higher scores on measures of mental and physical hardiness than nonmediators (Carson, 1993).

Patients vary greatly in their readiness to comprehend and benefit from acceptance strategies. The provider needs to consider numerous factors, including the patient's individual beliefs and cultural ideas, in constructing interactions that promote experiential acceptance. An individual's illness etiology beliefs may not support needed utilization of health care services and may make communication difficult during the health care visit (Cheung & Spears, 1995). Within the prevailing culture, unspoken societal beliefs may limit the practitioner's communication with patients who are suffering difficult disease processes, such as Alzheimer's (Herskovits, 1995). The health care provider is challenged to recognize and master experiential avoidance within himself or herself. At times, providers may ask patients about spiritual beliefs and illness causation (Patel, Musara, Butau, Maramba, & Fuyane, 1995). The patient's language is very important in treatment planning. Use of patient language in development of classification and treatment plans may help low back pain patients accept and commit to difficult treatment plans (Borkan, Reis, Hermoni, & Biderman, 1995). At times, nontraditional healers, such as Native American medicine men and women, may help primary care and behavioral health practitioners with certain patient groups (MacLachlan, Nyirenda, & Nyando, 1995; Van Blerkom, 1995). When a sense of control is not readily available through "quick cures," patient–provider interactions become more critical than ever.

5. Experiential Acceptance Facilitates Commitment to Behavioral Changes Needed to Improve Quality of Life.

Patients who struggle with control and with medical and mental problems have a lowered quality of life. They utilize more health care services. They have more family problems, and they experience more impairment to their functioning in the work place. Patients with comorbid anxiety and depression disorders report 2.33 days of work loss and 12.3 days of work cutback per 100 work days. Patients with anxiety, depression, and substance abuse report 0.87 days of work loss and 22.1 days of work cutback per 100 work days (Kessler, Nelson, McGonagle, Liu, Swartz, & Blazer, 1996). Actually, a person's survival may rest upon the ability to learn more active and less avoidant coping responses (Mertens, Moos, & Brennan, 1996). Integration of mental health and medical services may help the shrinking health care dollar stretch further by enhancing development and delivery of programs to improve survival and quality of life.

Patient mastery of experiential acceptance makes previously avoided behavioral change plans feasible. When a patient can tolerate the unchangeable discomfort associated with unwanted thoughts, feelings, and sensations, his or her ability to focus on behavioral goal setting is enhanced. Psychic and physical pain can actually help a patient clarify his or her values concerning how daily life is best approached. Most patients desire to have relaxing and enjoyable moments everyday, to have good relationships with loved ones, to make a worthwhile contribution as a worker, to make independent choices, and to achieve personal goals. As patients and providers accept the reality of pain, they can develop strong behavioral plans that move the patient, step by step, closer to these and other behavioral objectives. A high quality of life is characterized by both acceptance and commitment.

ACT-HC Objectives

The ACT-HC model proposes that health care outcomes can be improved by addressing experiential avoidance, as this is a prominent feature for patients with varying medical and mental diagnoses. Specifically, overall health status, appropriate utilization of health care resources, and patient satisfaction with care improve when treatment plans help patients (1) use experiential acceptance strategies and (2) identify and commit to use of effective methods for creating an optimal quality of life. In the remaining sections of this chapter, the authors provide further elaboration of this model to help readers who are (1) training primary care and mental health providers; (2) clinicians who are developing integrated programs for specific primary care population groups; and (3) researchers who want to design studies that add to the theoretical basis for health care service delivery.

ACT-HC: A MODEL FOR TRAINING

As a training model, the ACT-HC theory suggests directions for improving outcomes with all patients. Patients who under and overutilize care are key targets for improvement, as outcomes for these two groups are most problematic. According to this model, providers may improve care seeking among patients who tend to underutilize health care services by learning to (1) retain patients who use experiential avoidance strategies frequently, and (2) design interventions appropriate to the patient's gender, level of motivation, and cultural context. Training programs need to help providers develop the complex group of skills needed to achieve these goals. Initial training objectives must include assisting providers with recognition of their own use of experiential avoidance, particularly in clinical settings, and development of facility in creation of experiential acceptance in interactions with patients. The ACT-HC model also suggests specific methods for improving outcomes with patients who overutilize health care services. These include training providers to implement models of care that integrate primary care and behavioral health services, as programs for shaping use of services are most easily developed and implemented in an integrated setting.

The ACT-HC model encourages health care providers to use a functional analysis of provider and patient behavior in health care encounters. Providers, like patients, vary in their ability to tolerate thoughts, feelings, and sensations associated with lacking control. Table 10.1 summarizes ideal and problematic events in primary care episodes of care. In the ACT-HC model, an episode of care begins when a patient initiates care concerning a specific health discomfort and concludes when both provider and patient agree that the discomfort has been addressed adequately. All encounters involve a provider and a patient and three components of their interaction during the episode of care. These components include problem definition, treatment plan development, and treatment plan adherence.

Ideal Encounters

In the ideal episode of care, the patient articulates her or his problem clearly, asks questions that have answers, participates actively in planning treatment, understands the treatment plan, and has the skills and resources to implement plans made during the original and any planned follow-up encounters. In follow-up visits, the ideal patient keeps the appointment, reports

TABLE 10.1
ACT-HC Functional Analysis of Ideal and Problematic Primary Care
Encounters

Elements of Encounter	Ideal Encounter/High Control		Problematic Encounter/Low Control	
	Patient	Provider	Patient	Provider
Problem Definition	Articulates clear descriptions	Identifies organic basis	Presents multiple, vague complaints Presents highly anxious about discomfort	Orders multiple tests Finds no organic basis
	Asks questions	Gives specific diagnosis	Insists on diagnosis	Gives no diagnosis
Treatment Plan Development	Comprehends plan	Explains affordable, effective treatment	Does not understand/Is dissatisfied with advice	Gives general advice for coping
	Has skills & resources to implement plan		Lacks skills needed to cope with discomfort and perceived lack of control	Lacks skills needed to help patients address unresolved discomforts
Treatment Plan Adherence	Attends follow-up	Schedules follow-up	Insists on multiple appointments with multiple providers	No follow-up scheduled
	Has adhered to plan	Revises plan as needed; discusses prevention issues	Focuses on any inconsistencies in opinions from multiple providers	Difficulties coordinating care among multiple providers
	Satisfied with outcome	Schedules follow-up; ends episode of care	Adheres poorly to treatment plans	Episode of care continues without coordinated plan
			Changes primary care providers	Patient seen as difficult

adherence to the plan, and is satisfied with treatment outcomes.

Providers enjoy participating in ideal episodes of care. Under these circumstances, the provider identifies an organic basis for the problem or a nonorganic basis that is acceptable to the provider and patient. Also, the provider gives a specific diagnosis that is associated with an affordable, effective treatment. The provider schedules a follow-up visit, acknowledges the patient for successful adherence to the plan, revises the plan as needed, discusses prevention or maintenance of health issues, and ends the episode of care.

Problematic Encounters

In problematic encounters, the patient often presents with multiple, vague complaints. Also, the patient is anxious about her or his symptoms and insists on a specific diagnosis. The problematic encounter may worsen further if the patient does not understand or is dissatisfied with the provider's advice. In addition, the patient may lack the skills needed to cope with the discomfort and with her or his perceived lack of control over the discomfort. This may result in multiple appointments with multiple providers. Then, the patient may become confused, focus on inconsistencies in opinions from multiple providers, adhere poorly to treatment plans, and shop for other doctors and services.

Recommendations for Training

Primary care providers have a very difficult job, and they work diligently. On average, primary care providers work 52.8 hours per week (Howard, 1992). When they go through a week with numerous problematic encounters, they may struggle with their own perceived lack of control. Behavioral health specialists need to be prepared to help providers experience this very painful and difficult aspect of primary care work. Primary care providers welcome self-care workshops that emphasize acceptance and commitment strategies. When providers become highly skillful in these areas, they are empowered to use these strategies directly with more patients and to recommend behavioral health programs teaching these strategies to patients.

Behavioral health providers may also assist their primary care colleagues by helping them evaluate specific elements in problematic encounters with patients. Medical providers are accustomed to case discussions as a learning method. Their most difficult (and costly) patients are the high utilizing, multi-problem patients. Providers will welcome the ACT-HC model because it is simple, can be discussed briefly, has application to a wide range of patients, and helps generate functional analyses and specific interventions that are feasible in the primary care setting.

ACT-HC: PROGRAMS FOR PATIENTS

Educational and therapeutic programs can enhance health care outcomes by providing skill-development opportunities for patients who are perceiving a lack of control over mental or physical discomforts or both. We will describe three primary-care based programs developed to be consistent with the assumptions of the ACT-HC model. Prior to this, we will summarize the research literature concerning use of techniques consistent with this model with medical patients.

Acceptance and Commitment Treatments for Medical Patients

Numerous patient groups benefit from integrated programs consistent with the ACT-HC model. These include patients who are candidates for new and uncomfortable screening procedures, patients receiving a new diagnosis of a serious medical illness, and patients with chronic medical problems. Medical technologies continue to expand and new screening procedures may help prevent serious illness in large groups of patients. For example, there is a new flexible sigmoidoscopy for screening for colorectal cancer. Unfortunately, only 49% of referred patients attended the screening (Cockburn, Thomas, McLaughlin, & Reading, 1995). The referral process could be improved by addition of ACT-HC techniques to help the patient accept and prepare for the procedure. Early-stage interventions that encourage active behavioral coping and active cognitive coping rather than avoidance or passive acceptance of illness may help patients cope with a new diagnosis of illness. These programs may attenuate psychological distress caused by breast cancer and empower patients to improve their overall quality of life (Fawzy, 1995).

Integrated behavioral programs consistent with ACT-HC principals may improve outcomes for patients with on-going medical problems. For example, patients with diabetes mellitus who fear long-term complications showed significant improvements regarding fear, acceptance of chronic disease, and work after participating in a treatment consisting of imagined exposure, relaxation training, and analysis of dysfunctional health beliefs (Zettler, Duran, Waadt, Herschback, & Strain, 1995). Similarly, a group of patients suffering chronic idiopathic tinnitus showed improvement on multiple measures after participating in a cognitive–behavioral program to train them in coping with tinnitus (Kroner-Herwig, Hebing, van Rijn-Kalkmann, Frenzel, Schikowsky, & Esser, 1995). Patients with documented coronary artery disease also showed benefits from an acceptance-promoting stress reduction program, including increased exercise tolerance and delay in onset of ST-segment depression (Zamarra, Schneider, Besseghini, Robinson, & Salerno, 1996). The course of HIV disease may be improved by patient participation in programs that integrate behavioral care with traditional medical care. Patients who participated in a package of complementary therapies (including nutrition, stress reduction, exercise, and community involvement) lived asymptomatic lives that exceeded in quality and length the lives of those HIV-positive individuals not presented with the complementary treatments package (Kaiser & Donegan, 1996). Behavioral programs also improve adaptive pain beliefs and disability level among chronic low back pain patients (Newton-John, Spence, & Schotte, 1995).

Integrated behavioral programs in the primary care setting consistent with the ACT-HC model may also improve numerous outcomes related to family issues. Through thoughtful goodbyes and acceptance behaviors, children may identify the meaning and ongoing nature of loss, and resolve difficult feelings associated with the chronic illness and death of a parent. A positive outcome of loss may be an increase in self-esteem when children learn to identify and draw upon their own inner strengths (Semmens & Peric, 1995). When health care providers model acceptance, families with seriously mental ill members (e.g., schizophrenia) are empowered (Van Hammond &

Deans, 1995). Likewise, children with asthma may benefit from behavioral programs that help their families feel more "in control" (Meijer & Oppenheimer, 1995).

Acceptance-Promoting Programs for Older Primary Care Patients

As patients age, they are confronted with more and more discomforts, most of which are unwanted. These include physical discomforts (e.g., arthritis) and psychological discomforts (e.g., loss of loved ones). Health care can help prepare patients to age well by providing instruction in psychological acceptance strategies and methods for maintaining a high quality of life. For example, elderly patients who learned to change states of consciousness through on-going practice of specific mental techniques were able to improve systolic blood pressure, associate learning, word fluency, and internal locus of control (Alexander et al., 1989).

Over the past few years, behavioral health specialists have worked collaboratively with primary care professionals to develop integrated models of care for older patients. These programs include models to promote healthy aging starting in the fifth decade of life and cost effective, satisfying treatment of the frail elderly. They were developed to be consistent with ACT-HC principles (Robinson, Del Vento, & Wischman, 1997). The most recent program is called the Health Improvement Project (HIP). This program is designed for patients who go through a period of sustained high utilization of health care services. Our current definition is 2 years of utilization above the 70 percentile for the physician panel to which the patient belongs. Patients invited to participate in HIP are aged 57 and over. Of course, there is no upper age limit, and several patients are approaching birthdays in the ninth decade.

The HIP program involves collaborative work between a primary care nurse with a specialty in geriatric nursing and a psychologist working in the primary care clinic. The two "cross-train" each other in their respective disciplines and consult on specific cases as needed. The nurse provides the basic service and the psychologist offers back-up consultation and group services.

The Nurse Phone Program. The HIP nurse program includes a series of seven brief phone calls to patients over a 4-month period and two HIP plans written collaboratively with the patient's primary care team to address any problems in the health care process. The first four phone calls occur weekly and address specific behavioral skills. The nurse mails a 1-page interactive brochure to the patient after each phone call. The brochure summarizes the skill discussed in the call and the skill development exercise planned with the patient. The first call includes a brief evaluation of the patient's relationship with her or his primary care team and development of a written plan to address areas needing attention. The fourth call includes development of a written plan concerning the patient's efforts to improve her or his quality of life over the following 3-month period. Both of these written plans are shared with the primary care team and, then, placed in the patient's medical record. The topic and behavioral health message for each call is summarized in Table 10.2. The nurse initiates three monthly follow-up calls during a continuation phase which follows immediately after the more intensive beginning of four weekly behavioral health assessment and change planning calls.

The Body–Mind Tea Party. The HIP psychologist provides a weekly group to backup the nursing phone intervention. The nurse extends an invitation to the group to all patients in her first phone call, explaining that the group is optional. About half of the patients attend the group one or more times. About one-third attend the group more than three times. The group is a one-hour program. During the first 20 minutes, tea is served and patients share personal discoveries of community resources that embellish daily quality of life. During the remainder of the group, the psychologist provides a brief lecture on a health or wellness topic, demonstrates a skill for developing experiential acceptance or enhancing sensations of wellness and teaches the skill to patients.

TABLE 10.2
HIP Nursing Phone Calls

Week	Topic	Message
1	Self-Awareness	Self-awareness involves knowing your body and mind
2	Gently Pushing Physical Limits	Use it or you lose it
3	Making Connections	People live longer and better when their connections are stronger
4	Living Your Values	"Life is either a daring adventure, or nothing at all." *Helen Keller*
Monthly Calls 1, 2, & 3	Follow-up of Lifestyle Plan	Keep your commitment to yourself to live life well

During the last decades of life, patients are confronted with the need to make significant and large changes in their daily lives. The Health Improvement Program attempts to prepare patients to make these changes well and to use health care providers to assist them when needed.

For example, May was an early participant in HIP. When she started the program, she was plodding through her eighties with increasing health problems and waning hope for a decent quality of life. Seven years of caring for her frail and demented husband had drained her of personal resources and she had not bounced back after his death. She had moved to the basement of her home and lived in one room. While her son and daughter-in-law lived in the remainder of the house, there was little interaction between them and most interactions were experienced negatively by May. During the initial nursing phone calls, May indicated that medication had once been helpful to her. She was encouraged to restart a daily practice and to attend body–mind class. May did attend the class and found it helpful. She learned breathing exercises and used them to help her relax more during interactions with her live-in relatives. May also indicated an interest in returning to daily writing. She had two books in progress and had stopped writing over a decade ago. Over the course of the 4-month program, May sold her house and moved to an apartment near a large library where she could attend writing classes and obtain materials easily. She began to view a chair aerobics program several times each week on television and developed more upper body strength. At a 12-month follow-up, May indicated that she had submitted a book for publication and that she was attending a writer's group on a weekly basis.

Acceptance-Promoting Programs for Adults with Compromised Role Functioning

When patients present to primary care and report significant limitations in ability to function in one or more areas of life, integrated behavioral health services are useful. Over the past 5 years, we have offered a two-tier behavioral health service in the primary care setting. The first tier consists of one or more half-hour individual consultations. The second tier is a back-up group program which provides patients with opportunities to develop needed skills in a class environment in the primary care clinic setting. A brief series of individual behavioral consultation visits is adequate for many patients. For some patients, a more extensive experiential, educational program is needed to make specific skill gains required for optimal functioning at home, work, and in leisure or social activities. A general behavioral health consultation service, in combination with an ACT-HC group, will meet the needs of many adult patients presenting to primary care with mild to moderate role functioning problems.

Consultation Services. In an integrated behavioral consultation service, patients are seen for a single visit or a series of two or three visits. These visits are 15 to 30 minutes in length. The behavioral health specialist focuses on collaborative development of a specific, simple plan that involves a small behavior change that can be supported over time by the primary care team. Often, one or two follow-up visits help the patient orient toward an acceptance promoting strategy and commit to ongoing practice of key coping strategies.

For example, Elaine came to her primary care physician for a physical examination. During the visit, she revealed a 20-year habit of severe hand and toe nail biting. Her biting had increased recently and a current boy friend had encouraged her to seek treatment. Elaine agreed to see the behavioral health consultant in the primary care clinic. The consultant helped Elaine determine a framework for accepting her "excessive grooming" behavior. They developed an initial plan involving her (1) going for a manicure and (2) letting her boyfriend know that she was addressing the problem and that she would ask for his help if she needed it. At the follow-up visit, Elaine indicated adherence to the plan. She also indicated that she had signed up for a knitting class and that she planned to continue with the manicures. She also indicated an interest in becoming more assertive with her boyfriend. The behavioral consultant acknowledged her progress and helped her locate an assertiveness training class in her neighborhood.

The Quality of Life Class. The Quality of Life Class is a 7-week psychoeducational group series for primary care patients. The class is supported by a self-help book (Robinson, 1996). The topics covered in this class are summarized in Table 10.3. The format includes an initial 15-minute period where the behavioral consultant teaches a specific skill concerning acceptance-promoting strategies or creation of sensations of wellness. In the remaining 45 minutes, the consultant presents a brief behavioral health lecture that includes a summary of pertinent research findings, illustrates a specific skill by way of an example, and invites participants to complete a brief skill development exercise. After the class ends, the consultant remains available for 15 minutes to help requesting individuals develop specific behavioral health plans concerning application of the skill presented at that class. During the last class session, participants develop a behavioral plan requiring commitment to a life-style that represents their values on a daily basis. Copies of the life-style plan are placed in the patient's medical chart so that the primary care team can support the patient in their plan over time. The format for the class allows patients to attend a single class or all classes.

TABLE 10.3
Quality of Life Class

Class	Topic	Skills
1	Hoping . . . Planning . . . Doing	Building hope
		Making a behavioral health plan
2	Building Acceptance and	Accepting thoughts and feelings
	Making Value-Based Choices	Clarifying important values
3	Appreciating Your Mind	Learning to breathe & relax
	and Body	Embracing difficult thoughts
4	Solving Problems	Applying 7 steps
5	Responding To Interper-	Caring for yourself in conflict
	sonal Conflicts	Making conflict work for you
6	Expressing Yourself . . .	Making a personal assertion plan
	Assertively And Creatively	Planning creative activities
7	Continuing To Live Well . . .	Planning a value-based life-style
	Planning Your Life-style	

Many different individuals find the title of the service (Quality of Life Class) acceptable and the content helpful. For example, Linda decided to take the class to help her find more satisfaction in her life as a single mother. Linda had recently stopped using mind-altering drugs after 13 years of dependence and abuse. She struggled with depression and wanted to be employed and capable of independently supporting her daughter. During the series, Linda obtained a job and developed a plan to see supportive friends on a regular basis. Additionally, she developed a daily exercise plan and two playtime rituals with her daughter. At the end of the group, she integrated her behavior changes into a life-style plan, and reviewed this plan with her primary care provider.

ACT-HC: CHALLENGES FOR RESEARCH

Many factors are contributing to the current milieu of rapid change in health care. These include more sophisticated purchasers, developing technologies, and a challenged economy, among other factors. In entering the world of primary care behavioral health, one can easily find oneself in turf battles and come away feeling confused and isolated. To the extent that we can incorporate a theoretical basis into this context of change, we are empowered to move this process along with a larger picture perspective. Theory can help us rough out the picture, and science can help refine the images and update the colors in this picture.

The ACT-HC model is one of several possible roughed-out pictures that may help guide integration of primary care and behavioral health services. The ACT-HC model makes the following assumptions: (1) Patients want to be well. (2) Patients want to have satisfying, meaningful lives. (3) Primary care providers and behavioral health providers want to help patients be well and live meaningful lives. (4) Patients, primary care providers, and behavioral health providers struggle when patients fail to become well and live meaningful lives. (5) The quality of struggle may obstruct or enhance growth for patients, primary care providers, and behavioral health providers. Numerous hypotheses can be developed from these basic assumptions. Researchers are encouraged to grow this model slowly. The following two hypotheses warrant priority consideration for researchers wanting to develop theoretically-based studies in this new and growing area.

(1) A patient's utilization of health care services is correlated with the following four factors: (a) level of discomfort; (b) level of distress about the discomfort; (c) level of control desired over the discomfort; (d) level of confidence in health care provider/system. (2) Providers who model psychological acceptance help patients to accept and live well with distressing discomforts.

SUMMARY

Primary care patients face numerous unchangeable circumstances. Acceptance and commitment strategies may empower patients to live well under difficult circumstances and providers to acknowledge and work successfully within the limits of modern day medicine. The ACT-HC model may assist educators in developing training programs for primary care and behavioral health professionals and providers in designing simple, effective clinical programs for high risk primary care patient groups. Primary care providers and patients who have participated in programs conceived from the ACT-HC perspective report a high level of satisfaction with them. The authors hope that this model helps the odd group of bed fellows that are shaping the future of integrated primary care and behavioral health work together toward mutually desired goals. Researchers are encouraged to further illuminate a walk into health care in the next century by designing thoughtful studies that test key assumptions of this model.

11.

Life Skills Training to Ameliorate the Impact of Psychosocial Factors on the Development and Course of Medical Illness

**Redford B. Williams, M.D.,
Virginia P. Williams, Ph.D.**

Epidemiological research over the past two decades shows that several psychosocial factors impact negatively on the development and course of a wide range of medical illnesses, as well as on the costs of medical care in patients with chronic disease. Clinical research provides encouraging evidence that behavioral interventions aimed at ameliorating the impact of these psychosocial risk factors and the distress associated with them have real promise to improve psychological well-being and physical health, as well as to reduce medical care costs. Although there are many obstacles to be overcome, the research findings make a strong case for the development of behavioral

Acknowledgments. Preparation of this manuscript was supported in part by grants P01-HL36587 and R01-HL44998 from the National Heart, Lung and Blood Institute; 4060-AG11268 and P02-AG12058 from the National Institute on Aging; K05-MH70482 from the National Institute of Mental Health; Clinical Research Unit Grant M01-RR-30; a network grant from the John D. and Catherine T. MacArthur Foundation; and a research contract from the John E. Fetzer Institute.

interventions that can be implemented in primary care settings to reduce the distress, disease, and medical care costs associated with psychosocial risk factors.

In this chapter we shall first review briefly (other chapters in this volume provide more details) the research evidence that documents the need for and potential benefits of behavioral interventions to ameliorate the impact of psychosocial factors in medical illness. We shall then describe in more detail one such intervention, the LifeSkills Workshop, that we originally developed to teach the hostility control strategies presented in our book *Anger Kills* (Williams & Williams, 1994), and have subsequently refined it into a standardized, protocol-driven 6-session workshop product that can be delivered to patients in primary care settings with the goal of reducing psychological distress, improving coping skills, improving medical outcomes, and reducing medical care costs. Finally, we shall outline our plans for integrating the LifeSkills Workshop into a variety of primary care clinical settings.

PSYCHOSOCIAL FACTORS AND MEDICAL ILLNESS

In healthy populations, persons who score high on various measures of hostility have been found when followed up 20 to 25 years later to experience higher rates of coronary heart disease (CHD), cancer, and all-cause mortality than those with low hostility scores (Smith, 1992; Williams, 1994). Depression predicts increased incidence of both CHD and all-cause mortality in healthy samples (Anda, Williamson, & Jones, 1993; Barefoot & Schroll, 1996). Persons with low levels of social support also experience higher mortality rates when followed up over varying periods (House, Landis, & Umberson, 1988). And finally, lower socioeconomic status (SES) has been found in numerous studies to predict higher death rates (Pincus & Callahan, 1995).

These psychosocial risk factors do not occur in isolation from one another; instead, they tend to cluster in the same persons. Indeed, it has been proposed (Kaplan, 1995; Pincus & Callahan, 1995) that one factor driving such clustering is low

SES itself, with the clustering of psychosocial risk factors like hostility, depression, and social isolation in low SES groups playing a causal role in their increased health problems. Moreover, when two or more psychosocial risk factors are present, there is an enhanced impact on mortality (Kaplan, 1995; Barefoot, Williams, Siegler, & Schroll, 1995).

Among *clinical populations,* particularly CHD patients, psychosocial risk factors have been found to predict increased morbidity and mortality. Depression predicts increased mortality in CHD patients over both short (Frasure-Smith, Lesperance, & Talajic, 1993) and long (Barefoot & Schroll, 1996) follow-up periods. Social isolation predicts a two-fold higher 2-year recurrence rate among heart attack survivors (Case, Moss, & Case, 1992) and are threefold higher 5-year mortality rate among patients with angiographically documented coronary atherosclerosis (Williams, Barefoot, & Califf, 1992). Lower SES is also associated with increased mortality in CHD patients (Williams et al., 1992). In all these studies, the impact of psychosocial risk factors on increased morbidity-mortality was independent of the severity of the underlying cardiac disease.

In addition to their adverse impact on disease incidence and prognosis, psychosocial risk factors are also associated with increased *costs of medical care* in clinical populations. For example, among a sample of 6,000 primary care patients in Seattle, Washington, Simon et al. (1995) found that those with diagnosed depression had annual medical costs of $4,246, compared to only $2,371 among nondepressed patients. Among a sample of 381 consecutive patients in a cardiac rehabilitation program, those who were psychologically distressed (scores above the 90th percentile on the General Severity Index of the SCL-90-R) were 2.44 times more likely to be rehospitalized than nondistressed patients, with average rehospitalization costs of $8,556 for the distressed patients versus $2,035 for the nondistressed patients (Melek, 1996). And among a group of high utilizers of medical services in an HMO in the Northwest, 50% were found to be psychologically distressed (Katon et al., 1990). In these studies the higher costs were attributable to utilization of general medical services rather than to higher mental health costs. Even among high utilizers in a Midwestern HMO, those

who scored high on a brief depression screening instrument
had annual medical costs that were $1,498 higher ($5,764 vs.
$4,227) than those of high utilizer patients who were less de-
pressed (Henk et al., 1996).

The high utilization rates associated with psychosocial risk
factors have the potential to make a contribution to overall
medical costs that is anything but trivial, with the top 15 to 20%
of utilizers of medical services accounting for up to 80% of
medical costs in some studies (Pallak, Cummings, Dorken, &
Henke, 1995). Also, the potential savings are anything but trivial, as Cummings (1996c) has estimated that a 5% savings in the
annual U.S. expenditures for medical–surgical services would
amount to as much as $60 *billion,* with larger savings percent-
ages producing correspondingly larger dollar savings.

Given the adverse effects of psychosocial risk factors on
both morbidity-mortality and costs in patients with medical illness, behavioral interventions that are effective in ameliorating
these negative impacts are sorely needed. A considerable body
of clinical trials research suggesting this is possible already exists and offers encouragement that morbidity, mortality and
costs attributable to psychosocial factors can be reduced.

THE IMPACT OF PSYCHOSOCIAL AND BEHAVIORAL
INTERVENTIONS

In both CHD and cancer, randomized clinical trials of psy-
chosocial/behavioral interventions have documented clear
benefits with respect to prognosis of the underlying disease.
Friedman, Thoresen, and Gill (1986) found a 50% reduction
in CHD recurrence rates during the 3 years following a group-
based intervention that trained post-MI patients in behavioral
and cognitive skills relevant to reducing all aspects of Type A
behavior, including the toxic hostility component. In addition
to the specific skills patients learned in this trial, they also undoubtedly received social support from participating in the
group sessions. Frasure-Smith & Prince (1985) observed a similar 50% reduction in mortality among post-MI patients who

received a nurse-administered intervention that provided both social support and help in solving problems, compared to patients who received usual care. Ornish, Brown, and Scherwitz (1990) documented actual regression of coronary athereosclerotic lesions among patients who participated in a rigorous program involving exercise, low fat diet, a support group, and training in yoga. During the same period, patients randomized to usual care experienced a progression of lesions.

The evidence is equally encouraging for cancer patients. Spiegel, Bloom, & Kraemer (1989) randomly assigned women with metastatic breast cancer to either usual care or a cancer patient support group that provided, in addition to the social support, training in cognitive and behavioral coping skills. Women in the support group experienced an average survival of 36 months, which was twice that for women randomized to usual care. Fawzy, Fawzy, and Hyun (1993) showed that even a short-term, 6-session intervention totaling just 9 hours can produce long-term benefits in a study of patients with malignant melanoma. Compared to those receiving usual care, patients randomized to the group-based intervention that provided training in relaxation and various coping skills showed a 50% reduction in both melanoma recurrence and mortality rates.

In his review of the clinical research on psychosocial and behavioral interventions in patients with medical illness, Sobel (1995b) cited a number of studies that found such interventions to not only result in improved illness outcomes and quality of life but reduced medical costs as well. In a randomized controlled clinical trial of an 8-session group intervention that focused on provision of social support, training in coping skills, and increasing ability to perceive and express emotion, Kashner, Rost, & Cohen (1995) found that the intervention has the potential to achieve a 52% reduction in annual health care charges for patients with somatization disorder.

The most impressive evidence for the potential of psychosocial interventions to reduce medical care costs in patients with chronic illness comes from the "Hawaii Medicaid Project" that was conducted in the 1980s by Cummings, Dorken, Pallak, and Henke (1991; see also chapters 1, 2, 17, 18). Medicaid patients with chronic medical illnesses were randomized to either traditional one-on-one psychotherapy or to a structured 8-session targeted–focused group intervention that had as its goals to cope better with threats and transitions, to increase self-efficacy and sense of coherence, and to decrease learned helplessness. Compared to the 12 months prior to treatment, medical care costs for patients randomized to traditional psychotherapy actually *rose* by 17% in the 12 months following intervention. In contrast, among patients randomized to the targeted–focused brief intervention, medical care costs *fell* by 20%.

In the "Hawaii Medicaid Project," the findings were even more dramatic in an employed comparison sample of patients with chronic medical illnesses: medical care costs rose by 52% among those receiving traditional mental health treatment; in contrast, medical care costs declined by 26% among those who received the targeted–focused brief group intervention.

These studies suggest the real potential for dramatically large savings—in terms of reductions in both morbidity–mortality and medical care costs—to be derived from the application of psychosocial and behavioral interventions, especially those that are group-based, in patients with chronic medical illnesses. Moreover, these studies suggest that such interventions need not be long term or costly; rather, it appears that relatively brief, protocol-driven interventions that require only a few hours of health care professional time can produce long-term benefits.

Why, despite all the encouraging evidence for their benefits, have psychosocial and behavioral interventions not been adopted more widely? While many reasons can be enumerated (see chapter 2 for a more detailed discussion), several stand out. First, in its efforts to contain medical costs, the managed care industry has focused more on approaches to limit the supply of medical services, with little attention to approaches and systems that can reduce the need and hence *demand* for medical care services. Second, there is a perception, despite the evidence cited above, that such interventions would be costly, only adding to the costs of the mental health carve-out component of the plan. There is some reality behind this perception: if traditional one-on-one psychotherapeutic approaches are offered, the evidence from the "Hawaii Medicaid Project" suggests that *increased* medical costs might result. Another serious obstacle stems from the "not invented here" attitude so often found in bureaucracies, wherein solutions proposed from outside are often resisted by those within who feel a need to safeguard turf. A more benign version of this attitude holds that "until we see that your proposed solution works in our setting, we aren't going to believe it."

While some notable exceptions exist (see chapters 1, 2, 5) for the most part those working in the behavioral medicine field have not focused energies on developing low cost means of delivering their research-proven psychosocial–behavioral interventions in a format suitable for large scale applications in primary care settings. To accomplish this, we believe behavioral medicine should take an approach that will transform research-based interventions into *standardized products* that can be applied effectively and efficiently in primary care settings. Equally important for widespread dissemination and use by the patients who need them, *the packaging of psychosocial–behavioral interventions as health care products* opens the path for *marketing* them to the various managed care organizations that both control access to a growing proportion of patients and have the need to reduce demand for medical services.

An analogy from traditional biomedicine might be helpful here. Before the evolution of the pharmaceutical industry, physicians learned from one another to treat patients who suffered from "dropsy" (congestive heart failure) with various preparations they extracted from the leaves of the foxglove plant. We now know that the clinical benefits derived from these extracts were due to the presence of chemical compounds related to digitalis in the foxglove leaves. Some good was derived from these early efforts to extract active medicines from herbal sources. Yet only when the active agents in the foxglove preparations (digoxin, digitoxin, etc.) were identified did it became possible to manufacture standardized preparations. It was only then that the benefits of digitalis became widely available, in a form whose efficacy and safety could be monitored and managed, to the large population of patients in need.

Just as the development of the pharmaceutical industry was necessary to apply technology to the identification, production, marketing, and distribution of chemical compounds useful in the treatment of disease, we suggest that it may now be necessary to develop a "behavio-tech" industry to accomplish the same tasks for the psychosocial–behavioral interventions that research is now identifying as beneficial in the prevention and treatment of chronic diseases. It may be the case that those who have developed these interventions, often academicians working in university and medical school settings, are affected by intellectual barriers that cause them to resist "sullying" their hands with marketing and business pursuits.

A *New York Times* article by Gina Kolata (1996) illustrates what we mean. The Drug Abuse Resistance Education (DARE) program has been found in numerous studies *not* to be effective in achieving lasting decreases in drugs of abuse. In contrast, a program termed "Life Skills Training" by its developer, Dr. Gilbert Botvin of Cornell University Medical College, teaches adolescents behavioral and cognitive skills they can use to resist the forces encouraging them to take up drug use. This approach has been found in 10 rigorous evaluation studies to produce a long lasting 50% reduction in use of cigarettes, alcohol, and marijuana among teenagers taking the program versus those not in the program. Despite these marked differences in documented benefits, it is the DARE program that is being widely adopted and used by school systems around the United States, while the Life Skills approach has hardly been noticed by decision makers in school systems. The reason? The DARE program has been "aggressively marketed" by police departments (the program is delivered by police officers at no cost to the schools), while no one has taken up the cause of Life Skills Training. In the Kolata (1996, p. A17) article, Dr. Zili Sloboda of the National Institute on Drug Abuse was cited as saying, "Incredible as it might seem, the real reason that competing [with DARE] programs were rarely used was that school systems did not know about them, and the social scientists who designed them had *failed to market them*" (emphasis added).

There can be little doubt that those of us who have done

the research that documents both the adverse affects of psychosocial factors on health outcomes and the benefits of interventions to ameliorate the impact of those psychosocial factors, earnestly desire to see the fruits of our work applied to improving both the *physical* health of the American people and the *fiscal* health of the American health care system itself. Therefore, it would now appear that, just as our colleagues in departments of pharmacology have done with respect to new drug development, behavioral medicine researchers need to become active participants in development of the behavio-tech industry that will be required to achieve these goals. It was with this purpose in mind that we founded LifeSkills, Inc. to package the strategies taught in *Anger Kills* (Williams & Williams, 1993, 1994) into a product that could be made available to the largest possible number of patients.

THE LIFESKILLS WORKSHOP: BACKGROUND FOR ITS DEVELOPMENT

In the process of writing *Anger Kills,* we developed a workshop to pilot test the strategies to control hostility and anger that we were considering for inclusion in the book. The choice of strategies and the approaches we finally employed, in both the workshop and the book, were drawn from Redford Williams' (1994) research on the role of psychosocial factors in health and disease and clinical research experience in the application of behavioral approaches to the treatment of medical illness (Williams & Gentry, 1997), as well as Virginia Williams' training and experience in teaching and curriculum development.

The authors developed the LifeSkills Workshop not as a form of psychotherapy, but as a highly structured, time-limited *psychoeducational* experience that would provide participants with training in a sequence of skills that would enable them to cope more effectively with negative emotions and stressful life situations, to improve their relationships with others, and to increase the proportion of "positives" in their daily lives. In formulating the Workshop the authors drew upon a variety of clinical traditions, including behavioral therapy, cognitive behavior therapy, biofeedback–relaxation training, and skills training.

These authors have now presented this workshop over the past 7 years to scores of groups encompassing hundreds of participants in a variety of settings, including church groups, healthy persons interested in enhancing wellness, professional couples interested in improving their marriages, patients with a range of chronic diseases, and patients attending weight loss programs. Having used the experience gained in presenting these workshops, as well as in training workshops, the authors have presented their findings at meetings of the American Psychosomatic Society, the American Association for Cardiovascular and Pulmonary Rehabilitation, the Society of Behavioral Medicine, and the International Society of Behavioral Medicine.

While participant satisfaction ratings have been uniformly high, there have not been any systematic evaluations of short- or long-term outcomes. Given the similarity of the approach to those used in the clinical trials research cited earlier, it is believed likely that the LifeSkills Workshop can achieve comparable benefits; but controlled clinical trials will be needed to document this. Elements of the LifeSkills Workshop were employed in a randomized controlled clinical trial of stress management training among women employees in a local corporation. Compared to no treatment and education-only control patients, the working mothers assigned to the stress management group showed significantly larger increases in social support ratings following the intervention (Williams, Feaganes, & Suarez, 1996). The LifeSkills Workshop is currently in the process of being evaluated (with respect to patient satisfaction and well-being and medical care cost outcomes) in a Quality Improvement Study whereby it is being offered to high utilizer patients in the Department of Medicine's Primary Care Clinic at Duke University Medical Center. Negotiations are under way for other health care providers to conduct similar evaluations in a variety of managed care settings.

In its current form the LifeSkills Workshop is presented over 6 sessions. Each session is tightly scripted in terms of both structure and content, but the structure provides ample opportunity to deal with a broad range of problem areas specific to the personal experiences and needs of each participant. The following brief outline provides an overview of the content, format and approach taken.

THE LIFESKILLS WORKSHOP: OUTLINE OF STRUCTURE AND CONTENT

Ideal size

The ideal group size is 9 plus or minus 2. When larger groups must be accommodated, it is important to have two facilitators, so that smaller breakout groups can be formed to permit adequate practice of the in-session exercises by each participant.

Length of Workshop

The LifeSkills Workshop is conducted in 6 initial sessions of 2 hours each, with a 10-minute break in the middle. In clinical settings, we believe that up to four additional follow-up sessions over a 6-month period will help to maintain skills and gains and to provide ongoing social support.

Qualifications of Facilitators

Workshops can be effectively led by facilitators with a wide variety of backgrounds. In clinical settings it will be important for facilitators who are physicians, psychologists, social workers, or nurses to have additional training that will enable them to identify and manage severe distress that might arise in patients with underlying mental disorders. In wellness applications involving nonclinical populations, facilitators with some educational training and experience, but without clinical training, are also appropriate.

Target Groups

• High utilizers of medical care services.
• Patients with cardiac disease, fibromyalgia, or irritable bowel syndrome.
• Patients with any chronic medical illness.
• Healthy individuals with psychosocial risk factors (hostility, depression, social isolation) who wish to improve their chances of avoiding associated illnesses.
• Patients or healthy individuals who are at risk by virtue of high hostility, depression, or social isolation and are likely to fail in programs for smoking cessation, weight control, or other needed regimens. With respect to the latter application, the LifeSkills Workshop could be applied as an "off-the-shelf" stress management component that can be inserted in any of a variety of other disease management modules: e.g., self-management programs for diabetes, asthma, congestive heart failure, etc.

Life Skills Taught

Participants learn to understand themselves and others better via presentations and exercises focusing on the evaluation and management of negative thoughts and feelings and communication and empathy skills. Participants learn to act effectively via presentations and exercises focusing on problem solving, assertion skills, acceptance, and enhancement of the "positives" in everyday life.

Schedule of Sessions

The six sessions are sequenced so that the more basic skills are taught first, as they will continue to be applied as other skills are layered on in the latter sessions. When they have completed the 6-session curriculum, participants have available to them an array of tools they can use to evaluate and cope with any life situation that may be encountered. If one response strategy does not work, the participants will have learned to cycle back through the evaluation process and choose an alternative approach.

Format for Teaching Each Skill

Each skill is taught via a standardized sequence in which the Workshop facilitator explains the skill and then models its use. Participants then gain "hands on" experience in the use of such skills via both in-session exercises and homework assignments. Participants learn from one another by sharing their in-session exercises and the homework assignment experiences.

ACHIEVING MARKET ACCEPTANCE

In order for the LifeSkills workshop concept to gain broad market acceptance, managed care organizations must be convinced that the Workshop will improve patient satisfaction and well-being, improve medical outcomes, and decrease need and demand for and, hence, costs of medical care services. Managed care organizations can refer to the clinical trials described earlier in this chapter that have achieved such benefits using approaches very similar in content, structure, and philosophy to the LifeSkills Workshop. However, the best data in support of this concept will be clinical outcomes data, as being developed in the Quality Improvement Study currently under way at Duke University, as well as similar evaluations with other managed care organizations.

Managed care organizations have increasingly turned to external vendors for assistance in controlling costs as well as managing risk. The LifeSkills concept could lend itself well to such a risk sharing arrangement, whereby Quality Improvement Studies are conducted among high utilizer patients covered by the potential purchasers of the LifeSkills Workshop. The benefits of improved patient satisfaction and well-being and of reduced costs are evaluated, and then there is an agreed upon proportion of the cost savings to be shared with the Workshop developers and providers. This approach would be attractive to managed care organizations because it limits their exposure to costs while at the same time provides the opportunity to achieve significant costs savings.

Different HMO models are likely to prefer different approaches to the delivery of a product such as the LifeSkills Workshop. Staff-model HMOs may prefer that the Workshop provider train their personnel to lead the Workshop, providing all necessary materials (videos, workbooks, etc.), and providing ongoing quality assurance supervision. Network-model HMOs, on the other hand, are likely to prefer to rely completely on an outside company to deliver and monitor the Workshops. Under the first approach, the purchaser would assume more of the costs of administering the Workshop. The advantage of using the LifeSkills Workshop product for them would be the savings achieved by not having to develop the program from scratch, the benefits of using a proven product, and the marketing advantages to be achieved by having a product with broad recognition to increase satisfaction among current and potential members. Under the second approach, an outside company would assume more of the costs of administering the program, with the purchaser being able to engage the vendor in a manner that shares the financial risk and places a minimum of strain on its current resources and structure, an approach most likely to appeal to network-model HMOs.

We realize that the approach embodied in the LifeSkills Workshop is still in its infancy; much hard work has to be done, and many obstacles must be surmounted before the benefits of this training will be available to the millions of persons who stand to gain and the cost savings achieved. The enormous potential gains to patients with chronic diseases as well as the medical system itself indicate that the effort will prove worthwhile.

12.

The Lilly Family Depression Project: Primary Care Prevention in Action

Simon H. Budman, Ph.D., Stephen F. Butler, Ph.D.

It is generally agreed that prevention of disease and disorder is the ultimate goal of medicine. Many of the most effective primary prevention efforts, such as sanitation, have become so much a part of modern life, that they are practically taken for granted. Achievement of public health prevention goals have long included dissemination of information. At the turn of the century, for instance, health departments distributed fliers on "How to Keep a Safe Privy," and efforts to prevent venereal disease in military personnel overseas used brochures and graphically dramatic posters to get the word out (McGinnis, Deering, & Patrick, 1995). Education on the hazards of tobacco use, substance abuse, and unsafe sex reflect current efforts to save lives, not to mention dollars. The U.S. government has recognized the cost-effectiveness of prevention efforts and, in 1990, instituted a prevention agenda called *Healthy People 2000: National Disease Prevention and Health Promotion Objectives* (U.S. DHHS, PHS 1991). The focus of much of this prevention work is the dissemination of health information, considered the most cost-effective activity the government can do (Will, 1989).

Acknowledgment. The authors acknowledge with appreciation that this work has been supported by a grant from the Eli Lilly Corporation, Indianapolis, Indiana.

In this chapter, we describe a project called the Lilly Family Depression Project, implemented by Innovative Training Systems, Inc. (ITS), a research and consulting company based in Massachusetts. The primary goal of this project is to prevent depression in high-risk youth. The project targets children of depressed parents, between the ages of 8 and 12 years, by bringing together recently developed concepts on depression prevention with video technology. The result is an economical, easy-to-use, videotape-based program that is suitable for dissemination in primary care practices. The authors will also describe empirical tests of safety and efficacy of the program that are currently underway. The rationale and development of the prevention videotape program is presented and the field trial described. Beyond the specifics of this particular project, the Family Depression Project represents a model for conceptualizing, developing, and testing behavioral health prevention products that can be used routinely in primary care practices.

THE PROBLEM

By any measure, depression is a major public health concern. One in eight individuals may require treatment for depression in their lifetimes. Direct costs of treatment along with indirect costs, such as loss of productivity, are estimated to exceed $16 billion in 1980 dollars (Depression Guideline Panel [DGP], 1993a). Affective disorders in adults are among the most common mental disorders, and 11 million people, or almost 6% of the population, suffer from major depression each year (Greenberg, Stiglin, Findelstein, & Berndt, 1993). Rates of depression have been increasing in successive birth cohorts throughout the 20th century and the age of onset for depression has been decreasing (Klerman, Lavori, & Rice, 1985). Depression is now the most common clinical problem facing primary-care physicians (Katon & Sullivan, 1990). These disturbing statistics reflect the suffering of the individual patient, yet it is well known that affective disorder has long-term consequences for the spouse and children of the ill individual

(Beardslee & Wheelock, 1994). It has been estimated that, at any given time, 8% of mothers are depressed (Weissman, Leif, & Bruce, 1987). Since parental depression is a risk factor for affective disorders in children, millions of children are being exposed to risk factors for developing behavioral and emotional problems.

Psychopathology in Children of Parents with Affective Disorder

As recent reviews have documented (Beardslee & Wheelock, 1994; Downey & Coyne, 1990; Keitner & Miller, 1990; Rutter, 1990; Zuckerman & Beardslee, 1987), there is compelling evidence that the children of parents with affective disorder fare more poorly than comparison samples whose parents have not experienced affective disorder. These children experience not only high rates of depression, but other types of impairment as well. Thus, as a consensus from a variety of perspectives suggests (National Institute of Mental Health, 1993; Institute of Medicine, 1989; Shaffer, 1989), there is a need for preventive intervention strategies for children of parents with affective disorder.

An array of rigorous empirical studies of children, whose parents have an affective disorder, has shown that such children are at high risk for serious affective illness and other psychiatric disorders (Beardslee, 1990). In a random sample of patients at an HMO, Beardslee and colleagues (Beardslee, Keller, Lavori, Klerman, Dorer, & Samuelson, 1988) found the rate of affective disorder in children of parents with affective disorder to be 30% compared with 2% in children of parents without affective disorder. Using life table methods, these authors estimate that 50% of the children whose parents have an affective disorder will experience a depression by the time they are 19. The few existing longitudinal studies support the high rates of disorder in children of parents with affective disorders. For example, Hammen and colleagues (Hammen, Burge, Burney, & Adrian, 1990) evaluated children, age 8 to 16, of unipolar mothers, bipolar mothers, medically ill mothers, and normal controls every 6 months for 3 years. Using life table estimates, these investigators demonstrated that the cumulative estimated probability of an episode of major psychiatric disorder by late adolescence is 80% in the children of unipolar depressed mothers and between 70 and 80% in the children of bipolar parents. Children who experience episodes of childhood and adolescent depression are severely impaired (Kovacs, Gatsonis, Paulauskas, & Richards, 1989), and episodes of disorder in childhood are predictors of affective disorders in adulthood (Rutter, 1986).

In addition to studies of diagnosable disorders in the offspring of affectively ill patients, many studies focused on general difficulties in functioning these children exhibit (Beardslee, Schults, & Selman, 1987; Forehand & McCombs, 1988; Zuckerman & Beardslee, 1987). Investigators have noted that children whose parents had affective disorder expressed more negative views about self (Hammen, 1988), more concerns about guilt (Zahn-Waxler, Kochanska, Krupnick, & McKnew, 1990), lowered self-esteem (Hirsch, Moos, & Reischi, 1985), deficits in adolescent functioning (Forehand & McCombs, 1988), and interpersonal difficulties (Beardslee et al., 1987). Longitudinal studies (Forehand & McCombs, 1988) suggest that these deficits persist over time.

Role of Parental and Marital Functioning

Two main classes of mechanisms have been identified in the transmission of disorders between parent and child in affective illness: genetic and psychosocial mechanisms (Beardslee, 1990). At present, definitive studies do not exist to separate the relative influences of these two categories. Both frequently are present in families with parental affective disorders. In terms of psychosocial influence, however, poor parenting practices and marital discord clearly have the largest effect (Downey & Coyne, 1990; Rutter, 1990).

Interactional studies of young children and their parents have repeatedly demonstrated deficits in terms of parental responsiveness and interaction (Downey & Coyne, 1990). Depressed mothers are less effective than nondepressed mothers at disciplining and setting limits with their child (Kochanska et al., 1987). For older children, maladaptive interpersonal patterns between mothers and children have also been described as well as higher levels of criticism and verbal abuse (Gordon, Burge, & Hammen, 1989). Interactional studies of adults with affective disorders have demonstrated that family functioning is profoundly disturbed in a variety of ways, both in the acute phase of the disorder and thereafter (Keitner & Miller, 1990). Finally, parenting is impaired through decreased attention, less intensity of interaction, and an inability to focus on the child (Beardslee, 1990; Downey & Coyne, 1990).

Examination of children with an affectively disordered parent(s) suggests a wide range of outcomes in children are possible. A significant number show characteristics of resilience (Beardslee & Podorefsky, 1988). Self-understanding has proved an important component of resiliency (Beardslee, 1981, 1983, 1989). Beardslee and Podorefsky (1988) studied the role of self-understanding in resilient children whose parents had experienced affective disorder. They demonstrated that resilient adolescents were aware of their parents' illnesses, had spent a great deal of time thinking about them, and had developed an understanding of the illness. These adolescents reported understanding that they were not the cause of illness, which was essential to the process of moving on with their lives. They saw themselves as separate from their parents and from the parent's illness, and able to act independently. Such findings suggest the feasibility of an intervention targeted to enhancing the resiliency of high-risk children.

Preventive Intervention Efforts

There have been several efforts to prevent depression in adults, especially with people facing unemployment (Price, van Ryn, & Vinokur, 1992), those undergoing loss (Bloom, Hodges, Kern, & McFaddin, 1985), and those at high risk due to minority and poverty status (Munoz & Ying, 1993). Most efforts at prevention in adults use cognitive–behavioral approaches

(Lewinsohn, 1987; Vega, Valle, Kolodoy, & Hough, 1987). Few efforts, however, have been initiated targeting high-risk youth. Clarke and colleagues (Clarke, Hawkins, Murphy, Sheeber, Lewinsohn, & Seeley, 1995) targeted adolescents with elevated scores on self-report measures and decreased rates of disorder using short-term cognitive interventions. Seligman and colleagues (Jaycox, Reivich, Gillham, & Seligman, 1994) found that school-aged children with depressive symptoms improved with a cognitive and social problem-solving intervention. To date, only the work of Beardslee and his colleagues have directly addressed prevention in the nonsymptomatic offspring of adults with affective disorder.

Prevention of Depression in Children of Families with Affective Disorder

Beardslee and colleagues have developed an approach to primary prevention that is based on well-known concepts in psychosocial interventions. Two formats of intervention have been developed based on the assumption that worries about children were salient, of deep concern, and were largely unaddressed by patients' therapists and doctors. The first form of the intervention is a short-term, intensive focused, clinician-based intervention with long-term follow-up. The core elements of the intervention are: (1) assessment of all family members; (2) presentation of psychoeducational material about affective disorders and the risks and resilience in children; (3) linking the psychoeducational material to the family's life experience; (4) decreasing feelings of guilt and blame in children; and (5) facilitating the children's independent functioning in school and activities outside the home. The second format consists of a lecture and group discussion session presented to a group of parents with affective disorder. The same psychoeducational material is presented in both interventions. Parental affective illness is depicted as a family experience, along with recommendations for mitigating the effects on children of the affective disorder. Parents attend two, one-hour lectures followed by brief question and answer periods. Both interventions attempt to address misunderstanding and provide information.

The clinician-based intervention is quite intensive. It follows a specific format during 6 to 10 sessions. It includes separate meetings with parents and children, family meetings, and telephone contacts or refresher sessions at 6- to 9-month intervals (Beardslee, 1990). The intervention is conducted by professional clinicians who have undergone an extensive training program. Ongoing supervision is provided, and a manual is used both for training and ongoing work.

Both interventions target families with children between the ages of 8 and 15, and where one or both parents suffers from an affective disorder. The 8- to 15-year range was chosen because the beginning of adolescence is a period of heightened risk for affective disorder (Keller, Lavori, Beardslee, Wunder, Dils, & Samuelson, 1988). The aim of this prevention is to reach families and children before the onset of the disorder. From a cognitive developmental point of view, children aged 8 and older begin to function more autonomously and acquire the cognitive capacity to understand that they are separate from their parent's disorder (Beardslee et al., 1987).

Beardslee and his coworkers have tested the safety of the interventions (Beardslee & Hoke, 1992), and they are currently engaged in a longitudinal study supported by the NIMH Prevention Branch, following families exposed to either intervention for about 9 years. Overall, the sample of participating families is severely ill, with an average lifetime duration of illness for the identified patient of more than 10 years (Beardslee et al., 1993). Results (Beardslee et al., 1993) demonstrate the feasibility and safety of both prevention strategies. At about 18 weeks follow-up, families reported both the clinician-based intervention and the lecture were helpful, and no negative effects were noted. Subjects exposed to both interventions reported significantly decreased worry about concerns at follow-up. Neither the lecture nor clinician-based intervention created additional concerns. Both groups reported significantly increased knowledge about depression and risks and resiliency in children. The clinician-based intervention subjects reported more changes in attitudes and behavior, though the lecture and clinician-based interventions equally impacted such behaviors as "increased talking with spouse." Subjects receiving the clinician-based intervention reported improved understanding in the marital relationship and with their children as well as more strategies to deal with illness than the lecture only.

These results suggest that the short-term effects of exposure to the interventions had a beneficial effect on the families. Differences were observed in favor of the more intensive, clinician-based intervention, and these differences were sustained over 3 to 4 years of follow-up. The continuing follow-up for both interventions will be necessary to demonstrate that these proximal changes in family functioning translate into the hypothesized reduction of instances of illness in the samples. There is reason to believe that these interventions will in fact, result in prevention of disorder. Certainly, the effects of both the clinician-based *and* the lecture interventions are apparent 3 to 4 years after the initial assessment.

The relatively good showing of the lecture-only intervention highlights several powerful features present in the lecture that appear to have brought about changes in the families (Beardslee et al., 1996). First, the lecture sought to demystify the affective illness for these families, letting them know that they are not alone. Second, while the children did not directly participate in the lecture or group discussions, an effort was made to provide some tools to families who wished to have family meetings with their children. Thus, the lecture included discussions on how to talk with children about affective illness, and what steps to take to have a successful family meeting.

Role of Primary Care in the Detection and Treatment of Depression

The promising findings revealed in Beardslee's work suggest that a powerful, preventive intervention exists that can have important public health implications. Any public health impact is limited only by the extent to which the materials are disseminated to families. While the preventive work of Beardslee and colleagues is clearly relevant to psychiatric practice, there is reason to believe that primary care providers should not be overlooked. It is well known that the health care industry is rapidly moving away from reliance on referrals to specialists. Increasingly, primary care providers are encouraged to attend to and treat depression without referral to mental health specialists. Clinical practice guidelines for primary care providers to diagnose and treat depression have been created and widely distributed (Depression Guideline Panel, 1993a, 1993b). Although some have cogently questioned the advisability of this practice (Munoz et al., 1994; Rogers, Wells, Meredith, Strum, & Burham, 1993), the fact remains that most depressed individuals are seen only by primary care providers. The likelihood is that most patients with depression will never see a mental health specialist.

Trends away from using mental health providers and increasing emphasis on prevention come up against the problem that primary care providers have a notoriously poor track record at detection of depression in their patients. Only one-third to one-half of those with major depressive disorder are properly recognized by primary care practitioners (Depression Guidelines Panel, 1993a). Thus, the expectation that these practitioners will efficiently and effectively implement preventive interventions, without assistance, is highly unlikely. Given the importance of access to health information as a necessary condition to effective prevention (Harris, 1995), it is absolutely essential that prevention of depression in high-risk youth include methods that are likely to be used by primary care providers.

Extending the Depression Prevention Program to Primary Care Settings

Although Beardslee set out to develop a cost-effective and practical intervention, the clinician-based intervention is relatively intensive and may cost too much to be implemented on a wide scale. Even the lecture requires access to and the time of a knowledgeable person (Dr. Beardslee conducted the lectures himself), space for the lecture, and scheduling, all of which may be too time- and cost-intensive to be widely used. Based on this, researchers at ITS, in collaboration with Dr. Beardslee, began to consider creating a well-produced, psychoeducational videotape series based on the intervention principles developed by Beardslee and his colleagues.

Prevention Using Video Materials

The flexibility and personalization of the intervention provided by highly trained, professional therapists, as in Beardslee's clinician-based intervention, is likely to yield the greatest preventive effect, as appears to be the case in Beardslee's preliminary data (Beardslee et al., 1996). Accessibility to such personalized, intensive services is unlikely to be great in all parts of the country. Indeed, such specialized and novel services may never be very widely available, even if proven effective. And, Beardslee's data strongly support a relatively large effect of the lecture-only intervention. This suggests that if the prevention principles were presented in a videotape format, effectiveness would be comparable to the lecture only intervention.

There is increasing interest in the potential of modern video and multimedia technology to disseminate health information, literally to enhance "access by making expertise portable" (Harris, 1995, p. 14). Numerous examples in the literature demonstrate the potential of psychoeducational videotaped materials for public health prevention efforts. These efforts have targeted adult populations as well as adolescents and latency-aged children. For example, preventive materials have been shown to effectively educate high-risk adult and adolescent pregnant women in ways to reduce preterm births (Freda et al., 1990). Videotapes have been used successfully with seventh-grade students for smoking prevention (Telch, Miller, Killen, Cooke, & Maccoby, 1990), and to enhance self-protective behaviors of young children to prevent child abduction (Poche, Yoder, & Miltenberger, 1988). Recent concern with prevention of HIV infection has resulted in attempts to impart information and behavior change in high-risk populations. Successful use of videotape materials are reported for teens and parents (Winett et al., 1993), gay men (deKooning, Debets, Blom, & Sandfoot, 1993), prisoners (Gross, deJong, Lamab, Enos, Mason, & Weitzman, 1994), and even mentally retarded/developmentally disabled adults (Samowitz, Levy, Levy, & Jacobs, 1989). A particularly well-researched effort has examined the use of "self-administered" videotapes to teach parenting skills to parents of conduct-disordered children (Webster-Stratton, 1994). These videotapes teach parents to cope with interpersonal distress through improved communication, problem-solving, and self-control skills. Although the training is directed to the parents, the conduct-disordered children in these families showed an increase in knowledge of prosocial behaviors. Clearly, there is ample encouragement in the literature that psychoeducational videotapes or tapes on depression prevention principles could be effective.

Using video and interactive multimedia to effectively convey health messages requires exploiting the strength of the media. Dede and Fontana (1995) describe a program, aired on PBS entitled, *Drinking and Driving: The Toll and the Tears*. The impact of this program was so great that the toll-free phone line offering a discussion guide was clogged for weeks, and stations were asked to re-air the program "dozens" of times. Subsequent declines in drinking and driving incidents were attributed to this film, although no formal studies were conducted. In their analysis of the apparent effectiveness of this program, Dede and Fontana note that the program used high-quality production values. The film was not preachy but effectively organized dramatic information that grabbed viewers' attention. The documentary style of the program presented several personal vignettes of people who had been responsible for taking someone's life while driving under the influence of alcohol. At the end of the program, Kelly Burke, the film maker, revealed that after only two drinks, he caused an accident which took the life of a police officer. This disclosure contributed to an especially powerful emotional impact of the film. Dede and Fontana (1995) describe several "design heuristics" (p. 169), for generating video and multimedia efforts intended to have a public health impact:

- Touch the emotions of individuals to gain the audience attention and prepare them for a learning experience and eventual action.
- Use a team of professionals including video producers, graphic artists, computer programmers, content specialists, and instructional designers.
- The design life cycle should be an interactive process with representatives of the intended audience and health educators.

To this list, we would add empirical test of the product for effectiveness.

There are other reasons arguing in favor of videotaped prevention interventions. It is estimated that more than 80% of U.S. households have VCRs. Videotapes can be easily disseminated by a variety of clinicians and health care workers, including primary care providers. For families struggling with potentially stigmatizing illnesses, like AIDS or mental illness, videotapes provide a highly confidential exposure to psychoeducational material. The convenience of videotaped interventions may reach individuals who lack the motivation or means to attend a lecture or a more intensive, clinician-based experience. Finally, videotapes truly make "expertise portable" in a manner that can reach essentially anywhere in the country.

This general model was used by ITS in the effort to develop a videotape program to prevent depression and behavior disorders in high-risk youth, specifically children of people with depression. This program is called the Lilly Family Depression Project, and is presented next.

THE LILLY FAMILY DEPRESSION PROJECT: UTILIZING PSYCHOEDUCATIONAL VIDEOTAPED MATERIAL FOR PREVENTION OF DEPRESSION

Effective presentation of video material appears to be a promising medium for imparting information that supports health-enhancing life-style and behavior changes in high-risk populations. Taking into account the equally promising findings of

Beardslee and his colleagues (Beardslee et al., 1993; Beardslee et al., 1996) regarding the effectiveness of informational interventions for families with a depressed parent, the extension of this work by means of a high-quality videotape program seems a logical next step. A fundamental assumption of such a project is that there are important similarities among families dealing with parental affective disorder. These similarities can be addressed in dramatically presented and professionally produced psychoeducational video materials. Such a video-based program may be sufficient intervention for many families, although other families may require professional intervention. The materials should be designed to increase the likelihood that such families will pursue an appropriate referral. That is, the material should strive to destigmatize the effects of parental depression on the children and support seeking help for difficulties which may arise. Any video materials intended for wide distribution as a preventive intervention must take into consideration that some families may require more intensive intervention. Finally, any preventive intervention must be easily integrated into the ongoing practice of internists, pediatricians, and family physicians, as well as psychiatrists, psychologists, and other mental health specialists.

With a grant from the Eli Lilly Corporation, ITS began the Lilly Family Depression Project. Anticipating the principles outlined by Dede and Fontana (1995), ITS assembled a team of clinicians (psychologists and psychiatrists) with professional video producers, screen writers, and actors. Working in close collaboration with Dr. Beardslee, this team put together two videotapes. One tape, the Parent Tape, is about 30 minutes long and presents the stories of three families. The stories behind these families are very loosely taken from patients seen in Beardslee's program. Significant changes were made, however, to protect the patients' true identities.

Actors worked closely with the clinicians on the team to realistically portray scenes from families in a documentarylike film. In Family 1, the mother is very depressed, withdrawn, and irritable, while the father and two children struggle to understand and cope with mother's erratic behavior. Vignettes of Family 2 depict an African-American family, in which the

young, depressed father contends with recent losses and ne-
glects his young son's need for attention. Finally, Family 3 involves a depressed, single mother of a preteen. Wrapped in her
own doubt and worries, the mother forgets activities that are
important to her daughter. Each story is told in a way that
highlights the challenges and risks experienced by each family.
In a matter-of-fact and nonmoralistic way, the film outlines for
parents the effect that their affective disorder may be having
on the family, especially the children. Possible solutions are
presented to the various situations of the families and illustrated on the video. The scripts enacted on the tape include
emotionally dramatic material. The patients' stories are inter-
spersed, documentary-style, with scenes from an interview with
Dr. Beardslee. The interview, along with voice-over and high-
quality graphics, underscores messages about the importance
of destigmatizing depression, opening and maintaining lines
of communication with all family members, and encouraging
resilience in the children (Beardslee, 1989).

A particular innovation of this program is the inclusion of
a videotape directed toward the child or children in the family.
This tape, called the Child Tape, is targeted specifically to children between 7 and 13 years old. The tape is titled "Kenny's
Incredible Adventure" and is about 20 minutes long. Viewers
first meet Kenny, a boy of about 11 or 12, working on a soapbox
racer in his garage, where he addresses the camera directly.
Kenny is the boy in Family 1 of the Parent tape, a feature intended to provide continuity and depth to the characters. He
shares his story and worries about what was happening to his
mother. This includes his fear that perhaps he is somehow
responsible for what is not right in his home, a common concern of children. He is shown approaching his older sister, a
teenager, who remembers what is was like for her. He also talks
with his father and expresses his concern that mother might
not be at the "big race." In the end, his mother sees him race
his car. Kenny explains to the viewer what he has learned. With
the aid of his "computer" and high-quality animation, Kenny
shows what is wrong in the brains of people who get depressed,
how it is an illness like any other, and is no one's fault. He also

emphasizes how treatment has helped his mother, and how it is his job to stay involved in school and other normal activities. Careful attention has been paid to the quality of the video-tape and production values. Indeed, the video series has already won numerous prestigious awards for excellence in documentary- and educational-style videos. We concur with other authors (e.g., Dede & Fontana, 1995) that high-quality video production is essential for a truly effective, video-based prevention tool.

Included with the tapes is an informative pamphlet, which describes important points about depression and a step-by-step procedure for enhancing resiliency in children. Signs and symptoms of depression in young children are also included in an easy-to-understand manner, along with suggestions about how to get help for themselves and their children. Parents are cautioned to watch the Child Tape by themselves before deciding to show the tape to their children. This feature of the program is intended to send the message that the parent(s) know(s) their child(ren). They are empowered to decide whether or not their children should watch the tape. At the same time, the pamphlet also emphasizes the importance of helping their child understand what is going on, that what happens is not the child's fault, and to encourage the child's involvement in activities outside the family.

Safety and Efficacy: Design of the Field Trial

Research to confirm the safety and efficacy of health information materials is a crucial component of the developmental process. From our perspective, production of video and print materials is only the first step in constructing a truly useful prevention tool. Safety of the materials must be assured. This may be particularly true for materials targeting high-risk populations that may feel stigmatized, blamed, or otherwise upset or worried by the materials. While some prevention strategies may use fear, such as smoking or drug prevention, in a depressed population, which by definition is already hypersensitive to self-blame, carelessly produced materials could worsen a family's situation. In addition to safety, satisfaction with the materials by the families and providers should be examined. Although depression tends to render individuals dissatisfied with everything, it is still important to obtain some measure of the willingness of patients and their families to use the materials. Providers, too, should be satisfied with the ease of use of the tape and results of the tape for their patients.

Finally, measures of efficacy of the materials is currently underway. Prevention studies, however, are very difficult and expensive to run. With federal funding, Beardslee and colleagues are following families in their study for nearly 10 years. Such longitudinal follow-up is necessary to demonstrate that a particular intervention has a primary prevention effect. Essentially, a prevention study hypothesizes that a given event, in this case depression or behavior disorder, does not occur. The researcher runs the risk that the event of interest occurs sometime after he or she stops observing. Even in a high-risk population, the occurrence of a disorder at any given moment is more unlikely than likely. Such studies are, therefore, quite complex and extensive.

The authors attempted to design a useful, but by necessity more limited, efficacy study. This was possible because of Dr. Beardslee's prior work. His data show intermediary effects of the interventions on family functioning. Changes in family functioning, such as increased communication, theoretically should create an environment that is most likely to result in greater resilience in the child and decrease the chances of depression or behavioral disorders occurring in the child(ren). Thus, the field trial was designed to test the efficacy of the videotape series by detecting the kinds of effects Beardslee observed early in the tests of his interventions (the lecture and clinician-based interventions). Toward this end, similar measures of effectiveness were used, as well as similar procedures for subject selection, confirmation of depressive illness histories, and so forth. By demonstrating that the videotape series replicates the kinds of interim effects that Beardslee observed, we can extrapolate the preventive potential of the videotape, prevention materials.

Specifically, we have selected adult patients having any kind of depressive disorder (major depression, dysthymia, depression NOS) and who have at least one child in the targeted age range. Excluded are patients with bipolar disorder, psychotic disorders, or families in crisis (acrimonious divorce, acute and out-of-control substance abuse, etc.). Although Beardslee's work included bipolar patients, it was felt that it would be confusing to include material relevant to bipolar disorder and depression in one tape. For this reason, the Lilly Family Depression Project elected to focus on depression only. Families are recruited from an HMO in Maryland and a large psychiatric practice operating in New Hampshire and Massachusetts. After an initial assessment of the identified patient and spouse (children are not directly assessed), families are randomly assigned to an experimental or control group. The experimental group is given the videotapes and pamphlet immediately and reassessed at 6 weeks and 3 months. Control subjects are reassessed at 6 weeks, at which point they are given the materials and reassessed again 6 weeks later. Thus, the design involves both within- and between-group comparisons. It is hypothesized that families given the tapes will view them. Families who receive the videos and pamphlet will report (1) increased knowledge about depression; (2) increased knowledge of risks and resiliency in children (including recognition of warning signs); (3) destigmatization–normalization of illness; (4) decreased guilt and worry about concerns; (5) increased communication among family members; (6) increased understanding of other family members' experiences and feelings, and (7) adoption of new strategies (e.g., seeking information about depression, seeking help for children).

Progress of the field trial has been excellent. At the time of this writing, over 60 families have been recruited and studies are being run at the two sites (Maryland and New England). Although it is too early to analyze the data, early examination of comments by the participants suggests that, in general, the families find the tapes enjoyable to watch, informative, and realistic. Comments about the child tapes are likewise generally positive. The portrayal of the depression as a medical illness that can be treated is mentioned by parents as an important feature of the videos, as well as their upbeat, positive tone. Child viewers report liking the way Kenny directly addressed the viewer, and they seem reassured that family problems are not their fault. Several parents have spontaneously commented that the videos made it easier to talk with their children about their own situation, a major goal of the Lilly Family Depression Project.

As the field test continues, the authors are also learning more about developing such prevention programs for wide distribution. For instance, a few comments emerged regarding the fact that the three families depicted on the videos did not reflect that viewer's own situation. Since such coverage would be impossible, this feedback has prompted us to consider various modifications in the pamphlet's instructions on how to use the tapes. Although there have been no negative instances to date, we will be examining the data to identify particular sorts of families for whom the videotape series might not be sufficient. For example, in some instances, after viewing the tapes, parents revealed that they have "hidden" their depression from their child(ren). These parents were especially concerned that their child(ren) would be upset or confused watching the child tape. Again, such comments have resulted in consideration of further steps, such as telephone consultations with parents to discuss whether and how to approach their children or some other method of follow-up.

More complete results from the field trial are not yet available. Data collection is expected to be completed in early spring of 1997, and results will be published. Planned analyses include not only the within- and between-group comparisons described above, but also comparisons with data from Beardslee's investigations of the lecture and clinician-based interventions.

THE FUTURE

Once the field trial is completed and any modification of materials accomplished, plans include national distribution of the program (videotapes and printed material) to primary care providers, mental health providers, and HMOs. Clearly, dissemination of the program to suitable end users is the next major hurdle in achieving a genuine preventive effect. Toward this end, we have created a program that is simple for providers to employ and easy for families to access. As noted above, dissemination of health information is a highly cost-effective activity, and increasing access of families not only to VCRs but to the internet, promise to boost the cost-effectiveness of disseminating health information (McGinnis et al., 1995). We expect to continue data collection on families' use of and response to the prevention materials.

Trends in health care suggest that the primary care team will increasingly be called upon to prevent disorders in high-risk populations, detect occult disorders, and intervene in the most cost-effective way possible. Health care experts increasingly recognize that much of the illness addressed in the PCP's office is generated by or exacerbated by disturbances of emotions, behaviors or abuse of substances. As was noted above, few people now see specialists for these concerns, and fewer still will see specialists in the future. Innovative Training Systems, Inc. is dedicated to the development, production, testing, and distribution of a wide range of tools designed to help PCPs identify individuals at high-risk for mental health and substance abuse disorders and to help the providers effectively intervene. The Lilly Family Depression Project is just one of a variety of prevention and health-education projects underway or planned by ITS. Computerized, interactive multimedia programs are under development for screening and PCP intervention of, for instance, hazardous and harmful alcohol use (as opposed to later-stage alcoholism). Similar programs are targeted toward prevention of smoking in children, relapse prevention for alcoholics and drug abusers, and prevention of depression in patients with coronary heart disease. One recently initiated project uses multimedia, health education, and computerized monitoring to improve medication compliance in AIDS patients, for whom complex medication regimens can be effective, but only if compliance with the medication schedules is high. These projects and others reflect our belief that significant, future gains in health care will be the result of providing more complete and effective health information. However, such information must be carefully constructed and tested. As Dede and Fontana (1995) have put it:

> Significant changes in behaviors that lead to healthier individuals require the design of information systems that personalize wellness information, emphasize individual responsibility, and promote the internalization of knowledge and its immediate application in daily life. As long as information about health choices remains noninteractive, impersonal, and moralistic, improvements in citizen's decisions are unlikely. (p. 167)

The Lilly Family Depression Project exemplifies one effort to create and disseminate preventive health information in a manner likely to yield behavioral change. Families struggling with affective disorder and their providers now have a promising tool to help them learn to cope better.

PART IV

Informatics and Financing

13.

Health Care Informatics: Its Role in Behavioral Health's Successful Integration into Primary Care and the Larger Health Care System

H. Edmund Pigott, Ph.D., Bruce Meltzer, M.D., Deborah L. Heggie, Ph.D.

The behavioral health industry suffers from several related paradoxes which stymie its acceptance by, and successful integration into, the larger health care system. The authors contend that emerging information technologies will play an increasingly critical role in resolving these paradoxes, thereby maximizing the behavioral health sciences' influence within specific systems of care.

In competitive industries from retail sales to manufacturing, insurance, banking, and financial services, the essential success factor has become the ability to harness information technologies to lower costs and enhance the quality of products and services for targeted customer groups. The same will be true in health care as it rapidly evolves away from its cottage industry roots into a truly competitive industry. The authors believe that linking emerging information technologies with the behavioral health science's knowledge-base will form the basis for entrepreneurial innovation well into the 21st Century.

Behavioral health's first paradox is that despite 40 years of solid biopsychosocial research documenting treatment efficacy rates often exceeding those of many common medical procedures, behavioral health is still the orphaned child within the larger health care system. This reality is best exemplified by two facts: First, behavioral health consumers and providers lack parity in insurance reimbursement for proven and cost-effective health care services. The second is that the behavioral health delivery system provides care to less than 20% of those consumers who warrant our services (Regier et al., 1993). The other 80% are treated, mistreated, and most often left untreated by the larger health care system at great cost to the consumer, their families, their employers, and society at large. In fact, frequently occurring mental health diagnoses are missed in one half of patients treated in the primary care arena (Higgins, 1994; Spitzer et al., 1994).

The second paradox is a corollary to the first. Despite the wealth of empirically sound treatment outcomes research documenting the efficacy of defined interventions for defined conditions, the bulk of behavioral health's $75 billion in annual spending has little connection to this knowledge-base. This is best illustrated by the fact that 50% of total behavioral health spending continues to go toward psychiatric hospitalization despite over 25 years of controlled research documenting that other forms of care are more effective, less costly, have lower suicide rates, and result in up to 400% fewer psychiatric relapses regardless of the patient population studied (Black, Warrack, & Winokur, 1985; Kiesler & Sibulkin, 1987; Pallak & Cummings, 1992; Pigott & Trott, 1993).

Much of outpatient and substance abuse care fares no better. Few providers have the time, inclination, or proper training to synthesize and effectively translate research findings to differentially guide their treatment of individual health care consumers. Despite the wealth of clinically relevant research, few such findings filter down to inform actual practice on a wide scale and consistent basis. Even in their treatment of major depression, psychiatrists demonstrate wide variance in practice, with many prescribing subtherapeutic doses of antidepressants or prescribing minor tranquilizers instead (Sturm & Wells,

1995). With more subtle diagnoses, as well as complex comorbid conditions, the degree of variance in practice patterns only increases.

Historically, practitioners have overly emphasized the "art" of clinical practice while minimizing the behavioral health sciences' ability to meaningfully inform service delivery to specific behavioral health care consumers in their "unique" circumstances. This fundamental professional bias preserves practitioners' decision-making autonomy while protecting many from rigorously examining the soundness of their clinical decisions (Pigott, Alter, & Heggie, in press).

The final, and perhaps most profound paradox is behavioral health's failure to leverage its basic and applied research knowledge-base for maximum impact within larger systems of care. On the applied side, this fact is best illustrated by behavioral health's failure to exploit the pioneering research on the medical cost-offset effect by Follette and Cummings (Cummings & Follette, 1968; Follette & Cummings, 1967). Thirty years later, no health care organization has capitalized on the offset effect as the basis for financing and extending behavioral health services to health care consumers. This is the case despite repeated studies documenting that conceptually driven, differentially applied, brief and targeted mental health services lower overall health care spending more than covering the cost of behavioral care (Jones & Vischi, 1979; Cummings, Dorken, Pallak, & Henke, 1991; Melek, 1996). Rather, the medical cost-offset effect has been behavioral health's ongoing "great giveaway" to our own demise (Wiggins, 1997).

On the basic research side, extensive research has been conducted in how people learn by such psychologists as B. F. Skinner and Albert Bandura, among others. Few behavioral health care providers are familiar with this research. Fewer still have sought to apply this knowledge to enhance the actual health care delivery process itself. For instance, Bandura (1977a, 1977b) has shown that strategies which increase people's perception of personal effectiveness have a broad and profound influence on them. Such interventions increase people's belief in their ability to successfully execute whatever behaviors are required to produce desired changes in their lives.

Bandura has shown that enhancing individuals' "perceived self-efficacy" is self-reinforcing, and therefore will increase and generalize to other behaviors over time. Conversely, perceived personal ineffectiveness and dependency are progressive disorders. Despite such findings, the bulk of behavioral and general health care services are still delivered in ways which reinforce the latter, while undermining the former.

INFORMATICS: THE BIG PICTURE

As President Clinton indicated in his second inaugural address, America is going through a historic shift from an industrial to an information-based society. The speed of this shift has been accelerating during the 1990s and its implications for the creation and delivery of products and services in every industry are profound.

In competitive markets, tomorrow's leaders are those who have learned to better serve their customers by leveraging technology to become less labor, and more information intensive. As industries become more competitive, the percent of gross annual revenue spent on information technology increases on a proportional basis. Today, insurance, banking, and financial services invest 10% or more of gross revenue in information technology. Manufacturing and retail spend 6 to 8% of gross revenue on information technology and it is climbing (Hau, 1996).

The above figures are for each industry as a whole. Individual companies within each industry spend more or less. Successful companies tend to spend more on information technology, and spend it more wisely. WalMart in retailing, and Gateway Computers in manufacturing, are but two examples. Both have used such technology to reduce cost, enhance customer service, increase market share, and maintain profit margins in brutally competitive industries. In the 1980s, WalMart developed a point-of-sale and inventory control system which formed the basis for their competitive advantage and accelerated growth in the late 1980s and 1990s. The genius of WalMart's system was that it electronically linked each store's item-by-item sales to its various product suppliers. This enabled numerous efficiencies for both WalMart and its suppliers as well as more tailored product offerings to WalMart customers. Among others, these benefits include:

- Electronic commerce efficiencies in the placing and filling of orders between WalMart and its suppliers resulting in a virtual elimination in errors and a dramatic reduction in labor costs for all parties.
- "Just-in-time" production and distribution of products resulting in a significant reduction in excess inventory and its associated costs for WalMart and its suppliers.
- Tailored product offerings at WalMart stores based on each stores' customer buying patterns.

Gateway Computers is a manufacturer who has taken point-of-sale and inventory control software systems one step further by moving into direct sales as well. Besides electronically linking with its suppliers, at Gateway, a computer is not built until a customer's order is taken. This not only eliminates excess inventory, but allows Gateway to respond quickly to consumer's changing buying patterns and take market share away from more established firms such as Compaq, Apple, and Dell Computers, among others. In virtually every industry, the innovative application of information technologies has become the engine which drives ever accelerating change. Such innovation literally determines the winners and losers in today's economy.

HEALTH CARE INFORMATICS

In contrast to other industries, health care as a whole spends only 2% of its gross annual revenue on information technology with behavioral health spending even less (Hau, 1996). The overwhelming bulk of these expenditures is focused on billing, collecting, and paying claims, versus positively impacting the efficiency, effectiveness, and consumer satisfaction with, actual health care services. Due to health care's cottage industry roots, until recently "claims" was the only important unit of information to manage. Add in treatment authorization, network credentialing and an accounting package and you pretty much have the state-of-the-art in managed care information systems today. Such systems enable managed care organizations to fulfill their fundamental role as an arbitrageur, or broker, between buyers and sellers of health care services. The resulting database is more than sufficient for reporting functions to the employer/purchaser as well as "provider profiling" to identify those sellers who deliver too many (or too costly) units per episode of care or have high repeat claims rates (Pigott, 1996).

As a trillion plus dollar per year cottage industry consuming over 10% of America's Gross National Product, health care has been ripe for radical and ongoing change. Whereas arbitrage services were the first wave of market forces impacting health care during the 1980s, today the primary forces are health care's consolidation and industrialization which are moving it away from its cottage industry roots. Figure 13.1 reflects this industrialization and the resulting movement toward setting up integrated delivery systems which organizationally link primary (front-line), secondary (specialists and community hospitals), and tertiary (academic medical centers) care. The diagram includes the primary information system requirements necessary to enhance clinical efficiency and effectiveness within such systems of care. Generally, a basic premise of such systems is to use primary care professionals to provide the bulk of patient care while controlling access to more expensive services at the secondary and tertiary level. Patients, and their ill health, are basically feeders into a system designed to more efficiently return them to health.

Common Computerized Medical Record

A common computerized medical record is critical to achieve the promise of collaborative and efficient care within integrated delivery systems. As bit players in such systems though, behavioral health professionals are unlikely to play a significant

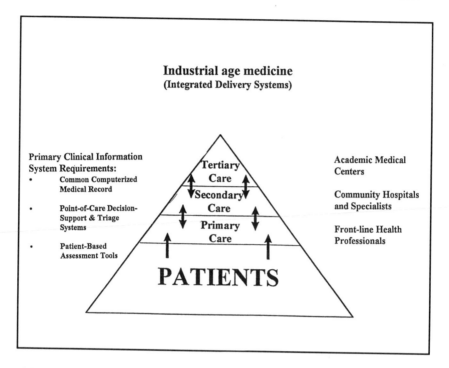

Figure 13.1. Industrial age medicine (Integrated Delivery Systems).

role in designing the delivery systems' electronic medical records. Rather, individual behavioral health providers can use the electronic record as a platform for improving collaboration and information exchange with patients' primary care physicians, specialists, ancillary providers, and care managers. While assisting in behavioral health's socialization and integration into larger healthcare systems and improving patient care coordination, the electronic record in itself does nothing to reduce the disparity between what is known from the behavioral health sciences and what is actually applied in specific health care transactions.

Point-of-Care, Decision-Support, and Triage Systems

Each month the National Library of Medicine processes over 33,000 peer-reviewed articles. While most of this "knowledge" is not relevant to a particular provider's care of a specific patient, some of it is (or should be). The information age has become more like the information deluge. Specialists can barely hope to stay current in their own narrowly defined area of expertise. Across the spectrum, the disparity between what is known and what is actually applied in specific health care transactions is due to a fundamental disconnection between the knowledge production and knowledge utilization sides of the health care business. This disconnection between science and practice in health care, Docherty (1996) observes, results in embarrassingly wide variations in practice patterns and large deviations from practice standards.

Due to their industrial-age model, integrated delivery systems have the potential to reduce such variance in provider practice patterns and bring some sanity to the care delivery and resource allocation process. Point-of-care, decision-support, and triage systems for front-line professionals are essential to bring such potential to fruition and avert disaster. Due to health care's increasing knowledge-base, having the least trained professionals responsible for specialty care triage decisions is short-sighted unless they are provided with the tools necessary to apply this knowledge in their clinical decisions. Besides the potential adverse health consequences to patients, in today's litigious environment, integrated delivery systems are toying with legal hari kari without such information system tools in place.

A recent review on the impact of point-of-care expert systems on provider behavior report generally positive effects (Johnston, 1994). Expert systems have also been shown to be useful in reminding clinicians of overlooked diagnoses and treatment alternatives as well as interpreting and filtering information (Berner, 1994). Within behavioral health, expert systems provide the opportunity to reduce the disparity between what is known and what is actually applied by explicitly linking critical patient variables to the differential treatment decision-making process. By taking a lead in this process, behavioral health can expedite its integration into primary care and the larger health care system. This process will involve developing better case identification procedures for patients warranting behavioral health interventions as well as defining and automating within an expert system format a host of key differential decisions such as:

- Which patients can have their initial medication evaluation performed by their primary care physician (PCP) or psychiatric nurse practitioner (PNP) versus those requiring a psychiatric consultation? Presently, two-thirds of all antidepressant and anxiolytic medications are prescribed by PCPs with no rational triaging mechanism in place (Strain, 1986).
- Which depressed patients require long-term antidepressant therapy versus just a 4- to 6-month medication trial?
- Which depressed suicidal patients can be managed safely with a "no-harm" agreement, telephone monitoring, and/or multiple weekly contacts to monitor their risk level versus those requiring an inpatient admission?
- Which substance abusing depressed patients should first have a 4- to 6-week period of sobriety and psychosocial treatment prior to initiating antidepressant therapy versus those who would likely benefit from an immediate trial on an antidepressant in addition to psychosocial treatment?
- Which behavioral health patients are appropriate for cognitive–behavioral therapy, versus interpersonal therapy, versus distress tolerance training, versus a trial on medication alone, or in some combination with one of the above?
- Which patients are appropriate for such interventions to be administered in individual therapy, versus marital–family, versus group therapy, versus referral to a self-help program, or some combination thereof?

By making explicit the criteria for various psychosocial and psychopharmacological therapies, research can proceed to clarify further which treatments, or combinations thereof, best help which types of patients (Litman, 1995; Pigott & Broskowski, 1995). Online access to such expert systems provides PCPs and PNPs with the tools to initiate relevant and timely treatment or refer to behavioral health specialists where appropriate to do so. Implementing such systems is not meant to imply that their findings should be rigidly applied. Expert systems by definition have limitations. There will always be clinical situations which require the professional to select (or deselect) other treatment components based either on additional data, or a different interpretation of the available data. In such circumstances, the use of expert systems forces professionals to be explicit and thoughtful about why they are making such "nonroutine" decisions. Forcing this thought process alone enhances the quality of care.

Another purpose of expert systems is to reduce variance in implementing health care's independent variables (i.e., the host of clinical and resource allocation decisions which collectively comprise treatment) so that dependent variables (i.e., the treatment outcomes) become more directly interpretable. By reducing variance in clinical decision making, integrated delivery systems are better able to reliably identify and repeat those clinical processes which result in superior outcomes while discarding less effective practices (Bultema, Mailliard, Getzfrid, Lerner, & Colone, 1996; Pigott et al., in press). Ultimately, the purpose of expert systems is to enable their rapid obsolescence through constant, knowledge-based updating. Implementing expert systems thereby helps unite and give focus to health care's knowledge production and knowledge utilization sides of the business. The behavioral health sciences can take a leadership role in this process.

Patient-Based Assessment Tools

Computerized patient assessment and outcome tracking tools are becoming increasingly important in health care. The importance of such tools reflects health care's shifting emphasis from solely tracking what is done for billing purposes (e.g., specific medical procedures and CPT codes) to also tracking what is accomplished (e.g., changes in functional health status) from such interventions (Ware, 1996). This is an arena where the behavioral health sciences can exert influence due to its expertise in designing and assessing the reliability and validity of such instruments.

For tracking changes in functional health status, the National Committee for Quality Assurance (NCQA) recently endorsed the SF-12 Health Survey as part of its accreditation criteria (Ware, 1996). In addition to tracking outcomes, the SF-12's mental health scale can be used to identify patients who may warrant behavioral health services. A number of such patient-based assessment tools have been developed to identify patients with behavioral health disorders presenting in primary care settings. These include the SDDS-PC (Broadhead, Leon, & Weissman, 1995) and PRIME-MD (Spitzer et al., 1994), among others.

By implementing patient-based assessment tools, integrated delivery systems can address the pervasive underdiagnosis of behavioral health disorders presenting within primary care settings. This will result in a huge influx of cases identified as warranting behavioral health services. Behavioral health professionals will need to work closely with their primary care colleagues to set up efficient triage and treatment systems to manage this inflow of patients thereby providing an ideal proving ground for documenting, enhancing, and getting credit for the medical cost offset effect.

INFORMATION-BASED HEALTH

Health care's next wave of change is its shift toward information-based health. The primary market force driving this shift is consumerism. Informed choice in choosing products and services based on their quality, convenience, and price is consumerism's foundation. Consumerism has transformed industry after industry from retailing and automotives to telecommunications, banking, and financial services, among others (Herzlinger & Freeman, 1996). Health care, consuming 10% of America's Gross National Product, will likely be the next industry to be so transformed by the consumer movement. As in other industries, the innovative application of information technologies is the essential success factor in this new environment.

Information-based health is premised on the simple fact that people, by what they do and what they don't do, can have far greater impact on their health status than that of all medicine combined. Whereas health care's industrialization through managed care and integrated delivery systems has focused primarily on gaining efficiencies in the supply of health care services, information-based health focuses on empowering consumers by providing timely, easily accessible, individually tailored and relevant information to assist them in their role as their own primary care provider.

Information-based health services provide the context for behavioral health to leverage its basic research knowledge-base for maximum impact. As consumers increase their access to such services, it is critical to fully integrate behavioral health into primary care. This will require the thoughtful design of an information technology and health care delivery infrastructure which reinforces people's personal effectiveness in managing their own health. Implementing such an infrastructure will have a dramatic impact on enhancing consumers' overall health status while substantially reducing the cost of obtaining it.

Information-based health services are not a futuristic pipe dream. Today, men with enlarged prostates use an interactive multimedia system to help them decide whether to have surgery or take a noninvasive approach to treating their condition. Persons with AIDS use home health computer workstations to better manage their own care while drug-addicted pregnant women get tailored health information via touch-tone phone access to a computerized voice-mail system (Ferguson, 1995). In Camden and Newark, New Jersey, multimedia health kiosks in public housing projects provide health care information and education 24-hours a day in both Spanish and English, while linking residents to their primary care clinic for teleconferencing with physicians and nurse practitioners for both routine and emergency care (Schneider, 1997). Ferguson (1995), reports that a panel of consumer health informatics experts predict that such "cyberhealth" information systems will turn patients into providers by offering customized health information at the touch of a button. The revolution is on. The behavioral health sciences have much to contribute if we seize the opportunity.

Figure 13.2 is a diagram reflecting this shift towards information-based health care services. Such services recognize the central role consumers play as their own primary care provider. Timely, readily accessible and relevant information presented in an easy to understand and apply format is the key service such consumers need to best manage their, and their family members, health. The health care provider role changes profoundly in this new environment. The nature of transaction between buyers and sellers of services moves away from one of "patients" buying health from "omniscient doctors." Such transactions will be replaced by ones where frontline professionals are more like partners or "coaches" providing advice, encouragement, and mutually agreed upon medical and psychosocial interventions in support of the consumer's own primary care provider role. When specialized expertise, and/or high technology diagnostic and medical procedures are required, consumers access such health experts in consultation with their health partners.

The role of information technology shifts in this new environment from an exclusive focus on improving the clinical efficiency and effectiveness of health care professionals to one which includes empowering consumers. The following are some examples of the necessary information system capabilities in this new era.

Telemedicine, Multimedia Health Kiosks, and Online Care

Health-oriented telecommunications and informatics redirects the traditional focus from intervention to prevention. Consumers become empowered with knowledge allowing them to assume greater responsibility for their health care and life-style decisions (McNamara, 1994). For the elderly, such technology

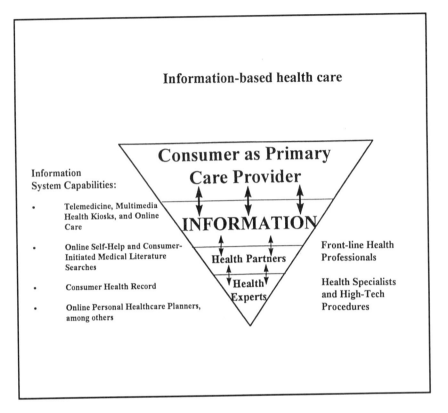

Figure 13.2.   Information-based health care.

has been used not only to enhance their functional health status but enable them to remain in independent living arrangements for much longer than would be otherwise medically advised (Celler, 1995).

Telemedicine originally focused on delivering care and information to underserved populations living in remote areas (McGee and Tangalos, 1994) or urban centers using multimedia health kiosks and computerized voice-mail systems (Ferguson, 1995; Schneider, 1997). Increasingly, such technology will be applied to other populations by making health kiosks accessible at work sites, clinics, and homes. In behavioral health, online psychoeducational support groups for specific conditions are now possible using interactive teleconferencing technology, among other uses.

Online Self-Help and Consumer-Initiated Medical Literature Searches

In general, health care professionals have underestimated the extent and impact of the self-help movement. Increasingly, the self-help movement is going online. Both America Online and CompuServe have active self-help forums and numerous self-help organizations have set up interactive forums on the Internet. Such condition-specific forums, combined with the availability of consumer-initiated medical literature searches, provides consumers with a rich knowledge-base for their primary care provider role.

Consumer Health Record

Developing consumer interfaces to computerized medical records is critical to reinforcing their primary care provider role. Such technology can enable seamless linkages between consumers and their behavioral and primary care health partners which support efficient information exchange and true collaborative care. It is essential for information within a consumer's personal health record to be presented in an attractive and easy to understand format if such efforts are to succeed.

Online Personal Health Care Planners

Personal health care planners use self-assessments to provide customized life-style and health care recommendations to consumers. Access Health, Inc. provides an example of one such online planner at their Internet web site (www.access-health. com). At Access Health's web site, consumers can take a self-administered health risk assessment which then electronically generates a customized set of life-style and self-care recommendations.

Personal planners need to be developed and empirically validated for a variety of health care conditions. In behavioral and primary care, such planners are a natural extension of patient-based assessment tools such as the SF-12, SDDS-PC, and PRIME-MD, among others. Once administered, presenting the assessment findings back to consumers in both a text and graphic format with reference to population norms, empowers consumers to make better informed decisions. Too often, consumers have received little, if any, feedback on the behavioral and medical assessments they take. Linking such assessment findings within an expert system format to the range of appropriate self-care, psychosocial, and psychopharmacological treatment options, will help consumers truly partner their behavioral and primary care providers in their own care.

SUMMARY

Health care is going through a period of rapid and fundamental change. Market forces, combined with emerging information technologies, are the engines which increasingly will drive this change process. This period of flux presents a unique opportunity to leverage the behavioral health sciences' knowledge-base by integrating into primary care and the larger health care system. Information technology can play a central role in this process and help ensure its success.

Like other industries, health care too will be restructured in ways that make it more responsive to consumer needs. This will require the thoughtful design of an information technology and health care delivery infrastructure which reinforces people's personal effectiveness in managing their own health as well as promoting information exchange and collaborative care between consumers and providers.

14.

The Effect of Capitation Paradigms on Collaboration between Primary Care and Behavioral Health Providers

Jeremy Kisch, Ph.D.

As the health care system evolves toward greater consolidation, with shrinking dollars and fewer players, the underlying fiscal structure contains both incentives and disincentives toward collaborative linkages among practitioners. Risk arrangements and the allocation of costs shape the dynamics in the relationship among providers, supporting or discouraging collaboration. Differing methods of reimbursement establish incentives that unify or separate primary from specialty practice. The interface of primary care with behavioral health care is especially complex. Understanding the interplay among risk sharing, cost-offsets and reimbursement is essential for building programmatic bridges among medicine, pediatrics, obstetrics and gynecology, and behavioral health care.

BACKGROUND ISSUES

Purchasers, providers, and consumers, each with their own needs and vested interests, compose the health care system.

257

The purchasers are composed of two groups: subscribers and sponsors. The subscribers are the employers and associations who purchase a plan of health benefits for their employees or members. They purchase this benefit coverage from an insuring health plan that underwrites the financial risk and responsibility for payment for the delivery of those health services. The sponsors, the health insurance companies who provide the reimbursement to networks of providers, have come to view themselves as managed care organizations (MCOs) or health service organizations (HSOs). Their mission is to enhance the health of their members by promoting and providing availability of medically necessary and appropriate services. As part of this mission, they seek to manage the provision of services to their members from provider networks assuring quality while containing cost.

Traditionally, consumers looked for ease of access to desired health services while being protected against catastrophic cost. Today, there is increasing expectation of availability and low cost provision of all health services. The payors of those services are looking for control of utilization and its attendant cost. The subscribers also want low cost with ease of access for needed services. The effect of these pressures has been a trend to find the lowest cost provision for those services. The practitioner feels the squeeze of those pressures maximally.

Purchasers and providers have conflicting economic needs. Purchasers need to contain costs to maintain their viability, while providers seek to enhance income. There are significant conflicts between the interests of the parties as they try to better serve their respective customers. In behavioral health this dissonance has fostered two divergent visions as to what constitutes quality care. Quoting different literatures, supporting research efforts that are not readily reconcilable, these camps each vie to reduce the influence of the other. The outlook of one group, closely aligned to practitioners, is committed to advocating for extensive services to the individual. The other stresses a utilitarian approach to serving the needs of the population.

Pivotal in this controversy is the role of medication and the value of generic psychotherapy. The discoveries of a host of effective psychoactive pharmacological treatments have greatly favored a population oriented, less labor intensive, ambulatory approach to psychiatric and chemical dependency treatment. The participation of primary care in behavioral health treatment and behavioral health integration within primary care is an essential aspect of this controversy, made more salient by prescribing practices especially as they relate to the newer antidepressants.

THE JEOPARDY OF BEHAVIORAL DYSFUNCTION

In the past health insurance was sold as a virtue of its service attractiveness rather than price. Insurance companies operated with the notion that losses from one year could be recouped by higher premiums the following year. Within the last two decades, increased cost led health care purchasers to become increasingly concerned with price. Premium increases now threaten loss of market share.

Insurance companies have long understood that utilizers of mental health services pose an underwriting hazard because they are also high utilizers of medical and other specialty services. The cause may be twofold: recipients of mental health services consist of individuals who readily utilize professional services and others who have significantly higher rates of co-morbidity.

Table 14.1 describes the greater utilization of health services in a health maintenance organization (HMO) by members with visits to behavioral health providers (BHP). Even moderate utilization of mental health services is associated with higher utilization of primary and specialty care. Members who had six or more mental health visits had greater utilization of primary and specialty care at more than 4 times the rate of total utilization.

Table 14.2 shows the higher cost of medical services in a preferred provider organization (PPO) for enrollees who received a behavioral health service whether by a primary care provider (PCP) or BHP. The cost of medical claims alone was 1.5 times greater for women and 2 times greater for men.

TABLE 14.1
Average Ambulatory Visits for Members with and without Mental Health Visits (MHV)

	No MHV	< 6 MHV	6+ MHV
Members	30,432	1922	1044
Av. MHV	none	2.34	13.5
Primary Care	3.29	4.41	4.98
Specialty	1.43	1.84	2.57
Ob-Gyn	.43	.72	.74
Total	5.15	9.3	21.8

1991 adult (age 23+), HMOdata

TABLE 14.2
Cost Comparison of Visits for PPO Members Age 23–64 with and without Behavioral Health Service

No BHV	$ Med V	$ Tot V	$ Med V	BHV	
29,220	1941	3877	2931	3217	Women
20,756	1723	4471	3396	1948	Men
49,976				5165	Total

Service reflected by cpt codes by both PCPs and BHPs

The close association of medical and behavioral health problems points to the importance of integrated programmatic efforts to address the problem of increased health jeopardy evidenced by behavioral health problems. These tables demonstrate that even within managed care delivery systems, utilizers of behavioral health services present significant demand on resources. Fiedler and Wright (1989, p. 147) have described the relationship of mental health visits to medical utilization as a *dose–response conundrum*. Proficient treatment programs are crucial to improving outcome as well as containing cost.

Despite retrospective findings that utilization of mental health services are associated with overall high utilization, there is prospective evidence pointing to an offset in medical cost by the application of behavioral health interventions (Friedman, Sobel, Myers, Caudill, & Benson, 1996; Pallak et al., 1995; Strosahl & Sobel, 1996). Intervention and treatment of members of the population who are symptomatic for mental illness and/or chemical dependency may produce a savings through reduced need for medical care. Specific interventions for high utilizers, evolving under a disease management protocol, have shown improved health, lower utilization, and decreased costs. While outcome research has yet to lay the medical cost-offset question to rest, the current prevailing wisdom is that a cost-offset can be obtained in a correctly designed program. The challenge is to find those best-practices and attempt to generalize their applicability (see chapter 1).

The paradoxical situation exists in which mental health services generally are associated with higher health care costs, but specific mental health interventions may result in a medical cost-offset. Strategies to control the cost of behavioral health services, while simultaneously fostering behavioral medicine interventions for disease management, offer a two-pronged approach to cost control.

THE ECONOMIC EQUATION, P x Q = C

Unit Price × Quantity of Units = Cost: cost of health care hinges around the price of a service unit and the number of service units delivered. In health care there is wide cost variability irrespective of differences in outcome. As a result of the chilling effect of higher costs and the absence of compelling evidence that there was any relationship between rising cost and value, numerous strategies came into being to control cost. The effort had led purchasers of health care to find means to better integrate the financing and delivery of health care. Since the midsixties, there has been a progressive evolution in methods for financing the delivery of health care. The result has been an emergence of continual change in fiscal and structural systems.

Managing *demand* for both hospital days and outpatient visits is one means to control cost. Initial attempts to control demand focused on utilization management techniques. Notions of medical necessity and appropriateness as guidelines to authorize treatment were one means to limit utilization. Managing the cost of *supply* is a parallel development. Progressively complex methods to control supply and demand have been developed. Contracted per diems, discounted fee-for-service, risk-withholds, risk-bands, and capitation are all strategies to control the cost of supply as well as the demand for utilization of services.

For a period of time, purchasers of behavioral health care, both subscribers and HSOs, often found it easier to carve-out the behavioral health benefit from the rest of their health insurance. By engaging a behavioral health managed care organization (BHMCO) willing to assume risk for provision of these services they could fix their cost. Allowing a third party a margin of profit to secure cost by managing demand and charges became good business.

A significant number of excess dollars are present to be recaptured through better management of care and leveraging of the provider systems. Aggressively competitive HSOs, to lower their own bottom-line, are trying to recapture the profits that BHMCOs have enjoyed. Models to lower cost by integrating primary and specialty care through risk-sharing incentives have become more widespread. These approaches are now being applied to behavioral health care as competition becomes more intense and margins for profit shrink.

There has been a progression in the organizational structure of managed care. Pagano (1995) described four stages of developmental maturation in the managed care delivery system. The introduction of the HMO represented the first phase. Increased penetration into the health care market by MCOs followed. A shake-out of marginal players with an extension of risk sharing arrangements characterizes the third stage. The fourth phase involves integration within the health delivery system (HDS). Paralleling this development is an evolution in the system of financing and reimbursement of health care with special emphasis on vertical integration within the delivery system.

These changes have impacted health care delivery generally, but behavioral health care traumatically. The emergence of complex integrated shared risk arrangements are precipitating consolidations and realignments in all aspects of health care delivery. They are a catalyst for integration of behavioral health with primary care, while part of psychotherapy practice may splinter off residing apart from health care.

THE INTEGRATION OF PRIMARY AND BEHAVIORAL HEALTH CARE

The presence of psychiatric conditions is an indicator of increased risk for both medical and psychiatric utilization. Depression is the most frequently diagnosed and highest cost psychiatric condition in commercial health coverage (Table 14.3). By diminishing the deleterious influence of anxiety and depression, either as a primary condition or as a comorbid factor alongside a medical condition, a medical cost-offset may be achievable. Encouraging primary care providers (PCPs) to play a larger role in the provision of behavioral health services while better linking behavioral health support to PCPs in managing difficult patients, is strategically advantageous to cost effectively serving a greater number of patients in need of treatment.

TABLE 14.3
Diagnosis and Cost Associated with Depression in a PPO

Total Number of Enrollees	86,916
% seen by a BHP	6.56%
% Dx of Depression	52.3%
Cost Associated with Depr. Dx	57.2%

Dx of Depression consists of Major Depression, single episode, MD Recurrent, Depression NOS

Primary Care Providers can make a *diagnostic* contribution through early detection. To the extent that these practitioners are willing to intervene through their *prescribing* privilege, they can achieve a further cost-offset. Sturm and Wells (1995) have shown that while there is a cost savings through primary care intervention in treatment for depression, those savings were

associated with poorer outcome. Outcomes, in terms of reduction of functional limitations, were superior when treatment
occurred in a specialty setting. There are a number of efforts
underway to demonstrate that specialty behavioral health providers can support primary care intervention into behavioral
health problems so as to achieve a higher quality outcome while
realizing lower cost (Katon et al., 1995).

On one side, primary care is being invited to play a larger
role in behavioral health care in order to achieve a cost-offset.
This can be considered an inverse medical cost-offset in that
behavioral health costs are being reduced through primary
care intervention. Behavioral health practitioners have a direct
medical cost-offset role to play by assisting PCPs in disease management. What are the incentives for both primary and behavioral health providers to act in concert within some framework
of integration and/or collaboration?

CAPITATION

It is necessary to understand *capitation* in order to understand
the practice patterns of providers within any delivery system.
Capitation is essentially the cost of the health care for an individual within an insured group. The concept is expressed in
terms of the cost per member per month (*pm/pm*). The term
capitation also denotes the prepayment to a provider to cover
possible health care services needed by an individual. These
payments secure the right of a member to receive services by
that practitioner when necessary.

The difference between the cost of health care and the
premium is the medical loss ratio. When the medical loss ratio
is 85%, which is considered a fair rate, then 85% of the premium is going directly to health services. The remainder may
be going to the administrative cost of the insuring entity and
to profit. There is both challenge and opportunity for part of
that profit to be channeled to providers as an incentive to better control costs.

Table 14.4 delineates elements in the global capitation for
a hypothetical health plan. Within the capitation of $134.55

TABLE 14.4
Capitation

Global Capitation		Behavioral Health Capitation	
Premium	$140	Hospital/	
Hosp	$ 39.10	Psych	$1.45
Hosp/Outpat	$ 22.50	Chem Dep	$ .35
Med/Surg	$ 48.20	Partial Hosp	$ .90
Prescrip	$ 12.50	Outpatient	$1.80
Adm	$ 12.25	Total	$4.50
Total	$134.55	[$4.50 present within $109.80]	
Income	$ 5.45		

pm/pm, a percentage is allocated for hospital service, primary care, specialty care, etc. Patients, in a given period, may utilize more or fewer resources than were budgeted to that component of service. More hospital days may have been used than projected or the number of patients requiring expensive tests might have increased beyond the expected level. On average the determined amounts should balance, so that expenses are equal to or less than the premiums collected.

In the above example, a profit of $5.45 pm/pm accrued. The health related cost of $109.80 pm/pm is a competitively low capitation for many parts of the country. This overall amount, $134.55, contains a medical loss ratio of 81.6%. The remainder represents administrative costs and profit. Milliman and Robertson, an actuarial company, publish capitation rates for regions of the country. The American Psychiatric Association (Melek & Pyenson, 1995) has published capitation tables developed by Milliman and Robertson specifically for behavioral health.

Table 14.4 also delineates the breakdown of capitated costs for behavioral health. The $4.50 pm/pm allocated to behavioral health is separated into outpatient care, inpatient care, and partial hospital costs. These behavioral health costs are contained in the hospital, outpatient, and medical–surgical parts of the global capitation. In this example, behavioral health constitutes 4.1% of the clinical budget. Actual capitation rates for behavioral health vary for specific populations and depend on geographic area, state laws pertaining to mandated benefits, and customary practice in local communities.

MANAGEMENT MODELS OF HEALTH SERVICE DELIVERY SYSTEMS

Capitating a group of providers for provision of services is one mechanism for both sharing risk as well as providing incentives to those practitioners to better manage the care they were providing. The most common group to be capitated were PCPs. But, capitation is not limited to PCPs. In a mixed model some specialists will receive fee-for-service (FFS), while others such as podiatry or chiropractic might be capitated along with the PCP. The capitation could be global, limited, or soft.

The global capitation is the total medical cost. The PCP can be capitated for all health services. Any referrals are charged against the PCPs' capitation placing them at total risk for the ambulatory and hospital health costs of the patient. Capitating the PCP for all services needed by the patient creates a strong incentive for the PCP to monitor that care scrupulously. Alternatively, the capitation might be limited and only for a specific specialty or arena of care. The PCP might be capitated solely for ambulatory services, freeing the PCP from risk for hospital charges. Some states by law limit the degree of risk a practitioner can assume.

When a practitioner is capitated, FFS charges are still calculated. In a soft capitation arrangement the provider receives FFS payment. The capitation is a target, not a reimbursement. If the capitation is not realized then the following year they may face a lower fee schedule, especially if the partial withholding of payments was not sufficient to offset the difference. In a hard capitation the practitioners are totally at risk. Sometimes, BHPs have a similar capitated arrangement.

Capitation needs to be understood in context to the organizational model it supports. Three basic models characterize HDS organization: indemnity/fee-for-service, health maintenance organizations, and preferred provider organizations. The effect of capitation is different in each of these organizations as is the nature of reimbursement and the relationship among clinical providers. The structural model of the HDS contains incentives for reimbursement that affect collaboration between different specialty providers.

Indemnity health insurance emerged from World War II as the dominant form of health coverage offering substantial reimbursement for FFS charges. It required two decades and a shift in federal legislation for the HMO to begin to rival indemnity insurance. It took only one decade for the success of the HMO to give impetus for the PPO to significantly compete with the HMO. Recently, variations of PPOs such as large primary care groups and physician–hospital organizations (PHO) have become highly aggressive competitive entities for market share. Both indemnity health insurance and HMOs have lost significant market share.

Table 14.5 presents aspects of four forms of health care organization, including the impact of capitation, the nature of reimbursement, and the organization of providers. PPOs are separated into two categories, one characterized as traditional and the other advanced. The advanced PPOs are a more recent development in which capitation and risk-sharing arrangements are integrated through both *vertical* and *horizontal* components of the HDS. Horizontal integration is used to describe links within a continuum of care in a single specialty. Vertical integration describes the linking of care across specialties, joining PCPs to specialists in a continuum of services and incentives.

TABLE 14.5
Dynamics within Four Health Delivery Systems

	Indemnity	HMO	PPO Trad.	PPO Advanced
Effect of Cap	None	Global	Mixed	Specific
Reimbursement	FFS	Fixed/Salary	Disc. FFS	Contingent
Deliv. Sys.	Independent	Collaborative	Competitive	Integrated

FEE FOR SERVICE

In a fee-for-service (FFS) system professionals practice independently from one another. The individual clinician is reimbursed for clinical services. Reimbursement is maximized by providing as many services as possible irrespective of the number of recipients. Most clinicians try to provide what they believe to be optimal service to the individual. The cost consequence of referral or varying styles of practice falls entirely on the purchasers and payors of health care. The risk imposed by capitation impacts on the insuring entity in FFS practice.

Within the fee-for-service/indemnity model the relationship between primary and specialty care is neutral. There are no financial consequences to the practitioner that are a direct consequence of collaboration. The boundaries of practice are solely the result of the prerogatives of the practitioner. Most primary care physicians have little affinity or interest in addressing mental health or substance abuse problems. Psychiatry and psychology traditionally practiced relatively independently from primary care referral. Within this system collaboration was weak and sporadic. A patient with emotional difficulty might consult with a primary care physician or might choose to contact a mental health specialist directly. Generally, medical and behavioral health practitioners had minimal involvement with one another. A few more innovative medical practitioners included a psychologist or social worker within their suite of offices.

Although a pattern of prescribing psychoactive medications for their patients developed, primary care physicians often failed to make diagnoses of depression, anxiety, and/or substance abuse and, when doing so, they underprescribed or excessively utilized benzodiazepines (Sturm & Wells, 1995). Conversely, many individuals seeking out some form of mental or substance abuse care did so without the awareness of their primary care doctor.

THE HEALTH MAINTENANCE ORGANIZATION

The HMO is an integrated health system providing comprehensive health care services, usually in a center that houses multispecialty practice. Typically out-of-pocket expenses, copayments, or deductibles are either low or nonexistent for HMO members. They are usually held harmless for authorized out-of-network services. The HMO promotes access to services to support health and promote early intervention.

Capitation affects the practice as a whole. The HMO setting facilitated collaboration between primary and specialty care. Primary care providers are salaried and do not receive a fee for the services that they provide. Specialists are either salaried or contracted and are not fee dependent for reimbursement. As a result, there is no incentive to provide unneeded services. The relationship within the HMO among providers is collaborative and the financial incentives all operate at a collective group level. There is a philosophy of care that emphasizes serving a population of individuals in a clinically and financially responsible manner.

Since providers receive fixed payment, their particular practice style affects the group as a whole but not themselves as individuals. As a result the incentives for the individual practitioner are weak. If a primary care provider refers a patient to a mental health provider, as opposed to managing the care directly, there is no direct financial consequence to the provider. Referral of behavioral health problems is facilitated by the practice setting of a multispecialty service center. The percentage of patients seen by behavioral service departments within HMOs, compared to FFS, is often as high as 8+% rather than the 5 to 6% in FFS. Like their medical colleagues with no direct incentives, HMO behavioral health clinicians often complain that referral rates relative to staffing levels are high and patient expectations outstrip resources.

Through an integrated management approach HMOs try to shape provider practice patterns. Even when HMO managers championed participation of primary care in behavioral health care, that emphasis was often not shared by providers. The PCPs were free to determine the boundaries of their practice comfort. The HMO practitioners believed that they had traded somewhat lower earning levels for the freedom to practice in a manner consistent with their own values. The cost of this freedom impacted on the organizational bottom line and not on the PCP.

THE PPO

The PPO became a more widespread phenomenon in the last decade serving as an alternative to both the HMO and FFS coverage. Initially PPOs were arrangements by which reduced numbers of providers were promised higher rates of referral for discounted fees. These providers contracted with an HSO directly or as members of an independent practice association (IPA). Similar to indemnity health plans, it offered members a choice of practitioners with some of the additional financial advantages of an HMO. Indemnity carriers could easily utilize a PPO arrangement to better control costs in the bid to dominate market share. Not all PPOs are derivatives of indemnity insurance companies. Some have developed from primary care networks and others from hospital networks.

Preferred provider organizations were less expensive to establish and more economical to maintain. Unlike the HMO that set up a medical center and hired staff, the PPO had modest start-up costs. The providers maintained their own offices and were affiliated by contractual agreement. In areas where membership had low density there was no problem of maintaining costly, low utilized sites. Most HMOs today have moved to mixed models utilizing PPO arrangements in expansion areas.

Carve-outs were often a common strategy alongside a PPO arrangement. Large corporations, finding that their behavioral health costs were escalating, carved-out behavioral health directly to a behavioral health company while contracting independently for their medical coverage. Even within the PPO there was a disinclination for PCPs to play an active role in relating to the emotional problems of patients or attempting to contain the cost of behavioral health care. Unlike medical–surgical specialties, it was more common to carve-out behavioral health. This was made easier by the fact that often within IPAs medical practitioners felt little loyalty to psychiatric colleagues. Large behavioral health managed care companies came to control a significant market share.

In a capitated carve-out arrangement the costs of behavioral health become independent from the rest of the medical capitation. As a result of cost-shifting incentives there are inherent conflicts that discourage a joint approach to patient management. When the PCP provides a behavioral health service in a nonintegrated capitated arrangement they assume the cost by providing a service for which the BHP received a capitated payment. There is a disinclination on the part of the BHPs to become involved with primary care as any increase in referrals from the PCP will not increase reimbursement. Not incidental in these offsets is the effect of referral on practitioner time and workload. Additional referrals mean more work without additional payment. Separate risk pools tend to have similar effects.

Table 14.5 distinguishes two types of PPOs in which the effect of capitation is different for each. In the first the impact of capitation is mixed. The limited and soft capitations that typify this type of PPO do not support a consistent PCP relationship with BHPs. Referral itself is a hand-off, sometimes referred to as "patient dumping," rather than a mutual endeavor.

The older traditional PPO is organized within specialties with the PCP serving as a source of referral. The PCP serves as a gatekeeper for referral, authorizing clinical services received by the patients. Reimbursement and incentives are largely FFS with a *risk withhold,* serving as an incentive to the practitioner to play a greater role in cost containment. The withhold is a percentage of fees placed into a *risk pool* to be returned contingent upon capitation targets being achieved. Withholds are typically 10 to 20% of the reimbursed fee and are returned based on performance of the specialty. A limited capitation, when present, is usually only for the PCP. Behavioral health providers, like most specialties, receive FFS. Within more aggressive PPOs, sometimes called exclusive provider organizations (EPOs), primary care and other providers have additional incentives to control specialty and hospital costs.

REIMBURSEMENT AND INCENTIVES

The driving vision for the health care system is to provide quality care, be responsive to individual needs, and maintain the health of the population, all at reasonable cost. The pressure has been to develop incentive systems that give the practitioner an interest in practicing both effectively and efficiently. Integrated systems in which a common capitation is present facilitates actualizing those goals.

The global effect of capitation in HMOs provided no direct rewards to the practitioner for quality practice. The move to nonintegrated systems separated the specific challenge for behavioral health from the broader challenges of health care. Specialty companies were able to better compete, often at significant profit, to provide this care. However, carve-outs stifle incentive to expand the range of practice. Providers who are locked into FFS at modest reimbursement rates and are micromanaged will have no motivation to innovate. The presence of significant profit resulted in the system's gaining efficiency by channeling incentives to the practitioner, and could thus compete against a nonintegrated system.

INCENTIVES, HORIZONTAL INTEGRATION

In the newer advanced PPOs capitation plays its most innovative and complex role. Providers have assumed direct risk-sharing with reimbursement incentives for successful cost management. The assignment of capitation and the role of risk withholds is critical to understanding the incentives and disincentives that underlie the relationship of network providers.

The risk-withhold (Table 14.6) is a negative means for creating practitioner incentive. A risk-withhold can be present for any type of provider. A portion of reimbursement is withheld flowing into a risk pool and returned if the capitation targets are met. When the risk pools are separate for each specialty the return of withhold is solely a function of the performance of that specialty. The second type of PPO, which is a newer development, is vertically integrated in that the risk pools associated with hospital, specialties, and primary care are all linked. This encourages PCP involvement as well as giving specialists

TABLE 14.6
Withhold Return to Providers Anchored in Capitation

Ret	360	240	120	528	408	288	168	48	0
Cap	4.20	4.30	4.40	4.50	4.60	4.70	4.80	4.90	4.94

Based on $4.50 capitation, $2.20 pm/pm ambulatory capitation, 20% withhold on FFS. Return in units of K.

an incentive to contain their own costs by diverting treatment from hospitals when possible. The cost-withhold can be anchored within pm/pm costs so that the amount returned is dependent on the degree to which the capitation is met.

In a traditional PPO withhold, BHPs are not at risk for the hospital cost. The BHP receives return of a percentage of the withhold based on the practitioner's contribution to the pool of funds. Table 14.6 presents a model for return of withhold in which the practitioner is partially at risk for hospital expenses. The withhold is anchored in the global $4.50 pm/pm captitation not the $2.20 outpatient portion. The withhold may be used to offset hospital charges if the total capitation exceeds the capitated target. The providers may profit if the combined hospital and outpatient utilization is less than the capitated target. By linking ambulatory and hospital performance the BHPs can exceed their outpatient capitation and still receive a return by holding down the hospital expenses. This form of risk integration creates outpatient practitioner incentive to control utilization of total resources.

If ambulatory care for 100,000 enrollees generates fees equaling the full capitation of $2.20 pm/pm, then $528,000 will have been collected into the risk pool [$2.20 × 100,000 × 12 (months) × 20% (withhold) = $528,000]. If actual costs come to $5,928 or $4.94 pm/pm, then no withhold would be returned. The practitioners will have funded that degree of loss. Any costs less than $4.94 will produce a return. A full refund of $528,000 will occur when costs are $4.50 pm/pm.

Further incentive can be created by a positive anchoring of the withhold in the captitation as well. If the total cost is under $4.50 pm/pm then the providers will receive a return not only of withhold but of the difference to $4.50. At $4.40 pm/pm there is an additional $120,000 to be shared by the providers in the delivery system. Most MCOs permitting an incentive would actually share or split the incentive return through a risk-band. In a soft capitation where the pm/pm is a target and not a reimbursement, the providers receive FFS and would not necessarily share in the profit.

Fee-for-service systems generally reward inefficiency since the reimbursement is based solely on visits. When FFS is the main method of reimbursement, many practitioners accept the withhold as a cost of business and do not expect to get it back. They are also aware that their efficiency may not be matched by colleagues. Conversely, if their colleagues do well and they practice inefficiently they will profit further. Incentive strategies have been devised to offset this inequity. Withhold may be returned based on number of patients seen, not sessions held. Unfortunately, this may induce a practitioner to increase the number of patients seen by underserving or avoiding problematic patients.

A further variation is to develop a *report card* so that return on the withhold or incentives follows an econometric model predicated on quality guidelines for an individual practice. There can be additional return for an exceptional number of patients seen, average length of care based on severity of diagnosis, management of highly vulnerable patients, patient satisfaction, etc. This may redress the tendency to disregard the withhold or to avoid clinically complex cases in order to see more patients.

Rather than have a capitated provider group totally at risk, a risk-band might be negotiated with the HSO. In this risk-band, Table 14.7, the behavioral health providers are totally at risk for 5% of charges above and below the $4.50 pm/pm capitation. This means that if they exceed the capitation rate of $4.50 by 5%, then they will be responsible for those costs up

TABLE 14.7
Shared Risk-Band on Capitation

50%	25%	+ 0	25%	50%	
4.0	4.05	4.275	4.50	4.775	4.95	5.00

±5% band on capitation of $4.50 pm/pm with 25 to 50% risk share.

to $4.725 pm/pm. If they better the capitation rate by as much as 5%, they will receive the full difference between $4.50 and $4.275. Beyond 5% of the capitation, the purchaser of the service will receive or contribute 25% of the profit or loss. At 10% beyond the capitation rate, there is a risk sharing of 50%.

A simpler model would be a 50/50 split between the HSO and the provider group at above or below 5%. These compensation strategies reduce the risk to the provider of an occasional adverse occurrence and create an incentive for bettering the capitation rate. It reduces incentive to under provide services by sharing unexpected gains with the insuring partner, the HSO. Risk bands can be applied differently depending upon the context. Sometimes, it may be advantageous to have a direct 50/50 split on both sides of the capitation. There may be reason to change the median point of the risk-band annually.

These types of risks can only be assumed by BHPs organized within a group. Individual practitioners would be financially incapable of sustaining this degree of risk or offering the necessary level of services. These types of risk arrangements are strongly influencing the reorganization of delivery systems into networks of group practices.

VERTICAL INTEGRATION

In the risk return model, Table 14.7, the BHP was linked with hospital performance. Both BHP and hospital are part of the behavioral health network of services. This is a type of horizontal integration. When PCPs share risk with BHPs, the care is being vertically integrated. The PCP receives incentives based on financial results from specialty and hospital performance.

Figure 14.1 outlines an integrated risk sharing system with behavioral health. Placing the PCP at risk for the performance of BHPs is still not widespread. In this relationship the PCP is capitated for primary care. A specialty provider, in this case behavioral health, is capitated for that area of service. But, the PCP is placed at risk for the specialty's succeeding in meeting the capitation rate. If the specialty exceeds the rate, then the

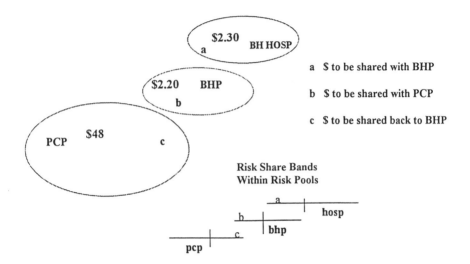

Figure 14.1. Vertical integrated risk share bands inside risk pool.

PCP shares in the vulnerability. If the specialty provider has lower than projected costs, then the PCP shares in the return. This provides the PCP with an incentive to offer care and not generate a referral since specialty care is typically more expensive than PCP care.

Similarly, the BHP is provided with a return if there are savings on the hospital capitation. This type of risk model creates incentives to provide care at lower cost and at the least intensive level. Conversely, failures in treatment that lead to higher costs work against the interest of providers. So there is compelling reason to refer early and whenever the patient's condition appears to be problematic. This model of placing PCP, specialty provider and hospital into an integrated linkage is present in PHO arrangements and is increasingly frequent in what has been termed the advanced PPO. In a PHO network the hospital is able to join the sharing of profit resulting from reduced utilization of hospital resources by its associated providers.

Those models that offer maximum incentives to the PCP to play a significant role both in practice and oversight have proved to be most cost efficacious. By linking hospital utilization with provider reimbursement in the continuum of care, an integrated service system matches utilization of resources with appropriate incentives.

Health maintenance organizations in fear for their own survival have begun placing providers at risk by taking a risk-withhold from salary and establishing risk-bands around capitation for return of the withheld salary. The risk-band serves as a further incentive for the realization of higher earnings. Usually there would be a 50/50 split in the risk-band. Poor performance, however, might result in lower salary levels or increased withhold the following year.

In summary, the combination of cost-withhold, anchored in the specialty capitation, linked within the continuum of care, supported through risk bands, and returned as an incentive to the provider based on report card profiling of practice, all represent a powerful set of tools to reward best practices and quality care.

MEDICAL COST OFFSET AND INCENTIVES

The description of cost-offsets and incentives have been discussed largely in the context of primary care participation with behavioral health treatment. There are significant numbers of patients who have primary medical diagnoses where psychological aspects may be impeding outcome. Gaining BHP collaboration with PCP treatment is clinically and financially advantageous.

When behavioral health interventions may lower general medical costs, the challenge is to provide incentives for that care to occur and to share those gains equitably. Melek (1996) has described two mechanisms, an aggregate and specific approach for BHPs to have an incentive return from medical cost-offsets. In the aggregate approach a fixed percentage that can accrue through behavioral health intervention is agreed upon. The BHP is at risk for that percentage and will profit when it is realized. Unfortunately, this approach of a fixed reduction in overall medical utilization occurring through behavioral health intervention is speculative and difficult to operationalize. In the specific approach, targets are set in the management of a specific disease entity. When these cost savings are achieved they are shared with the behavioral health providers.

While not tied specifically to capitation, this model of disease management is a current demonstration project between Blue Cross Blue Shield of Massachusetts and the American Psychological Association (Newman, 1996). The project is attempting to demonstrate specific cost savings by providing a psychoeducational program to women treated for breast cancer. These cost savings are related to lower medical costs brought about by reduced relapse resulting from more effective physician–patient engagement and a possible strengthening of the immune system through improved psychological adjustment. Through projections of decreased service utilization, specific cost savings are predicted which provide targets for evaluation of outcome.

Figure 14.1 shows vertical reciprocal risk-bands between the PCP and BHP. This reciprocity allows the PCP to share projected returns of behavioral health ambulatory and hospital costs that exceed rate targets. It allows the BHP to mutually share in medical cost offsets realized through behavioral health intervention. This type of vertical reciprocal integration is an ideal, first being developed for practice application.

OTHER SOLUTIONS

Despite the advantages of integrated service delivery within a global capitation, nonintegrated systems will continue to flourish. BHMCOs for numerous reasons, including the passage of parity legislation, will continue to be competitive. Within PPOs, and their PHO variant, behavioral health providers organized within a large group network often find themselves with a carve-out capitation separate from the medical capitation. Alternative solutions that facilitate cooperation between PCPs and BHPs become necessary.

The capitation calculations are derived within a specialty from the costs associated with clinical procedure codes and per diems, related to diagnoses. When a PCP diagnoses depression, and provides medication, the associated costs are not typically part of the behavioral health capitation. In a nonintegrated system, to the extent that new or additional problem patients are referred to BHPs, a cost shifting occurs which is not part of the original estimates. Conversely, increased consultation–liaison activities have no attendant reimbursement.

Considerable goodwill and cooperation need to occur so that patients will not be disadvantaged by the split in capitation. One mechanism is for the HSO to leave corridors present for cost sharing apart from risk sharing. Creating this corridor involves an enlightened attitude by both primary care and the purchaser, but it is ultimately to everyone's advantage. For example, a PCP who is managing a difficult chronic pain patient would benefit from a consultation with a BHP. A DSM-IV diagnostic code of 316, *psychological factors affecting a medical condition*, retains the case within the medical arena. A BHP can render a service that will not be charged against his or her own capitation. The fee generated will be assigned to primary care.

A number of diagnoses when associated with specific evaluation and management (E&M), codes can be designated to reside within primary care even though treatment is provided by a BHP. To the extent that office visits are reduced, the capitated PCP will gain and the BHP will have access to bill for services within the funding of the medical capitation.

Another method would be for the HSO to create contingency funds which can be drawn upon apart from any specific capitation. These funds might be accessed through case management when certain guidelines are met. Contingency funding is another mechanism to finance behavioral medicine programs that reside within no specific capitation but represent potential cost-offset health savings.

There are advantages within horizontal integration that are lost in vertical integration. There may be too much pressure for cost containment in vertical integration of risk-pools. Maximum pressure on the PCP to control utilization may simply make the practice of medicine intolerable. With independent risk-pools, each specialty has the opportunity to negotiate its boundaries, thus establishing practice guidelines for care within each specialty and with referral criteria. At one meeting a primary care physician mused, "Pay us fee-for-service and capitate everyone else and we will show you what can really be done."

The near future will present multiple challenges. Each attempt to enhance incentives comes with its own built-in problems, most specifically the tendency to undertreat and to avoid the complex patient. Medication should not be an intervention of choice replacing psychotherapy simply to lower utilization of labor intensive practitioner resources.

Despite elegant incentive designs, the reality of current clinical practice is a confusing amalgam. Practitioners are credentialed with numerous purchasing networks. A PHO formed by a single hospital network may still be participating with numerous HSOs and be involved in differing products. These may include FFS, capitation, an integrated Medicaid program, and a nonintegrated Medicare program. Providers within this single delivery system may not know each other. They may not know the basis for reimbursement of the patient in their office since billing and reimbursements may be handled by a management services organization (MSO).

These fiscal intricacies all need to be worked through by the HSO to minimize underservice of patients in jeopardy. The HSO must foster practitioner "buy in" so that prospective incentive systems do not become an unduly demoralizing influence on clinical practice. Nonetheless, within the chaos there is emerging a new dynamic organization for health care. Lowering practice barriers to encourage the integration of behavioral health and primary care fosters a more responsive patient focused health system to meet the needs of the greater good.

SUMMARY

The financing and organization of health care has been evolving toward more complex delivery and risk-sharing systems. A health system is optimal that encourages primary care providers to recognize behavioral health problems, to intervene within their competence, and to refer when service from a behavioral health specialist is warranted. In order for that to occur, there must be fiscal ability for behavioral health providers to collaboratively participate with primary care providers in treating behavioral and health related conditions. Managed care systems that have joint incentives and integrated risk-sharing models best facilitate this collaboration. The HSO must provide the leadership to foster linkages that support team work within the health delivery system.

PART V

The Behavioral Health Practitioner

15.

Collaboration in Action: Key Strategies for Behavioral Health Providers

**William B. Gunn, Jr., Ph.D., David Seaburn, M.S.,
Alan Lorenz, M.D., Barbara Gawinski, Ph.D.,
Larry B. Mauksch, M.Ed.**

Primary care medical practices vary widely from small, two-provider offices which operate independently to large multispecialty clinics which house a separate primary care division. Typically primary care medical specialties include physicians from specialties in family medicine, general internal medicine, pediatrics, and less often obstetrics/gynecology. Other health care providers, including physician assistants and nurse practitioners, also provide medical care in these settings. Nurses and office staff support these providers and ancillary services such as laboratory and x-ray are often part of the practice. Typically, behavioral health services are not an integrated part of these medical practices. Outside referrals to mental health as well as to other medical specialties are made routinely.

Most behavioral health practitioners receive little training or have no experience working directly in a primary care medical setting. Body and mind have been divided since the days of Descartes and most behavioral practice occurs in designated mental health settings or, if in a medical world, is established in specialty settings such as hospice, pain units, or rehabilitation programs.

This chapter will describe efforts to integrate medical and behavioral services in ways that the providers can practice more collaboratively. Best practices in integration or in collaboration with primary care will be described and examples will be given. The terms *integration* and *collaboration* will be used interchangeably. The chapter will address the *cognitive set, knowledge,* and *strategies* needed to collaborate with medical providers. It will be useful to behavioral health providers who wish to work in a primary care medicine context and for those already in these settings who wish to increase their effectiveness.

COGNITIVE SET

This section has been labeled *cognitive set.* It could also be called a *frame, belief system, paradigm,* or just plain *attitude.* The importance of considering a client's or patient's belief system during assessment and treatment is well known. It is one of the most critical elements in predicting change in treatment and has been the direct target of cognitive psychologists. The cognitive set of the practitioner is also important, especially in working with health care practitioners. The authors have learned in developing workshops which teach collaborative strategies to behavioral health providers, that these must include an experiential portion early in the workshop that is focused on flushing out the experiences and beliefs the providers have about physicians. Some of these beliefs are well entrenched. For example, a psychologist in one workshop described an abrupt manner in which a physician told her family of a death. This experience had led the psychologist to generalize to all physicians, rendering her less effective in collaboration. A social worker felt strongly that physicians as a group looked down on mental health providers and that he needed to constantly defend his position. This defense often resulted in confrontation between himself and the medical providers. Both these providers were able to discuss the issues which contributed to their belief system and adopt some different attitudes which led to more productive interactions.

This section will describe three tenets which are part of the thinking necessary for practitioners to be successful in working in integrated systems (Seaburn, Lorenz, Gunn, Gawinski, & Mauksch, 1996): (1) an integrative paradigm regarding health and mental health problems; (2) an ecological perspective on the interaction among professionals who collaborate; and (3) the treatment of patients and families as partners in care.

An Integrative Paradigm

During the 1950s and 1960s medicine made great strides in using technology and new medications to treat a variety of illnesses. One side effect of this advancement was to focus on the biological to the exclusion of the psychological or social etiology or consequences of illnesses. G. E. Engel (1993) developed the biopsychosocial model as an antidote to what he perceived as these reductionistic tendencies in medicine. This model connects the biological, psychological, interpersonal, and social factors as a larger framework of multiple systems interacting with each other.

The relationship among these systems is continuous and reciprocal. A patient who has diabetes must not only be evaluated in terms of blood sugar levels but also in terms of personal and interpersonal stress. In the same vein, a patient who comes into a mental health setting complaining of fatigue needs to be evaluated for hypothyroidism as well as depression or stress. The biopsychosocial model is a common approach for training health care professionals, particularly family physicians (Doherty & Baird, 1983; McDaniel et al., 1990). This approach is not as common in traditional mental health training programs.

The biopsychosocial model and systems theory enable both the health and mental health providers to conceptualize problems in an integrative manner. Such a dynamic model can stimulate dialogue and encourage providers to work together when looking for the complex connections and most potent leverage points for effective treatment. In addition, such cross-fertilization helps each professional understand the illness and disease experience of patients and families in a more complete way.

An Ecological Perspective

A second important way of thinking is to view patients, families, and problems in a truly ecological way. This is different from an interdisciplinary approach. Auerswald (1968), in distinguishing between these two related ideas, describes an interdisciplinary approach as one in which each profession presents its case for the etiology and treatment of a particular problem. While sometimes useful, this approach can become a competition about who can present the most articulate argument for his or her point of view, seeking to convert the most people to that way of thinking. In an ecological approach on the other hand, professionals are more interested in the process of the conversation and in hearing and learning from the perspective of others than in defending a position. In this approach the goal is for all involved to have a clearer vision of the problems and solutions through productive dialogue.

An ecological approach is to professional interaction what the biopsychosocial model is to illness. The biopsychosocial model focuses on the interface of professional disciplines with varying degrees of expertise in the treatment of illness. The ecological approach reminds us that the content of that expertise, while very important, is not more important than the capacity to "give and take" that expertise across disciplines.

Partners in Care

The third part of the cognitive set is a consistent orientation to include the patient and the family as active partners in the process. While building a relationship among providers is necessary for collaboration to be maximally effective, it is not sufficient without attention to the inclusion of the patient and family. Because patients as well as families experience the illness or disease, and since they often create their own best solutions, it is essential they be included in partnership. Kleinman (1988) suggests that patients and families be seen as "colleagues" and that the act of training patients and families as caregivers is a message of empowerment that is of symbolic and practical significance.

One trend in psychotherapy which parallels this tenet is the current focus on encouraging family strength and competence (Sprenkle & Bischof, 1994). Successful therapy depends as much on the resources of the patient and family as it does on the resources of the therapist (Karpel, 1986). Utilization of family strengths and resources is common in many approaches to family therapy, including solution-focused therapy (DeShazer, 1982), competency-centered therapy (Waters & Lawrence, 1992), narrative therapy (White & Epston, 1990), and family therapy of children and adolescents (Combrinck-Graham, 1990).

These three tenets make up the collaborative cognitive set. How behavioral health providers think about physicians and the medical system is critical in influencing the development of collaborative actions. Without a conceptual orientation toward collaboration, it will be difficult to apply the knowledge and develop the strategies necessary for the provider to integrate successfully so that the system of providers, including the patient-family, is much greater than the sum of its parts.

KNOWLEDGE

This section includes six different areas in which the behavioral health provider should be knowledgeable. The first area is background information on what is known about *types of patients, problems, and approaches* typically seen in primary care settings. The remaining five areas cover critical categories to consider in planning integrated efforts. They are *relationship building, developing common purpose, communication, financial arrangement, and location of service.* These five areas are included in the "key ingredients to effective collaboration," and are more fully described in *Models of Collaboration: A Guide for Mental Health Professionals Working with Health Care Practitioners* (Seaburn, Lorenz, Gunn, Gawinski, & Mauksch, 1996).

Patients, Problems, and Approaches in Primary Care

In a recent analysis of the 1978 Epidemiologic Catchment Area (ECA) study in the United States as a whole, mental and addictive disorders have a 6-month prevalence rate of 16% (Regier, Goldberg, & Taube, 1978; Regier, Narrow, Rae, Manderscheid, Locke, & Goodwin, 1993). However, for primary care patients who use medical services frequently (at least once in 6 months), mental and addictive disorders have a 6-month prevalence rate of 21.7% (Kessler, Cleary, & Burke, 1985). The high prevalence of mental disorders in primary care patients has been confirmed in studies of primary care populations, and thus mental and addictive disorders are more frequent in primary care settings than in the community as a whole.

One important subgroup of this population is the "distressed high utilizers" of medical care. The top 10% of medical users of health care are more likely than low or nonusers to have a psychiatric diagnosis (Katon et al., 1990), account for one-third of outpatient resources, and for half of inpatient resources. One-half of these high utilizers have mental health problems (Katon et al., 1990) and complex issues which are difficult to resolve. The term *distressed high utilizer* suggests that only the patients are distressed and that they are solely responsible for their high utilization. Providers, particularly those who feel solely responsible for "fixing things," may also be distressed. It may be more appropriate to refer to the situation by the term *overserviced-underserved* to better reflect the reality that all those involved are failing to find an effective way to meet the patient's needs.

In describing the demographics of primary care patients, Miranda, Hohmann, Attkisson, and Larson (1994) have determined that they are often more complicated than those seen in a mental health context. They are generally older, poorer, and nonwhite. They tend to be more resistant to a mental health diagnosis and treatment, and are more likely to drop out of treatment, whether this be prescribed medication or counseling. The majority of primary care patients with mental health disorders present physical symptoms rather than psychological symptoms. In addition these patients often have multiple, chronic physical and mental health disorders (Miranda et al., 1994). These differences should be taken into consideration in designing the structures of primary behavioral health care. Given the dynamics described, a collaborative approach is a reasonable alternative, providing cost effective and quality care.

One of the most prevalent problems in primary care is somatization. Patients with multiple physical complaints and no apparent physical disorders utilize up to 9 times the usual amount of medical care. These patients challenge the mind–body dichotomy that exists in our health care system. Physicians cannot easily refer these patients for psychological consultation because of the stigma attached and the fear that the patients would see such a referral as a dismissal of their concerns. Physicians themselves often report feeling frustrated and incompetent in providing adequate care. Behavioral health providers not working in a medical context will rarely see these patients and, if they do, they run the risk of downplaying the biomedical component of the patient's distress. Collaboration between medical providers and mental health professionals is essential for the adequate care of somatizing patients.

Smith (Smith, Monson & Ray, 1986; Smith, Rost & Kashner, 1995) at the University of Arkansas conducted two well-designed research studies using the integration of a single psychiatric consultation to primary care physicians for patients who display a moderate level of somatization. The intervention was a letter delivered to the physician making recommendations about limiting unnecessary testing procedures and conducting regularly scheduled outpatient visits. In both studies they showed significantly lowered utilization of inpatient and ancillary services with this population. Even though the results of this study are encouraging, the sample sizes were small and replications with larger populations need to be conducted.

Knowledge of the patient demographics and problems seen in primary care medical contexts is critical to understanding similarities and differences in a specialty mental health setting. Following are five key areas to address when integrating services.

Relationship: The Basis for Trust and Mutual Respect

The most important ingredient to effective integration is the overt emphasis placed on building relationships among providers. This is equal to the importance of building relationships with patients. A shared location (i.e., office space) cannot overcome a lack of attention to building a relationship. As with any new relationship, initial attention is given to building mutual respect by getting to know each other. By discussing ideas regarding etiology and change in various situations, mutual respect continues to build. Evidence of a strong professional relationship communicates to patients and families that there is a "treatment team" working with them.

There are rewards for working closely with the same group of providers over time. In Roanoke, Virginia, psychologist Susan Molumphy has worked in close proximity to Brambleton Family Physicians for 20 years. Molumphy and Wayne Grayson, a physician, have a particularly close collaborative relationship. They share a waiting room, which allows patients to come to a familiar setting and "blend into the crowd." Grayson and Molumphy describe their personal relationship as equally essential to effective collaboration. According to Grayson:

> We were just close. You need someone to trust that can counsel your patients through a tough time that you just can't do. I think family practitioners who have not cultivated a therapist they can

work with are not being all they can be or doing all they can to help their patients get well (Personal Communication, 1996).

Adds Molumphy:

> You learn to trust the fact that we are in this together. I can't practice medicine, but over the years you share so many patients together, you trust the physician's and your own intuition about who will need medicine. I can even make a recommendation about what medicine will be needed. Wayne trusts me to do that (Personal Communication, 1996).

Common Purpose: "Getting on the Same Page"

The central purpose of health care delivery is to effectively manage and treat each patient's concerns and to promote health in all members of the community. Whether it is called a "shared vision" or "mission" or "purpose," it is critical to clarify in general terms and in each specific clinical example the expected outcomes of patients, families, and providers. Making explicit the specific short-term goals of each party augments effective progress toward those goals. This strategy can be very helpful if conflict arises. It would be unrealistic to expect all parties to have identical goals. When the different goals appear to be the source of conflict, a review of the goals can help to resolve the conflict.

> A 65-year-old Hispanic woman lives alone in an apartment in the inner city. She sees her family physician on a regular basis to discuss her hypertension, which is currently managed with a combination of diet and medication. The patient has a tremendous amount of fear and anxiety regarding her medical condition, and she expresses concerns about her four children, each of whom is in significant distress psychologically or socially.
>
> The physician referred the patient to a psychologist who worked at the medical clinic. Although the patient was reluctant to see him at first, she agreed because he was in the same clinic. The physician assured her she was not going to see the patient less. She only wanted the psychologist's opinion as to the best way to manage the fears and anxiety. It was important at the outset to

clarify the differing goals. The physician wanted the patient to stay compliant with antihypertensive medication and become less anxious. The patient only wanted reassurance that she was not having a heart attack. The psychologist was interested in the patient's being able to connect her physical symptoms with the tremendous amount of psychosocial stress she was experiencing, and to use relaxation and cognitive strategies to provide relief. In a meeting with all three, these differing goals were stated and described.

The idea of developing a common purpose is a deceptively simple one. In the medical context it is not a question that is routinely addressed even though assumptions are made about what the expected outcome should be from a given intervention or encounter. Making these purposes explicit can be of great help.

Communication: How? What? When? Where?

Clear, concise, direct communication is essential for effective collaboration, especially in the early stages of the process. The cultures of mental health and health care can be quite different. It is often tempting to try to force the other culture to adopt certain forms of communication. However, this is rarely successful. Mental health and health care providers need to understand and respect each profession's unique rules for norms of communication. The same is true for communicating with patients and families.

Confidentiality is likely to be the most important dimension in communication. For physicians, nurses, physical therapists, and other traditional biomedical health care providers, the envelope of confidentiality is generally thought to contain all health care providers and the patient. Information is freely exchanged between nurses and physicians in the hospital about the most intimate details of the patient's life. Likewise, physicians are very forthcoming about a patient's life history with a mental health professional.

In general, there is a much stronger prohibition against disclosure of patient confidences enforced by mental health professionals. Protecting the particularly private nature of therapy is essential to cultivating a trusting relationship between therapist and patient. However, some disclosure is necessary if communication is to take place. Negotiating issues around confidentiality can be a balancing act that needs to be constantly and individually monitored. However, it has been found that when the patient or family member is asked for permission for health care professionals to talk together, they rarely refuse, assuming that more communication is better than the reverse. Difficulties develop among the providers if they do not acknowledge the differences in cultures on this issue. Negative assumptions about the other can be the result of not communicating about these differences.

One of the most frequent complaints from health care providers regarding behavioral health care professionals is the therapist's lack of follow-up to a referral. Even though they do not explicitly state they would like to hear what happens, it is expected that a letter with an assessment and recommendations will follow a patient consultation. A second related concern of physicians is the lack of specific advice given to them about how to approach a particular patient or family. They are often less interested in the dynamics and hypotheses around a situation than in the implications for them in their provision of care.

There are a variety of methods for communication among collaborative providers. Face-to-face communication, which allows for questions and immediate feedback, is often best. This form of communication is certainly facilitated by sharing a service location or being nearby. This can be a scheduled meeting, a luncheon discussion, or even a "bump in the hall" kind of interaction, in all of which brief updates are given spontaneously.

Charting is always an important consideration in integrating care. Clearly there are many advantages to sharing charts. Behavioral health notes can be kept either in a different section of the chart from the medical progress notes or included with the medical progress notes when appropriate. It has been found that having a short note in the chart giving specific, concrete, feedback to the physician on diagnosis and recommendations furthers collaboration. The behavioral health provider can also keep a second separate chart for more detailed history and information that requires a formal release for insurance or other requests for the chart.

Financial Arrangement: Alignment of the Reward System

One increasingly important ingredient in how collaboration occurs is the financial arrangement. The extent to which providers can integrate services often depends more on panel participation and capitation arrangements, who is approved to provide behavioral health services and who owns what health care company this week. For example, in a capitated situation, if behavioral health services are not included in the per member per month (pm/pm) rate, the physician is rewarded for referring the patient and avoiding involvement. Likewise, a mental health carve out provider is rewarded for referring back to the physician any medical problems and thereby also not being involved. Many plans will not reimburse primary care physicians for counseling procedure codes or mental health diagnoses. Clearly, the more that risk is shared across health and behavioral health domains, the more an integrated approach is possible.

It has been common historically for behavioral health and health care professionals to have parallel financial arrangements. When a professional in a private practice, a hospital employee or a staff member in a community mental health setting, each provider bills separately and maintains separate accounts and separate offices. Sometimes the providers are co-located and share support services, but are financially independent. In another variation, each provider is self-employed, but one of them (usually the behavioral health provider) rents space from the other. This financial arrangement has worked well with little scrutiny into the most cost effective care. With the advent of managed care models, the separation mitigates against collaborative efforts.

Today it is becoming more common for providers to be employees of a larger organization, such as a large group practice, a hospital, an integrated network, or a government funded clinic. Although there is less individual autonomy, there are advantages. These larger organizations have more bargaining power with the current HMOs and other third-party payors in asserting the need for an integrated model. One of the authors has recently joined a group practice that also provides family medicine residency education services. This practice wanted to secure some of the larger managed care contracts in the area but found that behavioral services were carved-out and the managed care company was not accepting new providers. The physician group made a strong, articulate argument to have both services included, citing some of the studies mentioned earlier. This argument was made both to the behavioral carve-out company as well as the medical director of the health care group to which the carve-out group had contracted services. Their requests were approved and they were asked to contribute data to support this model in the future.

Location of Service: The Importance of Geography

When the authors originally began looking at the key variables in successful integration, it was hypothesized that location of service was important but probably not as important as having a good relationship. However, it was shown over and over that proximity enabled a different level of collaboration to occur. Those who share an office, see each other every day, share charts, have financial incentives to work for high-quality service, tend to think alike, so that collaboration becomes a natural way of working together.

Various descriptions of integrated practices based on geography have been offered. Glenn (1987) refers to "together but separate" work as collaborative, but traditional. In this model, physicians have therapist colleagues in their practice, while the physician is clearly the leader of the working group. A fully integrated model was described by Dym and Berman (1986). They saw each primary care medical appointment together as therapist and physician, and viewed it as an opportunity for health and behavioral health to work together. Dym

described the new role for the therapist who is a working partner of the primary care physician. This will require new skills
with patients and families who do not come specifically for
behavioral issues. Therapists become part of a primary health
care team and develop relationships with patients and families
who come to the practice. All records are kept in a family chart
by all professionals and staff who encounter the patient and
family during visits. While this is appealing from an integration
perspective, this model is likely to be unrealistic from a financial perspective. A more middle-of-the-road arrangement was
described earlier in Sue Molumphy's practice in Roanoke. In
that perspective, medical and behavioral providers share in the
same space and practice as an integrated team.

Summary

The areas described in this section represent key categories
for practicing in primary care medical settings. Developing a
comfort level and confidence requires an understanding of patients and their problems in the traditional treatment setting.
This first step can be accomplished by shadowing a primary
care physician as he or she practices. An awareness of the importance of the relationship and a common purpose is essential
for patients seen jointly. Working out effective communication
patterns, a consideration of financial arrangements and working in close proximity also contribute to success.

STRATEGIES ACROSS THE "SPECTRUM"

We have used the concept of a spectrum to represent the range
of collaborative options available to mental health and health
care providers when working in partnership with patients and
families (Seaburn et al., 1996). The color spectrum as seen in a
rainbow comprises bands of color that are distinct yet maintain
some connection with each other. The spectrum of collaboration is similar where various "bands" of collaboration are distinct, reflecting different needs and functions. Each band is

also an extension of the others, allowing for flexibility of professional functioning and movement across the spectrum. The five bands are *parallel delivery, informal consultation, formal consultation, coprovision of care, and collaborative networking.* Each band requires different strategies of collaboration depending on the needs of the patient, family, and providers at the time. As the needs change the strategies also shift.

Parallel Delivery

In this band the division of labor is clear and the problems addressed do not flow into each other in any significant way. While this appears to be a split model where the physician deals with the biological factors and the therapist deals with the psychosocial factors, and does not represent true integration, there is cross-fertilization. In this band, providers benefit from the knowledge that a partner is involved and available, though each functions independently. Many questions asked of the patient and their family involves the other professional and little or no "splitting" occurs.

Sam and Barbara chose their primary provider when they moved into town and saw her for several years. They were seen not only for routine physicals, but the physician delivered their first child, Aaron. When Aaron was age 4, Barbara came in with concerns regarding her son's behavior. She and her husband disagreed strongly on the best methods for discipline and Aaron had grown increasingly difficult to manage. The physician felt comfortable asking Sam and Barbara about their previous methods of discipline and the impact of these on the marital relationship, knowing that a local therapist was available to help out if needed. After several conjoint visits, the physician suggested that Sam and Barbara set up an appointment with the therapist for additional help in managing their son's behavior. Although reluctant at first, they felt more comfortable when the physician described the therapist as competent and an easy person with whom to work.

Sam and Barbara contacted the therapist who worked at his separate location, and the family was seen together for the first visit. At the end of the session, the therapist asked permission to contact the physician. Sam and Barbara spoke highly of their physician and agreed that the two providers should talk.

The therapist had worked with two other families in conjunction with the physician. Interestingly, the therapist and the physician had never met face to face, yet each saw the other as caring, perceptive, and competent. The treatment plan was conveyed to the physician and all agreed to six treatment sessions over the next 3 months to work on specific behavioral goals. The family was satisfied with the treatment received from both the physician and the therapist.

Informal Consultation

This kind of consultation occurs when one provider asks the other for help in dealing with a particular situation. The patient or family is not seen directly and the consultation can occur in either the outpatient or inpatient context. The situation can be clinically related or personally related. For example, a physician could ask a therapist for help in developing behavioral strategies for dealing with a depressed patient or may simply discuss personal feelings of frustration toward that same patient. In the above case example, the physician had been working with the family for several years prior to calling the therapist for advice about how to proceed.

Most of these informal consultation encounters occur as "bumps in the hall" or "spot conferences" (Hepworth & Jackson, 1985) that last only a few minutes. This study showed that 92% of physician–therapist consultations in a primary care setting occur in this brief format, and that one-half are less than 5 minutes long. These consultations should not be devalued for their brevity. They are an important part of the choreography of primary care.

Requests for consultation at the group practice level can also be seen as informal consultation. Behavioral medicine providers are often asked to serve in the role as organizational consultants helping the group develop effective visions for themselves, strategies, and team skills.

Formal Consultation

Formal consultation differs from informal consultation in several ways. The level of documentation and record keeping is higher. The consultant usually receives a written request to have contact with the patient-family and make recommendations about etiology, diagnosis, and/or treatment. The consultant adds notes on the patient's chart if both are working in the same setting. If they are not, the consultant sends a written note to the consultee.

For all consultations, the consultee maintains responsibility for the case. The consultant's role is defined. It can be to differentiate a mental health diagnosis or to help the consultee develop a more effective relationship with the patient and family. The consultation may also facilitate the referral of a patient and family who are reluctant to enter therapy.

One of the authors who works in a primary care medical clinic recalls being asked to consult with a physician colleague about an elderly patient who he felt was severely depressed. The consultation question was to determine the right diagnosis and also to gain a better understanding about the relationship between the woman and her adult son. The physician was present for the first of two interviews. Recommendations were given to the family and the physician in both oral and written form. Postvisit discussion between the therapist and physician enabled the physician to clarify what steps he wanted to take with the family. The therapist was not directly involved again but kept up informal contact with the physician about the family.

Coprovision of Care

Coprovision of care often occurs with patients and families whose problems are confusing, complex, demanding, or long-standing. They are often the "distressed high utilizers" described earlier. They often have both physical and emotional complaints. They may be high utilizers of health care whose charts are thick, whose needs are extensive, and whose care is costly. They may have chronic pain, somatization disorder, chronic illness, as well as a full complement of psychosocial problems. The key element is that the biomedical and psychosocial problems are so interconnected that more intensive collaboration is the only way to provide effective care. Coproviders share responsibility for the patient's treatment, negotiating with each other and with the patient and family what role each will play in treatment and how communication will take place.

Coproviders also negotiate how fees will be handled. In fee-for-service situations, coproviders both may charge for visits with the patient. When they see the patient together, they may alternate charges, the physician charging one time, the therapist another, depending on the patient's insurance. In capitated systems, the providers are paid in advance to care for all their patients. As a consequence, any limits on collaboration due to financial arrangements disappear.

There is an ebb and flow to coprovision of care. At times the professionals may talk to each other several times a week, or the patient and family may see either the physician or therapist more often. The professional collaborators may need to see the patient routinely during periods of crisis, such as the diagnosis of a new illness or the exacerbation of parenting problems. This ebb and flow is determined by the needs of all those involved in the collaboration, the professionals as well as the patient and family. For example, with Sam and Barbara, if their son had had chronic asthma which flared at times of parental emotional distress, at such times, the physician and the therapist would need to be in close contact. Since therapy for the parents might increase parental tensions, the physician would be prepared for a flareup of Aaron's asthma.

Collaborative Networking

Collaborative networking recognizes that both a community of professional and natural supports may be needed to effectively care for some patients and families (Landau-Stanton & Clements, 1993; Seaburn et al., 1995). The behavioral health provider in a primary care setting, along with the primary health care or medical professional maintains central roles in this network. In conjunction with the patient and family, they coordinate overall treatment and they function as case managers, information interpreters, advocates, mediators, and the arrangers of other support services.

For example, if Aaron were felt to have attention deficit disorder with associated learning disabilities, the therapist and the physician would need to work closely with the school system to make sure the right evaluations are completed and resources provided. The parents might benefit from an additional therapy or a support group that discussed behavioral strategies to deal with these issues.

Collaborative networking requires the behavioral provider to develop strategies in the area of case management and network development. There is a continued search for appropriate resources for different problems and to maintain good relations with key agencies and community groups that may provide assistance. He or she realizes there is a larger system available to help when needed.

Summary

Flexibility is the most essential skill to develop. Professionals involved in integrated systems must move across a wide range of possible roles in order to interact effectively with other professional collaborators, patients, and families. In the case described above, the behavioral health provider functioned as a specialist, consultant, and coprovider of care. Such flexibility enables the behavioral health professional to adapt to the needs of any given situation.

The spectrum of collaboration encourages the behavioral health care provider to collaborate regardless of the practice setting in which he or she works. Although integration is much easier when professionals share space, the options described are based less on location of service than on the relationship among providers, patients, and families. It is the collaborative relationship that is central to providing effective care for challenging patients and families.

RECOMMENDATIONS FOR EFFECTIVE INTEGRATION FOR BEHAVIORAL HEALTH PROVIDERS

This chapter has outlined a developmental path for behavioral health providers working in medical settings. Following are some summary recommendations for integration:

1. Develop the cognitive set of being a partner in the medical context. Use "pull" marketing strategies which inquire about the needs of the medical providers rather than "pushing" one's own expertise.
2. Keep up with the literature and developments in collaborative care. Join organizations like the Collaborative Family Health Care Coalition and read journals such as *Families, Systems, and Health*. Most professional organizations have a special interest group focusing on medical issues.
3. Ask all new patients about their primary care providers and obtain permission to talk with them. Use the opportunity to develop relationships with the providers. Consider seeing patients part-time or full time in a primary care practice.
4. Develop working relationships with the staff of a primary care clinic. Consider yourself a consultant to the practice as well as to the individual providers.
5. Be accessible and available to the physicians and the practice. Be willing to be involved in hospital settings. Hospitalization is often a crisis time when people are most open to behavioral interventions.
6. Realize primary care providers will vary in their interest and skills in working collaboratively. Be flexible in accommodating this variability.
7. Avoid mental health labels in the early stages of involvement with patients, families, and medical providers. Realize there are a large number of patients in a primary care setting who will not respond initially to the idea of behavioral involvement.

16.

Partnerships with Primary Care Physicians: Reinventing Gatekeeper Relationships

James R. Moon, Ph.D., M.B.A.

The de facto mental health system in the United States has always been within the confines of the "family doctor's" or primary care physician's office. Estimates that more than 60% of all visits to a primary care physician have a behavioral health component that largely or solely motivates the office visit are well established. In this way, primary care physicians have acted as "gatekeepers." For many years, successful behavioral health practitioners in independent practice have known about the value of having a strong referral relationship with one or more of these family practitioner gatekeepers. During the past 15 years tremendous change has occurred in the medical field as health care undergoes alterations associated with industrialization. Behavioral health care, originally seen as an arcane specialty, has been "carved-out" for most of this period of industrial change. This carve-out phenomenon is rapidly ending as behavioral health technology becomes widely available.

Acknowledgments. The author would like to thank his colleagues for their support in the preparation of this chapter and their helpful comments and suggestions. Special thanks go to Susan Iskowitz, L.C.S.W., T. Russell McGrady, M.S., Jeff Reddout, Ph.D., Jim Seaton, L.C.S.W., and Mark Zwingelberg, Psy.D.

305

The next great opportunity for behavioral health providers exists in recognizing the value these services bring to the primary care physician's office practice. Behavioral health care providers can seize this opportunity by developing partnerships with primary care physicians and by reinventing and reengineering the professional relationship with these central gatekeepers. The experiences and plans of one such facility in central Florida are presented.

HISTORICAL BACKGROUND

The 1970s and 1980s have been described as "the golden age of independent practice" (Troy & Shueman, 1996, p. 56) for professional psychologists, and by inference, other behavioral health professionals. In the mid-1980s mental health benefits became a logical target of managed care initiatives. Managed behavioral health care grew rapidly, due largely to the successful reduction in mental health care costs associated with hospitalization (Cummings and Sayama, 1995). In fact, simply managing the hospitalizations through gatekeeper utilization reviews provided tremendous savings of health care resources and preserved benefits for policyholders. As more managed and solution-focused therapies were introduced, the cost-savings increased.

At first, the technology that drove these changes was known to a small select group. Then, in the mid-1980s managed behavioral health care ventures sprang up to offer services to the "client organizations," i.e., the large insurance carriers. The insurance carriers carved-out behavioral health care to managed behavioral health organizations such as American Biodyne, MCC, and others. The benefit structure for the patients of the better behavioral health care firms included no limits on the number of hospitalizations, no limits on the number of psychotherapy visits, and no copayments.

As the managed behavioral health carve-out model evolved, the technologies were more commonly available. The focus shifted from staff-model organizations to network-model organizations, and the "clinician" was often relegated to a case manager role. This produced several negative situations. First, the managed behavioral health care case manager (and thus the managed behavioral health care firm itself) was placed in an adversarial (and often antagonistic) position vis-à-vis the network provider.

Second, conflict ensued because financial incentives were not aligned. Managed behavioral health carve-out firms were paid a fixed amount per member per month (pm/pm). However, network providers were often paid in a discounted fee-for-service model by the managed behavioral health care firm.

The third and perhaps most significant negative consequence of the general shift to a network model is the managed behavioral health care firm's inability to foster and monitor the network provider's relationships with primary care physicians. In a staff-model behavioral health care organization, the center director can exercise administrative powers to ensure that the therapists keep in close contact with the primary care physicians. This administrative power is nonexistent in a network model.

BEHAVIORAL HEALTH BEYOND MANAGED CARE CARVE-OUTS

The role of the primary care physicians in delivering behavioral health care has always been large and critically important. It has been a relatively recent phenomenon for mental health specialists to evolve and lay claim to the ownership of behavioral health care (Matarazzo, 1994). Largely, the professional behavioral health guilds have been responsible for the increasingly independent practice of behavioral health care outside of traditional health care delivery systems.

As discussed earlier, even the health maintenance organization (HMO) movement has not been spared the separation of behavioral health care from the HMO's medical services delivery system(s) as behavioral health carve-outs occurred first in staff-model behavioral HMOs, then in an even more fragmented network-model behavioral HMO. The separation of behavioral health care from other types of health care is inherently inefficient and supports implicitly a mind–body dualism.

Philosophical arguments aside, the industrialization of health care will not tolerate inefficiencies, and the fragmentation of behavioral health away from other health care delivery systems will end. The "invisible hand" of competitive forces in the marketplace will work to drive out inefficient practices over time.

We have seen attempts to move behavioral health care from the purview of the primary care physician. However, despite the untold dollars and hours spent devising behavioral health care delivery systems, the primary care physician remains the primary de facto mental health care delivery system in this country. Indeed, the estimates consistently place at 60% or greater the percentage of patients that are motivated to seek help at a primary care physician's office due to problems that are solely or primarily of psychogenic origin (Cummings & VandenBos, 1981; Katzelnick, Koback, Greist, Jefferson, & Henk, 1997). The largest percentage of psychopharmacological agents (i.e., antidepressants and anxiolytics) is dispensed by primary care physicians (Jacobs, Kopans, & Reizes, 1995; Strosahl, 1996a). Many readers of this chapter, if they reflect on their own personal experiences with primary care, may take issue with these facts. This is because many highly educated professionals engage in an informal personal triage process and go to the appropriate health professional depending upon the particular symptomatology. *However, this is not the behavior of the typical health care seeking consumer.* The typical health care consumer goes to the primary care physician for any and every health care need (Strosahl, 1996a). Even if a system were devised whereby these psychogenically driven health care-seeking consumers could be directed immediately to mental health professionals, bypassing the primary care physician, we would need to effectively double the number of mental health professionals in this country. Since this doubling of the workforce is not likely to occur, it makes sense to work to improve the existing system to make it more responsive.

The answer, therefore, does not lie in further fragmentation of health care. Instead, behavioral health care must be reintegrated into established health care delivery systems. This reintegration follows a conceptual model for the reintegration process and necessitates two essential paradigm shifts related to behavioral health care and the model for behavioral health care delivery.

INTEGRATION OF BEHAVIORAL HEALTH CARE WITH PHYSICAL HEALTH CARE

A five-level model for describing the integration of behavioral health care with physical health care has been proposed by Doherty, McDaniel, and Baird (1996). At the most basic level, there is minimal collaboration or integration. Most private practices and agencies are at this level.

Level 2, called "collaboration at a distance," adds to the model periodic communication by phone and/or letter. An example of this level of integration would be when a mental health care provider discusses the depressive aspects of a diabetic patient with the primary care physician.

Basic collaboration on site is the third level of integration. At this level, the behavioral health and physical health care providers occasionally communicate face to face. However, there is not a strong sense of a treatment team, and there is no shared common language or an in-depth understanding of each other's practices. Health maintenance organization settings and shared-space medical clinics afford this type of integration largely due to physical proximity.

Close collaboration in a partly integrated system is the fourth level of integration. At this level, medical and behavioral health care specialists share biopsychosocial perspectives and there is a great deal of office systems infrastructure integration, e.g., common appointment scheduling, treatment team meetings, integrated treatment plans, etc. Some HMOs and hospice centers have achieved this level of integration.

Finally, level 5 depicts a fully integrated system in which there is close collaboration. All members of the treatment staff adopt a biopsychosocial approach and operate from within the same shared vision. There are efforts to balance power among the professionals by deemphasizing particular academic degrees while assigning influence and power based upon team members' roles and areas of expertise. An example of this setting is a modern hospice.

This model is a useful map to allow one to gauge where a particular treatment system is on the continuum of integrated care delivery. The model stops, however, at the tertiary care level. Clearly, the most successful integrated health care delivery systems will extend the level 5 integration into secondary and primary prevention areas. This move will provide integrated community wellness maintenance services and will involve a variety of other professionals, employers, community groups, and systems. An extension of the integrated model could involve employee assistance program (EAP) specialists, classroom specialists, and wellness specialists into the integrated mix of traditional behavioral health, hospice, home health, and primary physical health care specialists.

PARADIGM SHIFTS

There are two essential paradigm shifts which need to occur in order to move ahead in the reintegration of behavioral health into primary care.

Paradigm Shift 1

Behavioral Health in a Fully Integrated System is Not Traditional Psychotherapy in a Different Office Setting. If more traditional care is indicated, e.g., individual or group psychotherapy, referrals can be made. However, the majority of integrated behavioral health interventions will occur in 5- to 30-minute time segments in a primary care office. The nature of the intervention will not look like a traditional psychotherapy intake session. Instead, the session will be problem-focused, and relatively jargon-free. Most of the essential history will have been gathered and available in the chart. It will be essential for the behavioral health practitioner to quickly establish rapport, determine the reason the problem has been brought to the physician's office *now*, and develop a homework prescription that the patient takes from the office and follows. Usually, the follow-up session will be with the primary care physician who will ascertain whether the homework was completed and whether the problem has subsided. The modal number of 15- to 30-minute sessions with the behavioral health specialist will likely be one. The session will be very action-oriented and directive in nature. Bibliotherapy, audiotaped exercises, or other types of supplemental materials will likely be used to extend the therapeutic reach of the behavioral health professional. The progress note for this type of patient encounter is much more like a medical progress note, i.e., factual in nature and generally devoid of probablistic language (or minimal use of probablistic language so that the notes actually say something useful). Finally, the behavioral health specialist in a consultative role discusses the case with the primary care physician. This leads to the second essential paradigm shift.

Paradigm Shift 2

The Behavioral Health Care Specialist Uses Focused Behavioral Health Interventions to Further Enable the Physician–Patient Relationship. The important relationship is the physician–patient relationship. The relationship between the behavioral health professional and the patient is of minimal importance comparatively. The behavioral health care specialist has a new opportunity to be a catalyst for change in this context. In terms of who "owns the patient's case," the "ownership" resides with the primary care physician.

BRIDGES TO THE FUTURE: HOW DO WE GET THERE FROM HERE?

There are two bridges, conceptual and financial, to this new future of reinvented relationships with primary care physicians.

Both bridges must be crossed by most behavioral health provider groups. Behavioral health providers who already practice in a prepaid setting have a slightly shorter financial bridge to cross.

Conceptual Bridges

Approaches to Primary Care Physicians. Primary care physicians are generally receptive to the addition of behavioral health services to their practice mix. Most primary care physicians have had positive training experiences with behavioral health care providers in their medical training, and are prepared to accept focused recommendations from the behavioral health professional. A benefit to this approach is that the focus upon health and wellness maintenance places the physician and behavioral health specialist synergistically on the same page with the same overall goal.

There is a less obvious benefit that the behavioral health care provider brings to the primary care physician's office. Primary care physicians suffer from a high rate of burnout. This is not surprising given the demands placed upon primary care. Further, since most of the problems presented to the primary care physician have no definitive etiology (Shapiro & Koocher, 1996), the potential for burnout is obvious. The behavioral health professional can provide immediate consultation to the patient and offer an explanatory model to the primary care physician along with treatment alternatives. Further, over time, the behavioral health professional can teach many of these techniques to the amenable physician, broadening the physician's skill set (Cole & Raju, 1996). Both of these services will have mitigating effects on primary care physician burnout.

Approaches to Managed Care Organizations. This conceptual bridge is more difficult to traverse. Conceptually, if earlier intervention reduces the total cost of a care episode and if behavioral health care can be introduced sooner rather than later, there should be greater savings from the medical cost offset phenomenon (Pallak, Cummings, Dorken, & Henke, 1995). However, most behavioral managed care organizations have developed a pricing structure based upon expected penetration rates (number of new cases identified), average number of outpatient sessions, and/or the number of expected hospital days per 1,000 subscribers. Placing behavioral health care in the primary care physician's office threatens to "blow the capitation rate" due to the increased number of cases likely to be found.

Managed behavioral health care firms as well as other payor sources will need to be included in the integration plans to overcome these inherent barriers. This method of overcoming barriers, variously called "cooptation" or "coopitition," is used in other strategic business settings (Brandenburger & Nalebuff, 1996; Kotler, 1997).

Education of the Health Care Consumer. Today's health care consumer expects to go to the doctor, get a pill, and get better. Many bacterial and viral diseases are treated within this model. However, life-style diseases such as smoking, overeating, and stress-mediated diseases do not respond to the "just take a pill" approach. Similarly, chronic conditions such as chronic pain, arthritis, diabetes, multiple sclerosis, etc., are generally not cured as much as they are managed (Caudill, Schnable, Zutermeister, Benson, & Friedman, 1991). For these conditions the patient must be educated regarding the management vs. cure expectation. Patients who can manage a chronic condition are more likely to be satisfied than patients who expect to have their chronic condition cured. Behavioral health care professionals, especially those who practice brief intermittent therapy, have long been accustomed to having a limited focus approach while avoiding the concept of "cure" (Cummings & Sayama, 1995). Thus, the health care team must anticipate the challenges a patient (and/or the patient's family) faces when seeking treatment in the new integrated model. To this end, the physician–patient relationship can be used to motivate, enthuse, and educate the patient regarding the consultation with the behavioral health professional. Similarly, the behavioral health professional must be prepared to take a more directive and prescriptive approach in the treatment room to keep the patients motivated and engaged in participating in their own health care.

Education of the Employer. Employee Assistance Programs (EAPs) have long been a fixture in the modern corporate structure. They offer brief interventions to troubled employees and generally help to maintain the well-being of employees, reducing the cost of absenteeism and turnover for employers. Since employers often purchase medical benefit plans for their employees it is important to educate the employer, perhaps through the EAP mechanism, about the integration of behavioral health into the primary care setting. A side benefit of taking this approach is the possibility that the employer will invite the behavioral health care specialist to the worksite to present stress-management workshops, smoking cessation programs, etc. This invitation is more likely to be extended if there are financial incentives attached to overall lower utilization of the health plan (Sobel, 1995b; Friedman, Sobel, Myers, Caudill, & Benson, 1995).

Financial incentives are an important aspect of the continued industrialization of health care. There are key financial bridges that must be crossed in the effort to integrate behavioral health care into the primary care physician's practice.

Financial Bridges

The payor sources in health care comprise a complex array of payment strategies and methodologies. It is important for treatment providers either to know how much it costs them to provide a unit of care or be able to find or develop this information by doing a comprehensive cost analysis. Once the provider knows the cost of providing a unit of care, the appropriate business and negotiation strategies can be developed regardless of the funding sources. Further, by engaging in a *target* cost analysis the provider can more competitively negotiate contracts. A target cost analysis allows the provider to structure the practice based upon the current payment rates for particular units of service, e.g., 45-minute outpatient session, partial hospitalization day rate, etc. The providers then know in which areas they can effectively compete on price and which business opportunities must be abandoned due to the inability to provide quality service at that rate of reimbursement. Also, by knowing the cost to provide any particular unit of care, larger provider groups know where they can adopt a "loss leader" strategy and where such strategy would not be a good business approach.

Essentially, there are just a handful of payment schemes. These schemes can be grouped into two broad categories; fee-for-service and prospective payment. The fee-for-service can be via cash-only payments, indemnity insurance, performance contracts, and/or discounted fee-for-service. Fees are paid subsequent to the delivery of services. Prospective payment is either via a case-rate or capitated (pm/pm) scheme. Here payment is made before services are delivered. The latter two prospective schemes put the provider at some level of financial risk since the payment for service is set prior to the delivery of care. Prospective payments make the most sense in an HMO model of care since treatment and financial incentives are aligned. However, most providers would prefer fee-for-service since the provider does not assume any financial risk and encounters minimal amounts of paperwork. Realistically, provider groups need to plan to operate in a prospective environment if they hope to be successful in a world where health care is increasingly industrialized.

It is currently a challenge to practice in a financially successful manner where the goal is to integrate behavioral health into primary care. The least complex payment model (but the most difficult to find) is the fully integrated practice which accepts prospective payment from one payor source. An example of this model is the Group Health Cooperative of Puget Sound (see chapter 4). In this fully integrated model, payment is negotiated as a blended capitation rate.

Most provider groups, however, have a much more complex task regarding payment for services. It is not uncommon to find larger provider groups operating in an environment that has a full range of payment schemes. In this environment it is essential for the behavioral health group and the primary care group to be fully aware of the payment challenges. It is also important for the provider group to understand each patient's policy benefits and limitations. This information must be communicated clearly to the individual treatment providers and to the patients, who are often largely unaware of the limits and restrictions of their mental health coverage. While it is certainly the ideal situation that quality care be provided without regard to payment sources, the business reality is that choices must be made to maximize the amount of quality deliverable care within a particular benefit structure. Providers who routinely ignore this simple business reality will not remain in business.

In an indemnity situation where the patient's insurance pays for a percentage of the health charge while the patient pays the balance, billing for behavioral health services rendered in an integrated environment is generally not a problem. It is relatively simple to establish medical necessity and to find appropriate DSM-IV diagnostic codes that are reimbursable by the insurance company.

In a discounted-fee-for-service situation where fees are paid to network providers from a behavioral health carve-out firm, some problems exist. Behavioral health carve-out companies generally are wary of an integrated approach to health care since their capitation rates are based on assumptions that are violated in a more integrated approach. In this situation, the behavioral carve-out firm stands to lose a great deal if the case-finding rate (or penetration rate) significantly exceeds the projected amount. Clearly, there are financial incentives for behavioral health carve-out firms to resist any attempt to increase penetration rates beyond the assumptions made in their pricing algorithms.

The reverse is true for primary care physicians in this model of payment. That is, if a primary care group is already capitated, there are strong financial incentives for the primary care physician to refer the patient to the most appropriate level of care. Often, this will mean a referral to behavioral health due to behavioral health's demonstrated ability to reduce overall medical costs. Thus, behavioral health providers who are network providers for a behavioral health carveout firm must strategically work with a behavioral health carve-out firm prior to any attempts to integrate services with primary care. If the behavioral health group fails to do this they may find themselves out of the provider network and/or not able to bill and collect for behavioral health services rendered in a primary care setting.

These are the challenges currently faced in today's real world of behavioral health care delivery. A case illustration of the ongoing evolution of a behavioral health provider group in Winter Haven, Florida, highlights some of the challenges and opportunities faced by behavioral health care specialists as they attempt to navigate the changes in health care.

THE WINTER HAVEN EXPERIENCE

Winter Haven, Florida, is a small town of approximately 30,000 in Polk County, a county of approximately 440,000. The county is located in central Florida midway between the urban centers of Tampa-St. Petersburg and Orlando-Daytona Beach. Polk County is geographically about the size of Rhode Island, and, despite being home to nearly half a million inhabitants, is considered to be largely rural. The predominant industries are citrus, phosphate, and cattle. Winter Haven is the second largest population center in the county after Lakeland, and is perhaps best known as the home of Cypress Gardens (Florida's oldest theme park) and the winter home of the Cleveland Indians baseball team.

Winter Haven Hospital (WHH), a not-for-profit division of Mid-Florida Medical Services, is a medium size hospital which provides a broad range of quality medical services to Winter Haven and eastern Polk county. Within the organizational structure of WHH is the Behavioral Health Division (BHD), a behavioral health provider group consisting of over 130 licensed and non-licensed behavioral health and support staff. The Behavioral Health Division has been actively involved in bringing behavioral health benefits to the citizens of Polk County, while partnering with other divisions within WHH and Mid-Florida Medical Services to provide a variety of integrated services. BHD has also been active in the formation of an innovative public-private partnership and was part of a group which was awarded a contract for a Medicaid-waiver demonstration project. However, it was not always this way.

In the Beginning (1991–1994)

Although there were extensive behavioral health services available through WHH prior to 1991, they were traditionally administered in a fee-for-service, cost-plus pricing model. Managed behavioral health care had made virtually no significant appearance prior to 1991. WHH owns one of the two community mental health centers in the county. Historically, the WHH community mental health center serviced residents in eastern Polk County. Beginning circa 1991, the leadership of the region's five community mental health centers (two in Polk County, two in Hillsborough County, and one in Manatee County) began to explore the possibilities of forming a partnership to compete for Medicaid dollars. Florida, like other states, was considering a capitated waiver method to pay for Medicaid services in an attempt to curtail the rising spiral of Medicaid behavioral health costs. A variety of pilot projects, like the Biodyne-Hawaii project had demonstrated that significant cost reductions could be realized by managing the delivery of behavioral health services (Pallak et al., 1995) to a Medicaid population.

This innovative group of mental health leaders approached a variety of private managed behavioral health care firms to explore the possibility of a public–private partnership to deliver quality behavioral health services to Medicaid recipients under a capitated payment structure. Finally, Options, Inc. of Norfolk, Virginia was selected as the private partner. In March 1996, the 5 years of planning and preparation were rewarded as the Medicaid waiver project went "live" in a five-county area of west-central Florida.

In a somewhat parallel fashion beginning in late 1993, a series of internal studies and recommendations suggested that there would be substantial benefits from coordinating the efforts of the various behavioral health service groups operating as distinct departments within the WHH structure. There were four separate departments providing overlapping behavioral health services in distinct and separate organizational structures. These departments included the community mental health service, the Department of Psychology, a private practice model outpatient psychotherapy service called Clinical Counseling Associates (CCA), and an inpatient program for adults, children and adolescents called Center for Psychiatry (CFP). As these four departments were brought under one divisional control, some very interesting synergies began to emerge.

And Then There Was Light (1994–1996)

In order to be "user friendly" within a managed care business environment the internal restructuring relied heavily on models which had operated successfully in the managed behavioral health care industry, especially the Biodyne model which was heavily influenced by Dr. Cummings' work at Kaiser Permanente (Cummings & Sayama, 1995; Cummings & VandenBos, 1981). One of the primary initial considerations was to determine as closely as possible what it cost to deliver any particular unit of care. This task was more daunting than initially realized and consumed many staff hours.

Another early task was to determine performance standards for staff in terms of how many sessions of therapy needed to be delivered. Since initially all of the operation was in a fee-for-service (and discounted fee-for-service) reimbursement system, determining productivity standards in terms of revenue generation (billing) was straightforward. However, as movement into capitation and case-rate (prospective payment) reimbursement systems were anticipated, it was no longer meaningful to use billing amounts as a measure of productivity.

A productivity system was devised that relied neither on billing nor total number of patients seen. Instead, the productivity system involved variously weighted therapeutic encounters, no show rates, and percentage of caseload in various treatment modalities. In this system, the weighting for each "therapeutic encounter unit" as a measure of productivity can be changed as market conditions change. In addition, the caseload turnover rates can be monitored to ensure that patients do not get stuck in ineffective treatment modalities. The technical foundation for this change relied heavily on the adoption of solution-focused therapy techniques, especially the model of Brief Intermittent Psychotherapy Throughout the Life Cycle articulated in Cummings and Sayama (1995).

It was during this period that the corporate culture began to change. Mental health care delivery had changed very little prior to this period. Maintenance of the status quo was the norm. A new climate of change was introduced and staff were encouraged to take calculated risks in developing new programs and interventions. Metaphorically, it was as if the organization decided to stop playing baseball, where everyone knows his or her position and responsibilities, and instead play soccer. Soccer is a game which is very fluid. Unlike baseball, change occurs rapidly in soccer, with the goal remaining clear despite the fluid change. Each soccer player shifts position from moment to moment in an attempt to move the ball toward the goal. In soccer, it is important to rotate players in and out, taking advantage of fresh energy and particular skill sets. It is also important to anticipate where the soccer ball will be, while maintaining the flexibility to make last minute adjustments. Soccer, like behavioral health in the 21st century, is not "your father's baseball game."

In addition, the management team adopted the philosophy of "doing the right thing." It is very seductive in an era of shrinking dollars to adopt a philosophy of cost-containment. However, in "doing the right thing," quality of care remains high and increases the opportunities to deliver cost-effective treatment. "Doing the right thing" sometimes reveals philosophical differences in staff's treatment approaches, but the goal remains constant. A cost-containment philosophy of care can place dollars at a higher priority than patient care. This can produce gains over the short run, but it is a losing strategy over the long run, as lesser quality behavioral health firms have discovered.

Taking a solution-focused approach also bridges the gap in revenue sources. Several members of the BHD management team who had taken solution-focused approaches while in independent practice knew that solution-focused approaches produced very satisfied patients who now served as excellent referral sources. These management team members could attest to the fee-for-service potential of focused psychotherapy as well as the prospective payment potential of focused psychotherapy. Thus, revenue streams were generally preserved as the Behavioral Health Division reinvented and reengineered itself. The solution-focused model lends itself very well to the next step of behavioral health/primary care integration.

Staff were involved as much as possible in the change process and, not surprisingly, very little staff turnover occurred during this transitional period. Attention to staff turnover is critical, since recruitment and training costs are high. Leadership tasks during periods of rapid change have been clearly articulated by Kotter (1996), who provides guidance to managers involved in the change process.

And It Was Good (1996 and Beyond)

Some natural synergistic alliances began to form as other parts of the Mid-Florida health care system, including its wholly owned HMO/TPA subsidiary changed and evolved. Paramount was the development of outpatient Family Health Center (FHC) offices. These offices may well be the sites of future behavioral health care in the community. While full integration has not yet occurred, a number of meetings between BHD and FHC have resulted in partial integration with promising early results.

Not surprisingly, initial negotiations between behavioral health and medical staff were characterized by the "turf" and professional boundary violation issues commonly seen in medical organizations. One of the first tasks was to recognize that the medical care delivery system was changing and that the change was being driven by powerful external economic forces.

It was necessary to foster an internally cooperative approach. Relationship-building was a critical by-product of the initial meetings. As a group we knew that as many relevant interests as possible needed to be included in meetings. Invariably, especially early on, one or more parties would be unintentionally excluded from the process. When this was discovered, the excluded party would be included and briefed on the progress to date. While at times this process seemed laborious, it was often the quickest and most efficient way to reach a desired goal.

There have been a variety of responses to the changes thus far. Some key staff are more receptive than others. Diversity of staff opinion is not an impediment to change if the diversity results in powerful and creative ideas. Diversity also allows for an informal check and balance system to develop. As one key leader is fond of saying, "You can't change just one thing." This is balanced by another key leader who cautions, "You can only change one thing at a time." Indeed, managing this balance has been a challenge.

Other changes have taken place including the creation of a single point of access (which will ultimately provide financial as well as clinical triage), multiple delivery sites, and a commitment to ongoing staff training for staff at all levels of the organization. Staff have been sensitized to the need for excellence in customer service where the customer is broadly defined. Finally, a state-of-the-art computer system was purchased and installed to help manage the tremendous data handling requirements that industrialized health care brings.

Similarly, the support of Mid-Florida for employer health programs, wellness in the workplace programs, hospice, home health, and EAP programs offers some natural synergies in the integration of behavioral health and primary care. There is much exciting work to be done and there will likely be some "bumps" in the road ahead. However, the future in health care appears to belong to those integrated systems that can preserve the community's health and wellness in an efficient and effective manner. The mission of BHD is consistent with the Mid-Florida mission, "to optimize the health status of the community . . . ," and the vision of providing "solutions for healthy living through caring, responsive, innovative services."

SUMMARY

Health care is currently undergoing dramatic reengineering. Old paradigms are giving way to new integrated models for care which emphasize doing the right thing at the right time. As various approaches to health care delivery evolve and mature, it is likely that several large payor sources will contract with regional provider groups that provide a broad and comprehensive system of quality care.

An important part of the new delivery system will be the integration of behavioral health into primary care. Exactly how this will happen is currently being determined at a variety of locations throughout the country. It is likely that no one standard model will prevail but that each region will develop similar systems with unique components to deliver behavioral health care where it is most needed in primary care.

17.

The Behavioral Health Practitioner of the Future: The Efficacy of Psychoeducational Programs in Integrated Primary Care

**Nicholas A. Cummings, Ph.D., Sc.D.,
Janet L. Cummings, Psy.D.**

In the past 20 years, and especially during the last decade, there has been a surprisingly rapid emergence of psychoeducational programs that combine treatment, information dissemination, and behavioral techniques directed at inducing life-style changes, all within a time-limited group model. Early research, to be discussed below, strongly suggests that these programs are effective with a number of psychological and medical conditions and may replace much of the work that is currently conducted in one-on-one psychotherapy. Not only does the research indicate that many of these targeted group models are more effective with a surprisingly wide range of emotional reactions and physical diseases, they also cost significantly less than does individual psychotherapy, and even brief individual psychotherapy, for the same conditions.

In this era of cost containment, when psychotherapists' practices are experiencing serious economic downturns, any efforts to render psychotherapy more efficient are viewed with suspicion and even alarm by practitioners. Yet several psychotherapist researchers who predate the current cost-conscious climate have held that the responsibility of the practitioner is to render our interventions more effective and efficient for the sake of the patient, and that effective therapy results in cost-containment without making economics the primary focus (Balint, 1957; Budman & Gurman, 1988; Cummings, 1977; Cummings & Follette, 1968; Cummings & VandenBos, 1979; Davanloo, 1978; Erickson, 1980; Follette & Cummings, 1967; Hoyt, 1995; Malan, 1976; Sifneos, 1987). Effective–efficient practitioner driven psychotherapy systems are seen as the quality solution against which business driven systems cannot successfully compete (Cummings, 1996b). Cummings and Sayama (1995) make explicit that the therapist's obligation is to bring relief from pain, anxiety, and depression to the patient in the shortest time possible. This requires honing one's skills and striving to make this outcome a reality with every patient that is treated.

Several movements converged to produce the current enthusiasm for psychoeducational programs: brief psychotherapy, time-limited group therapy, and skills training. It is worthwhile to trace the historical precursors to the present movement, and to examine a few examples of research through which psychoeducational programs are being developed. This discussion will review the necessary characteristics and ingredients of successful psychoeducational programs and present several diverse, but effective models.

HISTORICAL PERSPECTIVE

Time-Sensitive Psychotherapy

Early efforts to render therapy more efficient and effective were largely directed toward individual therapy and have not abated. Alexander and French (1946) were considered outlandish when they suggested that in many instances psychoanalysis could be concluded within 150 sessions. They angered the psychotherapeutic community with their contention that Freud discovered brief psychotherapy when he eliminated Bruno Walter's psychic pain in his conducting arm in just 6 sessions and "cured" Gustav Mahler's sex problem during a 3-hour walk.

Bloom (1991) traced the history of short-term therapy and concluded that the field has never been hospitable to the notion of time-sensitive approaches. Most psychotherapists not only prefer long-term therapy, but they continue to see patients as long as they are willing to come in, and as long as insurance will pay for it, ignoring what might be identified as therapeutic drift. Bloom indicates that recently, many psychotherapists have escalated their hostility to short-term therapy as these techniques have impacted negatively on their previously flourishing practices.

Origins and Development of Group Therapy

Balint (1957) unleashed a storm of controversy when he envisaged group psychotherapy as filling the gap created by the shortage of psychotherapists. Since that time, critics of group therapy have continued to see this method as an expedient, while advocates take strong issue with that attribution. Actually, long before Balint, Freud (1955) outlined a group therapy model that is still quite meaningful. He stated that, in a way, all psychology is essentially group psychology, and group psychology is the original and oldest psychology. He spoke of a group of two, and thus was able to link individual and group psychotherapy together. Freud emphasized that a collection of people is not a group, but it can develop as such with the introduction of leadership. Traditional group therapy has consisted of "open groups" in which patients who are generally comparable in goals and problems enter a group, participate for a few months to a few years, and then move on. The group and the group leader have a perpetuity of their own. Most often group members are recruited from the psychotherapist's individual therapy practice, but a smaller number of prestigious group therapists who exclusively conduct groups receive referrals from a broad array of colleagues.

Historically, group psychotherapy received its greatest impetus in the United Kingdom after World War II. Following a lukewarm reception throughout most of the world's psychotherapeutic community, the nationalization of health care in Great Britain created a demand for group therapy because the need for treatment exceeded the number of practitioners who could provide one-on-one therapy. Within a relatively short time clinical research demonstrated that group therapy was not only expedient, it was also effective (Balint, 1957).

More recently the perpetual nature of traditional group psychotherapy has been challenged. Two highly respected long-term group psychotherapists discovered that 40% of their patients left before the end of the first year, 75% left before the end of 2 years, and 90% left before the end of 4 years (Rutan & Stone, 1984; Stone & Rutan, 1984). Only 10% of the group therapy patients fulfilled the traditional notions of perpetuity. Similarly, Klein & Carroll (1986) found that in a community mental health center 52% of patients entering group therapy left by the twelfth session, and the mean number of sessions for all patients was 18.8, while the mode was a single visit. Following a number of similar researches, Budman & Gurman (1988) developed their generic model of short-term experiential group psychotherapy. Its demonstrated effectiveness, along with its markedly increased efficiency, have made it an attractive alternative to more traditional models.

Much earlier clinical research revealed that certain conditions are more responsive to group therapy than to individual therapy. For example, early work at Kaiser Permanente indicated that group psychotherapy was highly effective with addictions, while individual psychotherapy was relatively ineffective (Cummings, 1979). Addicts require the group culture of enforced abstinence as a potent force, a feature absent in one-on-one therapy where they seem to settle for becoming a "comfortable loser" (Peele, 1978). For different reasons, agoraphobics were found to recover much more rapidly in specially designed groups, benefiting from the reinforced desensitization as well as the realization that others share their fears and that they are not "insane" or about to have a fatal heart attack

(Hardy, 1970). Since these early reports, there has been a proliferation of groups designed to address specific conditions. A number of trends are rapidly converging to forge the new group psychotherapies.

From Skills Training to Psychoeducation

Paralleling the development of short-term group therapy, and actually preceding it, is the large body of research in skills training. This has been reviewed extensively by O'Donohue & Krasner (1995), beginning with Jacobsen's relaxation training at the beginning of the century, through the social skills training of both children and adults, assertiveness training, parenting skills training, marital skills training, and even such issues as self-appraisal skills training and employment skills training. Throughout these groups, skills were emphasized. However, they never really became part of the health system (until at least very recently), and the term *psychoeducational* only rarely appeared and was overlooked in favor of skills training.

Third-party payors took the experimenters and clinicians who were involved in skills training at their own word, concluding they were not treatment per se, and excluded such approaches from insurance reimbursement. With a few notable exceptions (see, for example, chapter 11), it remained for the emergence of organized health settings, and particularly capitated ones, before there was a widespread use of these kinds of groups which, once in an organized behavioral health care setting, began very quickly to be known as psychoeducational programs.

The Influence of Organized Settings

It is not surprising that, given the rapid development of protocols for individual psychotherapy, there is a decided movement toward the rapid development of group protocols. There is a new definition of group cohesion, for now groups are being formed in direct response to patients suffering from a specific psychological or medical condition, including severe mental illness and chronic physical disease. Programs addressing chronic populations have been especially useful and popular in the emerging integration of behavioral health and primary care.

Currently there are available over 200 psychoeducational programs targeting specific populations. Examples range from survivors of incest to bipolar disorder, and from hypertension to rheumatoid arthritis. Unfortunately, only a few are the results of either empirical research or clinical demonstrations. Many seem to resemble pop psychology, while others have been subjected to rigorous study. In the future, only the latter will be part of the repertoire of our mental and behavioral care delivery systems. Managed care companies and HMOs have no incentive to finance ineffective therapies in which reliving childhood trauma is supposed to undo adult personality problems (Seligman, 1994), or to subject themselves to malpractice suits resulting from unsound treatment techniques. They do have a need for effective and efficient group therapy protocols, empirically derived.

If some clinically driven organized settings are harbingers, there are drastic changes about to take place in the delivery of behavioral health services. In its seventh year of operation nationally, American Biodyne's mental health and chemical dependency services were only 25% individual psychotherapy; another 25% was time-limited group therapy, while fully 50% were psychoeducational programs emanating from empirically derived protocols. The behavioral care system at the Santa Teresa Kaiser Permanente Medical Center is rapidly approaching a similar experience (see chapter 6).

Research is beginning to demonstrate the optimal number of group sessions for each condition (Budman & Gurman, 1988). The group protocols are as few as 5 sessions and as many as 60, again depending on the specific psychological or medical condition being addressed. Most experienced HMO therapists find a length of 60 sessions excessive, and prefer allowing the one or two patients from each group who could benefit from additional treatment to repeat the series rather than prolong the original series. In addition to parsimony, this also has the advantage of having one or two group members in the new group who are "seasoned" by a previous group experience.

It is difficult, if not impossible, for solo practitioners to attain the critical mass necessary to form a number of specific groups. On the other hand, organized delivery systems such as HMOs and managed care networks can offer a wide array of specific, time-limited groups. There are solo practitioners who specialize in a circumscribed population, such as patients suffering from repressed memories of child abuse or multiple personality disorder, to name only two of the most common. The danger here is the tendency of some such practitioners to overly diagnose the condition that absorbs their interest, and represents the majority of their practice and livelihood. Organized settings, having the capacity to address the universe of psychological conditions, have no incentive to overly diagnose certain conditions. One delivery setting has available over 70 specific group protocols (Cummings, 1985b) as covered benefits, making it unnecessary to funnel patients into a small repertoire of special groups.

PSYCHOEDUCATIONAL PROGRAMS

The senior author and his colleagues first began experimenting with psychoeducational programs in the late 1960s and early 1970s at the Kaiser Permanente Health Plan in the San Francisco Bay Area (Cummings & VandenBos, 1981). Those early years required seeking out or developing sophisticated programs, because there was a paucity of information and data. Four highly developed group protocols were available: (1) the agoraphobia desensitization program having wide dissemination throughout the Terrap National Network (Hardy, 1970) and adapted by the authors for their use; (2) a highly successful internally generated program to teach abstinence life-styles to addicts (Cummings, 1979); (3) a relaxation program which was the precursor to a more sophisticated stress management protocol that came later; (4) a smoking cessation program that attracted many referrals, as the Surgeon General had just issued his first warning on smoking.

During the ensuing years, more programs were empirically developed as a result of highly encouraging early determinations of effectiveness. By the early 1980s, there were 68 psychoeducational programs in various stages of development ready to be field tested in the Hawaii Medicaid Project (Cummings et al., 1993; Pallak et al., 1994). The research methodology employed to construct these protocols was the medical cost offset outcome methodology previously and extensively reported (Cummings, 1994). Although efficiency and effectiveness of these programs were demonstrated in Hawaii, these findings were part of an overall evaluation revealing the superiority of a prospectively reimbursed, organized, and focused psychotherapy system over the traditional, disjointed fee-for-service system of local solo practitioners. An additional study was needed which would render a direct comparison between individual therapy effectively delivered as the control group, and a comparable population diverted from individual psychotherapy to specific psychoeducational programs as the experimental group.

Methodology

Two new Biodyne Centers established in the same city in the late 1980s were designated for the study. Center A (experimental) implemented several psychoeducational programs and every patient who presented during two successive periods of 6 months, and who fell into any of five categories, was assigned to the corresponding psychoeducational program. These programs with designated patients were as follows: (1) adult children of alcoholics; (2) agoraphobia and multiple phobias; (3) borderline personality; (4) independent living for chronic schizophrenia; (5) perfectionistic personality life-style.

In center B (control), every patient falling into any of the above five categories was routinely assigned to individual psychotherapy for two successive periods of 6 months each. All of the study patients in both centers were followed for a period of 2 years after their 6 months in treatment. Although there was not a randomized assignment of patients to the control and experimental conditions because this would be tantamount to denying available services in center A, the two groups from the two centers were comparable in all demographic characteristics (age, gender, socioeconomic level, education, ethnicity). Further, this arrangement permitted direct comparison between individual psychotherapy and psychoeducational programs which was not possible within the randomized assignment of patients in the Hawaii Medicaid Project.

As noted, there were two different periods of patient selection of 6 months duration each in both centers. All patients had a 2-year follow-up after the initial 6 months. The total time of experiment was 3 years, but only $2^1/_2$ years for each particular group. Because center A was larger, there were 151 patients in the experimental group, while smaller center B yielded 84 patients for the control group.

Results

The results are shown in Table 17.1, which reveals that for these five categories, the average number of psychoeducational sessions (experimental group) was only two more than the average number of individual sessions in the control group. Not even taking into account the cost differential (individual ratio 1:1 between patients and therapists, psychoeducational 1:8 to 15), this resulted in a 90% reduction in demand for individual therapy, a 95% reduction in hospital days, a 97% reduction in emergency services (including emergency room visits and drop-in sessions), a 70% reduction in prescriptions for medication, and an 85% reduction in return visits.

For illustrative purposes, these findings can be translated into economic terms. Assuming an hour of individual psychotherapy costs $100, the cost of $1^1/_2$ hours of a psychoeducational program per patient would be $150 divided by the

TABLE 17.1

A Comparison in the Use of Various Behavioral Health Services between an Experimental Group Assigned to a Psychoeducational Model, and the Control Group Assigned to the Traditional Model

	N		Group Sessions		Individual Sessions		Hospital Days		Emergency		Perscript		Return Visits	
	Ex	Co	Ex	Co	Ex	Co	Ex	Co	Ex	Co	Ex	Co	Ex	Co
ACOA	38	12	570	46	76	132	1	11	6	8	16	24	53	38
Agoraphobia	23	8	460	0	46	122	14	21	9	37	26	28	38	63
Borderline	42	29	840	109	5	609	3	145	0	289	38	87	22	493
Indep. Living	22	18	422	315	21	72	26	183	4	51	41	68	251	488
Perfectionism	26	17	390	0	24	401	0	19	0	23	14	39	13	208
TOTALS	151	84	2682	480	172	1336	44	379	19	398	135	246	377	1290
MEANS			17.8	5.7	1.2	15.9	0.2	4.5	0.1	4.7	0.9	2.9	2.5	15.4

Legend:
ACOA: Adult Children of Alcoholics 15-session program
Agoraphobia and Multiple Phobias 20-Session program
Borderline Personality Disorder 20-Session program
Independent Living for Chronic Schizophrenics 25-Session program
Perfectionism Leading to Disabling Episodes 15-Session program
Note: Group therapy sessions for the control group were in traditional (i.e., nonpsychoeducational) groups, while group sessions for the experimental group were all in psychoeducational programs.

average patient group of 10, which equals $15 per patient. What is startling, this $15 per patient unit investment then goes on to save between 70 to 97% in hospitalization, individual therapy, emergency room visits, medication prescriptions, and return visits.

Discussion

These results do not indicate that all patients would do better in psychoeducational programs rather than individual therapy. Quite the contrary, what these results reveal is that for certain psychological conditions, a well-designed, empirically derived psychoeducational program may well be the treatment of choice. It must be emphasized that a good psychoeducational protocol is not the product of armchair speculation, but the outcome of fastidious empirical research (see again the description of the research methodology in Cummings [1994]).

Case Illustration

Loni was a 38-year old married mother of three children. Her husband was a highly paid vice-president for a large corporation, while she ran a successful financial planning business out of her home. She delighted in her three beautiful children who were excelling in school, her attentive executive husband, and a business that allowed her to set her own hours. Her large home in exurbia reflected a high degree of success and her excellent taste. She could not understand why every $1^1/2$ to 2 years she would be unable to cope and would need psychotherapy.

The first breakdown came in college when Loni was unable to turn in her term papers and other homework assignments because she saw her work as inadequate. She became suicidal and was successfully treated in the university counseling center. Since that time, she experienced 11 more episodes, approximately $1^1/2$ to 2 years apart, necessitating treatment which was always effective within 2 to 4 months. These episodes were typically bouts of severe depression, or disabling obsessive-compulsive symptoms. Twice she became agoraphobic, and struggled to leave the house.

Loni was a perfectionist, the perfect daughter of a perfectionistic father. When she became dysfunctional again at age 38, instead of treating her depression, she was referred to the Perfectionistic Lifestyle Group. Highly resistant at first, she quickly took hold and by the 15th and last session, she had drastically altered her life-style. She no longer subjected herself to unattainable standards, and her husband's perfectionistic demands, which sometimes seemed to replicate those of her deceased father, no longer bothered her. She became more relaxed with her three children, and especially toward the daughter she heretofore was certain "would turn out neurotic like me." As of this writing, it is over 5 years since her last recurring episode.

CHARACTERISTICS AND UTILITY OF
PSYCHOEDUCATIONAL MODELS

Psychoeducational programs serve three functions with varying degrees among the various programs as to which is the primary function in a specific model: treatment, prevention, and management.

Treatment

The surprising feature of psychoeducation is that it can be therapeutic, and for some conditions, more effective than traditional modes. Our preliminary results indicate that the greatest therapeutic effect is most likely to be with life-styles which reflect the patient's overscrupulousness: perfectionists, agoraphobics, adult children of alcoholics, and other conditions in which the patient suffers from overbearing neurotic guilt. These patients keep their appointments, engage themselves attentively, respect the authority of the professional, and always do their homework.

A lesser therapeutic effect is seen in personality disorders, such as borderline personalities, addicts, and other patients who are rebellious, challenge authority, are likely to thwart appointments, and avoid homework assignments. These are the patients who do not suffer from direct feelings of guilt, and their main distress is the result of their own chaotic life-styles. It is important that personality disorders not be placed in groups where the patients are neurotically guilt-ridden, as they will literally wreck the group and drive the other program participants to despair. This often happens because personality disorders can become depressed, phobic, or anxious, while borderline patients can mimic just about any psychological condition. The primary diagnosis of personality disorder must prevail over the dual diagnosis reflecting the secondary condition.

In chronic physical conditions such as asthma, emphysema, diabetes, rheumatoid arthritis, essential hypertension, and other diseases, the goal is not to cure that which cannot be cured. This does not mean that reduction in pain and morbidity are not in themselves therapeutic; the emphasis, however, is in disease management.

Management

It is precisely with these kinds of intractable conditions, both medical and psychological, that management is important. In the psychological conditions (e.g., borderline personalities, addicts, chronic schizophrenics, impulse disorders, and most "Axis II" patients), every practitioner is painfully aware of the constant, clawing demands and acting out that are so characteristic. Yet these patients, including the borderline personality, become manageable and less vulnerable to the consequences of their own emotional lability, constant rage, and impulsiveness. (For a full description of the borderline protocol, see Cummings & Sayama [1995, pp. 241–248]).

The independent living programs are conducted in various critical places in the environment, and teach chronic schizophrenics how to accomplish such frightening tasks as purchasing underwear, ordering a meal, or buying a bus ticket without being overcome with psychotic anxiety. Although the psychotic thought disorder is incurable, the patient suffers fewer and fewer "crises" which provoke acute exacerbations of the kinds of ideation and behavior which result in restraint and hospitalization.

With chronic medical diseases, psychoeducational programs can increase coping, especially regarding the management of pain and physical limitations, as well as enhance compliance with the medical regimen.

Prevention

The remarkable finding is that for appropriate patients assigned to appropriate psychoeducational programs, the demand for more intrusive services is significantly, if not dramatically, diminished. This is true prevention: services are no longer needed (i.e., the "demand" side in health economics), as contrasted with reducing services as found in most cost-containment (i.e., the "supply" side in health economics). Those patients who are prone to abuse hospitalization or emergency rooms by threatening suicide, such as borderline personalities, learn to manage their lives without such drastic recourse. Chronic schizophrenics who require frequent and sometimes protracted hospitalizations, learn to avoid the exacerbations which trigger this need for hospitalization or restraint by medication.

Reducing costs by reducing demand is certainly more desirable than rationing care, and is the very essence of both prevention and cost-containment. In fact, the impetus for developing the independent living programs was a direct result of the discovery that the first capitated behavioral health Medicare contract of 140,000 covered lives, along with the elderly, had 8,000 persons in their thirties who were on social security by virtue of disabling mental illness. Their average hospitalization rate of nearly 50 days a year could have bankrupted the coverage for the entire cohort of which the vast majority were elderly social security recipients. A series of independent living programs rescued the entire contracted system by drastically reducing the need for hospitalization (Cummings, in press).

Hospital days utilized can also be reduced in populations suffering from chronic medical conditions, along with significant reduction in emergency room visits and invasive procedures (Mumford, Schlesinger, & Glass, 1982; Schlesinger et al., 1983).

ELEMENTS OF PSYCHOEDUCATIONAL PROTOCOLS

There are a number of elements that psychoeducational programs have in common, although not every protocol will contain each and every one of the following:

An *Educational Component* from which the patient learns a great deal about the medical or psychological condition, as well as the interplay between one's body and emotions.

Pain Management for those populations suffering from chronic pain. This includes help in reducing undue reliance on pain medication and addressing any problems of iatrogenic addiction.

Relaxation Techniques, which include meditation and guided imagery.

Stress Management, adjusted to meet the needs of specific conditions and populations.

A *Support System* which includes not only the group milieu, but also the presence of "veterans" who have been through the program. A useful modification of this element is the pairing of patients into a "buddy system" that allows them to call each other, meet for desensitization or other homework, and generally be there for each other in time of need.

A *Self-Evaluation* component which not only enables the patient to assess how well he or she is doing psychologically, but also teaches the patient to monitor such critical features as blood pressure, diet, insulin, and other signs important in chronic illness.

Homework is assigned after every session. The homework is carefully designed to move the patient to the next step of self-mastery, and may include desensitization, behavioral exercises, planned encounters with one's relationships or environment, readings, and other assignments which are critical to the well-being of the patient. The homework is never perfunctory. It is always relevant to the condition being treated and well timed to enhance development.

Timing, Length, and Number of Sessions vary from protocol to protocol, reflecting the needs of each population or condition, and in accordance with research and experience.

Treatment of Depression for those patients whose severely altered mood is interfering with their ability to participate in the program.

Self-Efficacy (after Bandura, 1977a) refers to the belief that one can perform a specific action or complete a task. Although this involves self-confidence in general, it is the confidence to perform a specific task. Positive changes can be traced to an increase in self-efficacy brought about by a carefully designed protocol that will advance the sense of self-efficacy.

Learned Helplessness (after Seligman, 1975) is a concept that holds helplessness is learned and can be unlearned. Some patients with chronic illnesses fall into a state of feeling helpless in the face of their disease. A well-designed protocol will enable a patient to confront and unlearn helplessness.

A *Sense of Coherence* (after Antonovsky, 1987) is required for a person to make sense out of adversity. Patients with chronic physical or mental illnesses feel not only that their circumstances do not make sense, but neither does their life. The ability to cope often depends on the presence or absence of this sense of coherence, and the protocol should be designed to enhance it.

Exercise is an essential component of every protocol, and is the feature that is most often neglected by patients. Exercise helps ameliorate depression, raises the sense of self-efficacy, and promotes coping behavior. The patient should be encouraged to plan and implement his or her own exercise regimen, and then to stick to it.

Modular Formatting enables a protocol to serve different but similar populations and conditions by inserting or substituting condition-specific modules. An example of this is the chronic illness self-help program discussed below.

PSYCHOEDUCATIONAL PROTOCOLS

As of this writing the senior author has identified approximately 200 psychoeducational–psychotherapeutic protocols, many of which have an impressive empirical base (Beck, Steer, & Garbin, 1988), while others reflect extensive clinical experience and judgment (Beckfield, 1994). Some are proprietary and for sale, while still others are in the public domain even though they may be in use within specific settings (see chapter 6; Cummings & Sayama, 1995).

Two examples will be discussed. The first illustrates the modular format whereby mixing and matching one basic protocol serves a number of chronic diseases. It is based on the Arthritis Self-Help Course first developed by Lorig in 1978, and subjected to considerable later research and experience (Lorig & Fries, 1990). It was extensively utilized in the 7-year Hawaii Medicaid Project (Cummings et al., 1993) and subsequently within the American Biodyne behavioral care system nationwide.

The second example is illustrative of a single-purpose, but highly effective, bereavement program for widowed older adults that was developed and subjected to research verification in a cohort of 140,000 managed Medicare recipients in Florida (Cummings, in press).

The Chronic Disease Self-Help Program

Target Population:	Adults suffering from asthma, emphysema, diabetes, ischemic heart disease, hypertension, rheumatoid arthritis.
Sessions:	8 2-hour sessions spaced as follows: six weekly sessions followed by two monthly sessions.
Group Members:	8 to 10 adults in each group, with each group limited to one medical condition.
Specific Education:	There is one educational module for each of the six conditions, and the appropriate module is inserted for each group. Each patient learns a great deal about his or her medical condition. Although comprehensive, it is presented simply and with clarity.
General Education:	This educational component imparts knowledge as to how emotions and stress affect the body, and what kinds of psychological factors exacerbate a physical condition or act as triggers for relapse.
Self-Evaluation:	Patients are taught and encouraged to monitor their own important signs and

	their own medication. Each monitors his or her pertinent signs (e.g., blood pressure, blood sugar, etc.).
Exercise:	Exercise is mandatory and tailored to the patient's condition. Each patient is encouraged to design and implement his or her own exercise program and to stick to it.
Pain Management:	Extensive use is made of the best of pain management techniques, along with
Relaxation:	Relaxation techniques, guided imagery, meditation, and stress management.
Readings:	Self-help books on both the medical condition and psychological factors are assigned throughout the program. Patients are encouraged to discuss how what they read applies to themselves.
Support System:	The group is structured to be highly supportive. In addition, the patients are paired into a "buddy system" and encouraged to meet during the week, do their homework together, and practice their exercises together.
Homework:	Homework is given at the end of each session. There are two types: general homework which addresses common problems, and special homework designed to help the patient with difficult problems.
Self-Efficacy:	Much of the content and homework of the program is designed to restore confidence in performing specific tasks originally restricted by the patient's physical limitations, increasing coping behavior by reducing the sense of helplessness, and restoring the sense of meaning to life in spite of one's circumstances.

| Depression: | Patients who are suffering from clinical depression of the magnitude that prevents full participation in the program are referred for treatment of that severe mood disorder. After the depression has improved sufficiently, the patient may undertake the program. Since some degree of depression may accompany many patients with chronic medical conditions, it has been found that the milder depressions are best treated within the program. |

The Bereavement Program for Widowed Older Adults

Target Population:	Widowed older adults (over 62) who have recently lost a spouse, usually after many years of marriage.
Outreach:	An aggressive outreach program within the health plan identifies the patient shortly after the death of a spouse. Empathic telephone contact invites the individual to the first session only.
Sessions:	Total of 14 sessions of 2 hours each, and spaced as follows: four semiweekly sessions, followed by six weekly sessions, and concluding with four monthly sessions.
Group Members:	At least five and not more than eight patients are assigned to each group. An even number is desirable as the patients are paired in a "buddy" support system.
Screening:	In addition to the usual bonding, the first session is used to screen out patients who reveal severe depression rather than uncomplicated mourning.

Reactive depression reflecting internalized rage for years of marital unhappiness interferes with the healing process of mourning and is treated separately.

Medication:
Patients are helped to use antidepressants sparingly or not at all. These medications retard the process of healing and prolong and even postpone bereavement.

Education:
The patient learns a great deal about the process of mourning and its painful, but healing sequence. The grieving person is encouraged to cry, is given permission to spend a lot of time alone inspite of well-meaning friends, and rewarded for reflecting on a lifetime with the deceased, recalling all the good and bad moments. It is normal to miss the deceased very much!

Self-Efficacy:
The patient learns to cope with being alone, and if the widowed patient was unduly dependent on the deceased in certain matters (finances, initiative, etc.) he or she is taught to unlearn the helplessness.

Support System:
The pairing into a buddy system is particularly important for these patients who at times would rather be with someone who is also mourning than to be with well-meaning friends who often do not know what to say. The patient is also taught how to make friends more comfortable by releasing them from their self-imposed duty to make the mourner feel better. This results in making it possible for patient and friends to comfortably spend more time with each other.

The Veteran:	One or two patients who complete each group need additional support and wish to go on to a second group. They are encouraged to do so. Additionally, the presence of one or two "veterans" in each group is additional help and support to the newer patients. Their ability to say, "I remember when I felt exactly as you do, and this is what I did," is of inestimable value.
Homework:	Since these patients spend a lot of time alone, appropriate reading assignments are welcomed. Not as welcomed is the homework to exercise, and they often must be cajoled into getting out and doing brisk walking. Once they try it, however, they feel so much better that they become fairly consistent in exercising. Mall walking early in the morning is a common older adult activity, so these patients do not feel out of place engaging in that form of exercise.

At the appropriate time homework involving a *moderate* amount of social activity is assigned. This must be carefully tailored to the needs and abilities of each individual.

SUMMARY AND CONCLUSIONS

Several historical movements have converged to make the current interest in psychoeducational programs possible. The development of brief psychotherapy, the emergence of time-limited group psychotherapy, and decades of research in skills training all joined with the rapid emergence of organized settings where the critical mass existed, and the need in primary care was apparent.

Over 25 years of research in three disparate prepaid, organized health settings have demonstrated that selected psychological conditions respond well to empirically derived psychoeducation programs, and for these patients such programs are the treatment of choice over individual psychotherapy or more traditional group psychotherapy. The programs are directed toward faulty life-styles and do not replace the need for either individual or group psychotherapy. These psychoeducational programs are utilitarian in that they accomplish treatment, patient management, and prevention of future need, with varying degrees among the various programs. Finally, psychoeducational programs yield true cost-containment by reducing the need for more costly and intrusive services, such as individual therapy, hospitalization, emergency services, medication, and return visits. Rationing of care is thus avoided.

Although psychoeducation will never fully replace individual psychotherapy, years of experience with health delivery would predict the following proportions of psychotherapeutic services in the not too distant future: 25% individual psychotherapy, 25% time-limited group psychotherapy, and as much as 50% psychoeducational programs (Cummings, 1996c). Several health care settings are already reflecting this configuration.

18.

Holistic and Alternative Medicine: Separating the Wheat from the Chaff

Janet L. Cummings, Psy.D.,
Nicholas A. Cummings, Ph.D., Sc.D.

Because of advances in modern medicine during the 20th century, homeopathic and naturopathic medicine had nearly vanished in the United States. However, the past few decades have seen a revival of these and other alternative medical treatments. It is currently estimated that Americans make 425 million visits per year to homeopaths, massage therapists, herbalists, and other alternative practitioners (Griffin, 1996), spending about $13.7 billion per year on these alternative treatments (Langone, 1996). The American consumer expects modern medicine to be able to cure every ailment and alleviate every pain, and when it does not he or she often turns to holistic and alternative techniques such as colonic irrigation, meditation, hypnotherapy, aroma therapy, various forms of massage, and herbal remedies.

The recent revival of holistic and alternative treatments has many primary care physicians (PCPs) nervous, especially because of the large number of fads and cults available to the public in the name of health care. Most of the techniques remain unverified, and their proponents often rely on charismatic gurus and testimonials from the "cured" to lure the public.

Certain persons are particularly vulnerable to these fads and the allure of charismatic gurus. Persons with thought disorders, for example, often cling to fads or cults in an attempt to gain control over their thought disorders (Cummings & Sayama, 1995). When one fad no longer gives ample control over the thought disorder, the individual will often abandon that fad in favor of whatever new movement is on the horizon. Although this strategy for controlling a thought disorder eventually stops working, individuals with thought disorders meanwhile flock to fads and cults of various sorts. Even though not everyone who follows the latest fads has a thought disorder, those with thought disorders are particularly vulnerable to fads and likely to become involved in those with no scientific validity whatsoever.

Persons with somatization disorders are also vulnerable to health care cults and fads. For such persons, the attention given to them as one of the "cured" may be alluring enough that they are willing to trade in their psychologically induced symptoms for the chance to give testimonials before audiences of others wanting to be healed. These persons provide anecdotal, although not scientific, evidence of the effectiveness of these health care fads.

If alternative medical treatments were simply of no effect, PCPs would have little reason to be nervous about them. However, some of these treatments are not only ineffective, but dangerous. Griffin (1996) cites some examples of these dangers:

1. The FDA lists nine herbs sometimes used in holistic treatments which can cause serious problems such as kidney failure and stroke.
2. Some nutritional supplements, including fat-soluble vitamins, minerals such as iron, and niacin, can be toxic in large doses.

3. Colonics can be dangerous in that they may deplete necessary electrolytes.
4. Treatments involving intense heat may be dangerous to pregnant women, young children, the elderly, and people with high blood pressure or heart disease; they may also exacerbate circulatory problems in diabetics.

Perhaps more dangerous than these direct effects is an indirect effect of alternative treatments. The promises made by proponents of these techniques for cures without medication side effects or the pain of surgery may keep patients from getting medical treatments which have been proven effective in treating their conditions.

Despite the dangers inherent to some alternative treatments and the danger of relying on unvalidated techniques while rejecting validated ones, many alternative treatments have merit, especially when used as adjuncts to traditional medical treatments. It is the purpose of this chapter to discuss the effects of belief on illness, to outline some examples of validated alternative techniques, and to provide an in-depth example of an incurable illness which can be most effectively managed with a combination of traditional medical and alternative techniques.

THE PLACEBO EFFECT AND THE IMPORTANCE OF BELIEF

Freud discovered that patients often feel better with catharsis, but that the effect of catharsis is not always long-lasting. Temporary relief from stress is not the same as a cure, and it is important to distinguish between temporary relief or "feeling better" and actual changes in disease states.

The early history of medicine may actually be research on the placebo effect, as treatments such as lizard's blood, crushed insects, leeches, blood letting, and blistering were reported to effectively treat diseases (Kemeny, 1996b). These substances and practices probably did no more than to create the expectation of a cure.

The placebo effect has been well-documented and well-known since Beecher (1955) published his classic article, "The Powerful Placebo." Since that time, the placebo effect has been generally accepted by health care practitioners and the magnitude of the placebo effect has been generally accepted as about 35%.

Placebos may be used deliberately when a practitioner knows there is no pharmacological or other physiological basis for a treatment but hopes the patient will improve simply because of his or her belief in the treatment. Placebos may also be used unintentionally when a practitioner believes that a treatment is effective even though it does not act upon the disease (Kemeny, 1996b).

The incidence of placebo response generally varies from 10 to 70%, with symptom relief sometimes as high as 100%. The average placebo response across a number of studies of a number of diseases is 35% (Beecher, 1955; Kemeny, 1996b). Some diseases are more influenced by placebos than others (Kemeny, 1996b; A. K. Shapiro & Morris, 1978). In cases of severe pain, placebo can be up to 50% as effective as an injection of morphine and has been shown to cause endorphin release. Placebo has been shown to heal gastric ulcers in 40 to 70% of gastric ulcer patients and to be 50 to 75% effective in stopping acute upper gastrointestinal bleeding. Angina is 30 to 40% responsive to placebo treatment and about 40% responsive to mock surgery. Rheumatoid arthritis benefits about 80% by placebo, and about 85% of high blood pressure patients will show significant drop in blood pressure with placebo alone (Kemeny, 1996b).

Surprisingly, the best predictor of the magnitude of a placebo effect is the provider of the treatment rather than the treatment itself, and the relationship between the practitioner and the patient is crucial (Kemeny, 1996b; Shapiro & Morris, 1978). The more the practitioner believes the treatment will work the better he or she is able to instill that belief in the patient. If the practitioner is enthusiastic, optimistic, warm, and caring, the effectiveness of the placebo is markedly increased. Perhaps the charisma and enthusiasm of some of the alternative therapy gurus, along with the personal attention they give their followers, can explain their ability to "cure" some patients with techniques which in and of themselves have no ability to heal. Furthermore, group healing ceremonies performed by shamans and other faith healers serve to heighten the patient's arousal and build the expectation of healing, thus maximizing the placebo effect.

The situation which surrounds the use of a placebo also impacts the effectiveness of the placebo (Kemeny, 1996b; Shapiro & Morris, 1978). The practitioner who conveys the image of being an expert authority by wearing a white coat and having modern-looking medical equipment displayed in the office elicits a greater placebo response than the practitioner who appears informal and less "professional." Not surprisingly, doctors generally get a higher placebo response than nurses do when administering the same placebo for the same condition.

The appearance of the placebo itself can affect its usefulness (Kemeny, 1996b; Shapiro & Morris, 1978). The more the placebo looks and tastes like real medicine the greater the healing effect. Furthermore, a mild active substance which produces some transient feeling of internal change will have a greater placebo effect than a completely inert substance. For instance, a pill which does nothing other than produce mild nausea will have a greater placebo effect than a pill which does nothing at all.

Medical practitioners using even the most advanced medical techniques can take advantage of the placebo effect and utilize it to increase their patients' responses to their treatments. By appearing as "professional" as possible, by conveying belief in the treatment's effectiveness, and by demonstrating care and concern for the patient, practitioners can give their patients the best chance possible of responding well to appropriate treatments. A number of studies of a number of conditions and treatments demonstrate that patients improve more when medical professionals appear both to believe in the treatment and care about the patients (O'Brien, 1996).

K. H. Cooper (1995) cites a number of well-controlled scientific studies which demonstrate the benefits of spiritual beliefs on health. In asserting that spirituality can positively impact health, Cooper distinguishes between *extrinsic* belief (such as membership in a particular religious organization, rote recitation of a liturgy, or intellectual affirmation of a set of beliefs) and *intrinsic* belief (as evidenced by profound spiritual commitment, devotion to a transformed life, and heartfelt prayer). He further defines intrinsic belief in terms of two key elements: (1) a leap of faith initiating a life-changing belief, and (2) the belief that the body's ability to be healthy grows gradually with personal discipline.

Cooper (1995) lists six characteristics of persons who demonstrate positive health benefits from their spiritual belief:

1. They believe that their bodies are good and worthy of being treated as a creation of God.
2. They believe they have a personal responsibility to help *prevent* the onset of disease.
3. They believe they possess a natural inner power to promote the healing of disease.
4. They are open to receiving spiritual support from others.
5. They have a relatively firm and stable philosophy of life.
6. They are willing to stay committed to a personal fitness program, despite the changes and new findings that regularly occur in the scientific research.

Those individuals who experience the healing power of their spiritual beliefs, therefore, are those who take an active role in maintaining good health rather than those who passively wait for a higher power to heal them. Their health cannot be attributed to the placebo effect alone, but to the active role they take in their own healthy life-styles, as well.

The studies which Cooper (1995) cites demonstrate the positive health benefits of *intrinsic* belief. These benefits include: decreased depression, less smoking, less alcohol abuse, fewer medical complications in maternity patients and their newborns, decreased incidence of colon and rectal cancer, improved coping with breast cancer, higher self-esteem and emotional maturity, reduced levels of stress, lower blood pressure, increased survival following a heart attack, and greater ability to maintain healthy eating habits and overcome obesity.

Peterson and Bossio (1993) see optimism as contributory to good health. They define optimists as active participants in their own health who believe that their expectations impact their health. Therefore, these optimists take concrete steps to improve their own health as a result of their expectations. Peterson and Bossio cite longitudinal and experimental research demonstrating that people with this type of optimistic attitude are healthier overall.

Ninety-nine percent of physicians assert that belief heals, and Benson and Stuart (1992) see healing as a three-legged stool which includes medicine, surgery, and belief. They define belief in terms of the patient's taking responsibility for his or her own health. According to Benson and Stuart, a balance of medicine, surgery, and belief is necessary for the treatment of disease and maintenance of optimal health.

Practitioners who utilize only unvalidated techniques which rely on placebo or belief alone often do a terrible disservice to their patients by denying them the healing which modern medicine and surgery afford. On the other hand, practitioners who fail to understand the power of patients' beliefs rob their patients of this healing force. While it may be unethical for health care professionals to advocate particular unvalidated alternative techniques or to impose their religious–spiritual beliefs on their patients, they would do well to encourage patients to develop their own belief systems and to use whatever religious–spiritual beliefs they have in the service of good health while continuing to seek the most up-to-date medical care available.

The exception to the physician's insistence on verified alternative treatments may be seen in the approach to the dying patient. Such patients for whom surgery, radiation, chemotherapy, or other drastic treatments have failed, who are awaiting imminent death, may be comforted by the belief that an alternative technique, such as a certain combination of herbs, will accomplish what the intensive medical treatments failed to do. This may be part of nature's way of helping the patient remain optimistic while dying, and it would be unfortunate for the physician to insist on scientific validity in the face of the patient's need for optimism.

BEYOND BELIEF TO VALIDATED ALTERNATIVE TREATMENTS

Although many alternative treatments work simply because of their placebo effect, others have been scientifically validated for use with particular conditions. Those treatments with empirical evidence can be of particular use as adjuncts to traditional medical treatments, although most holistic and alternative medical techniques have yet to be validated and most of the field of alternative medicine remains unverified.

Although it would be impossible to address every available holistic or alternative treatment individually, a selection of treatments which have been validated for certain conditions will be offered as examples in the remainder of this section.

Nutrition

A high-fat diet is associated with susceptibility to certain cancers, particularly breast, colon, and prostate (Kemeny, 1996a; Gershwin et al., 1985). Although these cancers certainly have other risk factors (such as family history) associated with them, diet is one risk factor which falls within individual control.

Nicholson (1996), for example, reports that the risk for breast cancer drops significantly in women who consume 30% or fewer of their daily calories from fat. He also reports that breast cancer is nearly unheard of in women who consume 10% or fewer of their daily calories from fat.

Nicholson (1996) offers scientific evidence that substances found in certain plant foods also serve to reduce breast cancer risk. These substances include fiber, indoles, flavonols, vitamins C and E, beta carotene, and selenium. According to Kemeny (1996a) and Gershwin et al. (1985), sufficient intake of vitamin A lowers the risk for lung and other cancers. Vitamin C intake of more than 60 mg per day is associated with lower rates of stomach, esophageal, pancreatic, breast, cervical, and lung cancers. Vitamin E is also associated with reduced risk for cancer. Iodine deficiency is closely associated with cancer of the thyroid. Selenium (a trace mineral) protects against colon, rectal, pancreatic, breast, and prostate cancers; it may also protect against cardiomyopathy and other cardiovascular diseases (Badmaev, Majeed, & Passwater, 1996).

Soffa (1996) offers some preliminary evidence, although still experimental, that menopausal symptoms in some women can be effectively treated via nutrition without the need for estrogen replacement therapy. For example, hot flashes can be reduced by avoiding caffeine, alcohol, spicy foods, carbonated beverages, and excess sugar. Thus, such holistic treatment may be able to control menopausal symptoms without the increased risk for breast cancer associated with estrogen replacement therapy.

Although a low-fat, high-fiber, vitamin-rich diet alone is unlikely to cure existing cancer, it certainly can substantially lower the risk for new cancers. Even though surgery, radiation, chemotherapy, and other advanced medical techniques may be necessary to treat existing cancers, a healthy diet can provide better prevention for cancer than anything else modern medicine has to offer.

Exercise

Exercise can diminish certain types of pain by strengthening muscles, increasing endurance, releasing endorphins, and giving a sense of control over the pain (Kemeny, 1996b). For example, O'Koon and Morrow (1995) report that regular exercise relieves general body pain as well as specific joint pain in arthritis patients. It also strengthens the muscles and other structures around individual joints, which provides stability to the joints and relieves pain. It helps keep bones and cartilage strong, which in turn lessens arthritic pain.

Regular aerobic exercise can help relieve symptoms of depression in patients with minor depression, major depression, and premenstrual depression (Byrne & Byrne, 1993; Sachs, 1993). It likely releases endorphins and norepinephrine, and gives a sense of accomplishment and mastery to the patient (Kemeny, 1996b). Aerobic exercise can also serve to lessen symptoms of anxiety, perhaps by reducing excess levels of blood glucose, epinephrine, and oxygen (Byrne & Byrne, 1993; Hardy, 1970).

Although exercise alone may not relieve the pain of arthritis completely, it certainly can lessen the pain and reduce the need for analgesic medication in many patients. Even though exercise alone may not cure severe depression or anxiety, it can relieve minor cases of depression and anxiety without the use of psychotropic medications. In more severe cases, it can serve as a very helpful adjunct to pharmacologic and psychotherapeutic treatments.

Regular exercise provides a buffer against stress and helps prevent stress-related illnesses such as high blood pressure. However, it is unclear whether it helps prevent illness through its physical effects, psychological effects, or both. Also, it may be that people who exercise regularly are less likely to adopt unhealthy ways of coping with stress, such as smoking, overeating, and alcohol abuse (Sachs, 1993).

Although excessive exercise can actually decrease the functioning of the immune system, regular moderate exercise has been shown to increase immune cells for a period of time after each episode of exercise. However, it is unknown whether or not this increase is large enough and long-lasting enough to significantly increase the body's ability to fight infectious diseases (Sachs, 1993).

Massage Therapy

According to O'Koon and Morrow (1995), the kneading motion of muscle massage relieves arthritic pain by bringing warmth to the affected areas via increased blood circulation. It also can smooth out muscle knots and help joints attain their full range of motion. Massage has been scientifically demonstrated to lessen pain in children with rheumatoid arthritis or burns and in adults with fibromyalgia, perhaps because it raises levels of natural pain killers, or enkaphalins (Griffin & Gallagher, 1995).

Massage can shorten the time it takes for the body to recover from strenuous exercise. The pressure and warmth associated with massage cause the cells to release histamine. Histamine prompts the nearby capillaries to dilate, which increases blood circulation to the muscles. Therefore, the muscles receive more oxygen and nutrients, and metabolic wastes and toxins are removed more quickly (Griffin & Gallagher, 1995).

Because massage switches off the sympathetic nervous system, it has a calming effect on the body. Therefore, people who receive massages have an easier time falling asleep. Research has shown that fussy babies, restless children, adults under stress, and adults with chronic fatigue syndrome all sleep better after a massage (Griffin & Gallagher, 1995).

It is possible that massage therapy can help ward off colds and other viruses. There is strong scientific evidence showing that massage increases both the number and activity of certain immune cells called natural killer cells. This increase in immune functioning is likely due to the reduced levels of the stress hormones cortisol and norepinephrine brought about by massage (Griffin & Gallagher, 1995; Kemeny, 1996a, 1996b). However, even though these measurable changes in the immune system occur, it is not yet known whether or not these changes are large enough or long-lasting enough to actually increase resistance to viruses (Kemeny, 1996a, 1996b).

Massage therapy does not have to be expensive. Massages given by volunteers, such as parents to children or spouses to one another, can yield the same results as those given by trained professionals (Griffin & Gallagher, 1995).

Acupuncture

Although acupuncture was developed in China approximately 5,000 years ago, it is estimated that 9 to 12 million treatments are performed in the United States each year, accounting for about $500 million annually in health care expenses (Harvard Medical School, 1995). Acupuncture has been used to treat a large number of illnesses, including allergies, anxiety, arthritis, asthma, back pain, digestive problems, dizziness, fatigue, headaches, high blood pressure, neck pain, premenstrual syndrome, sciatica, sexual dysfunction, stress, tendinitis, urinary tract problems, viral infections, and vision problems (Harvard Medical School, 1995).

However, only a few of these uses have been scientifically validated in controlled studies (Harvard Medical School, 1995). In these studies, subjects have been randomly assigned to a treatment group (which received acupuncture) or to a control group (which received "sham acupuncture," or a procedure resembling acupuncture in every respect except that the needles were inserted in the wrong places) (Harvard Medical School, 1995).

These studies have demonstrated that acupuncture has significant effects in treating the following four conditions (Harvard Medical School, 1995):

1. *Menstrual cramps.* Nine months after treatment, subjects in the treatment group showed 91% reduction in symptoms, whereas control subjects showed only 40% reduction.
2. *Chronic low back pain.* In one study, 81% of treatment subjects and 31% of control subjects showed improvement one month after treatment. Nine months later, 53% of treatment subjects and no control subjects reported significant pain relief.
3. *Neck pain.* 80% of treatment subjects and 13% of control subjects demonstrated significant improvement 12 weeks following treatment.
4. *Alcohol abuse.* Several studies demonstrate that treatment subjects have fewer drinking episodes and hospital detoxification than the control subjects.

Research shows that acupuncture triggers the release of chemicals with pain-relieving properties (enkephalins and endorphins). It may also trigger the release of the neurotransmitter serotonin, which is associated with decreased depression (Harvard Medical School, 1995). In addition, acupuncture may stimulate nerves in a way that they sense the presence of the needle rather than the presence of pain (O'Koon & Morrow, 1995).

Relaxation, Hypnosis, Guided Imagery, and Meditation

These techniques have the following three features in common:

1. They shut down the activity of the sympathetic nervous system, decrease the stress response, and create a state of relaxation.
2. They create a distraction from pain, focusing the attention on pleasant images instead of on the pain.
3. They have been demonstrated to boost the immune system by increasing both the number and activity of natural killer cells. However, it is not known whether or not these changes in the immune system are large enough or long-lasting enough to reduce susceptibility to infectious diseases (Kemeny, 1996a, 1996b).

These techniques do help patients manage chronic pain by relaxing the painful areas and by creating a pleasant distraction from the pain (O'Koon & Morrow, 1995). However, they do not cure pain. The exercises must be repeated on a regular basis in order to remain effective.

These techniques are also useful in the management of anxiety, including panic disorder and generalized anxiety disorder. With continued practice of these techniques, patients become more adept at diminishing the stress response and creating a state of relaxation. Even though these techniques must be practiced regularly for a period of time in order for anxious patients to learn to use them proficiently, the learning that occurs eventually allows patients to relax themselves quickly without performing the complete exercise (Hardy, 1970).

Biofeedback

This technique involves teaching the patient to relax by controlling his or her body's reactions to pain and stress. Special monitoring equipment attached to the body measures heart rate, blood pressure, galvanic skin response (GSR), temperature, and muscle tension. Using this feedback, a trained professional helps the patient learn to gain control over these physical responses (O'Koon & Morrow, 1995).

Schwartz and Schwartz (1993) outline five types of biofeedback and their uses:

1. Electromyographic (EMG) biofeedback measures muscle tension and is used for tension headaches, physical rehabilitation, chronic muscle pain, incontinence, temporomandibular joint (TMJ) pain, and general relaxation.
2. Thermal biofeedback, which measures skin temperature, is used for Raynaud's disease, migraines, hypertension, anxiety, and general relaxation.
3. Electrodermal activity (EDA) measures very minute changes in sweat activity and is used for anxiety and hyperhidrosis (overactive sweat glands).
4. Finger pulse biofeedback measures pulse rate and force. It is used for hypertension, anxiety, and cardiac arrhythmias.
5. Breathing biofeedback measures breath rate, volume, location, and rhythm. It is used for asthma, hyperventilation, anxiety, and general relaxation.

Some researchers are experimenting with biofeedback for conditions believed to be due to irregular brain wave patterns, including attention deficit hyperactivity disorder (ADHD) and certain types of epilepsy (Schwartz & Schwartz, 1993).

Although most of these uses for biofeedback have been studied scientifically, two uses have been particularly well documented using controlled studies: muscle tension headaches and Raynaud's disease (Schwartz & Schwartz, 1993). Overall, about 50% of tension headache patients improve by 50 to 80% in controlled research studies, with 70% of patients improving by 50 to 85% in biofeedback clinics. Raynaud's disease involves a constriction of blood vessels in the fingers and toes, thus giving the patient the uncomfortable sensation of cold extremities. Controlled studies show that most patients (up to 92%) can reduce their symptoms by at least two-thirds and maintain the benefits on 2-year follow-up.

Social Support

It is generally accepted that thoughts, either positive or negative, can have an impact on physical health for better or for worse (Azur, 1996). The effectiveness of psychoeducational programs in preventing and treating disease has been outlined elsewhere in this volume (see chapter 17). The effectiveness of psychotherapy in treating somatization disorders and in offsetting medical and surgical costs is also well documented (Cummings, 1991a, 1991b, 1993, 1994, 1996a, 1996b; Cummings et al., 1993; Cummings & Follette, 1976; Cummings & VandenBos, 1981; Strain, 1993). However, the impact of support groups and social support in general on disease is also noteworthy.

Spiegel (1993) cites a number of studies which demonstrate the health benefits of social support. For example, one study found that the number of social supports which subjects had could predict the probability of mortality over the next 9 years. Other studies confirm that socially isolated people are two to three times more likely to die during the time of the studies than those who are least socially isolated. Another study shows that married cancer patients have significantly lower mortality rates than unmarried cancer patients, and a number of studies demonstrate that married people are substantially healthier and have lower death rates overall than single, widowed, or divorced persons. In general, social isolation is as strong a risk factor for death as is smoking or high serum cholesterol.

Spiegel (1993) cites several reasons why social support may positively benefit health:

1. Those who believe that others care about them may be more likely to take active steps toward staying healthy.
2. People who interact well with friends and family may also interact well with their health care providers, encouraging their providers to do all possible for them.
3. Social support may directly reduce the levels of stress hormones in the body, thus enhancing the functioning of the immune system.

Spiegel (1993) sees two reasons why support groups may be effective: (1) They counter isolation. (2) They allow people to feel as though they can help each other, which makes them feel competent rather than helpless in the face of their own illness.

Although support groups have been utilized for a number of medical conditions, their usefulness in treating breast cancer patients is particularly well studied. For example, Spiegel (1995) and Spiegel et al. (1989) studied support groups for women with breast cancer which provided a socially supportive environment, encouraged expression of feelings, and encouraged the adoption of new meaning and goals in life. These researchers discovered that women with breast cancer who attended such a support group for breast cancer patients lived twice as long as women with the same illness who did not attend a support group. Patients who attended the support groups showed improved psychological adjustment, better coping skills, better compliance with treatment regimens, and enhanced immunological functioning compared to controls who did not attend a support group (Sleek, 1995).

BLENDING MAINLINE AND ALTERNATIVE MEDICINE: THE TREATMENT OF MITRAL VALVE PROLAPSE AS A COMPREHENSIVE EXAMPLE

Mitral valve prolapse (MVP) is a congenital heart defect which causes a variety of physiological symptoms and seems to predispose the individual to the development of anxiety disorders.

Mitral valve prolapse is usually inherited and present at birth, but can also be caused or worsened later in life by rheumatic fever; it is incurable in the absence of high-risk surgery (Jeresaty, 1984). It is a condition in which the heart mitral valve is too elastic due to a lack of collagen synthesis. The valve consists primarily of procollagen, the chemical precursor of collagen, rather than of collagen (Dean, 1985).

The mitral valve separates the left atrium from the left ventricle. The valve opens to allow blood flow from the atrium to the ventricle and closes to prevent the backflow of blood when the ventricle walls contract to force blood into the aorta and out to the body (Dean, 1985). The elasticity of the prolapsed mitral valve causes some backflow of blood from the left ventricle to the left atrium when most of the blood is being forced into the aorta. Because some blood is backflowing with each heartbeat, a reduced amount of blood is leaving the heart through the aorta to the body. The body compensates by increasing adrenalin secretion to speed up the heart rate, thus ensuring that sufficient blood and oxygen leave the heart and enter the body (Edell, 1987).

Eighty percent or more of mitral valve prolapse patients exhibit some symptoms, including migraines, sweating, tense muscles, stomach cramps or nausea, chest pain, palpitations, breathlessness, and fatigue (Edell, 1987). Some may experience more serious complications, such as arrhythmias severe enough to necessitate drug treatment (Jeresaty, 1985). Mitral valve prolapse seems to predispose patients to the development of anxiety disorders, perhaps because the elevated adrenalin levels prime the system for panic attacks and perhaps because the symptoms which MVP causes, although usually benign, can be frightening to patients.

Although many MVP patients never seek treatment for their symptoms, those that do tend to be high medical utilizers. Because these patients do not understand their symptoms, the symptoms can be quite frightening and prompt repeated visits to physicians and emergency rooms.

Traditional Medical Treatments for MVP

Although pacemakers are used in a few severe cases to control arrhythmias (Campbell, 1982), beta-blockers are commonly prescribed to reduce heart palpitations (Merrill & Swain, 1982). However, these drugs do little to control anxious symptoms (Rosenbaum, 1987). Benzodiazepines are effective in controlling the anxiety associated with MVP, but are being used less and less frequently due to their addictive properties (Rosenbaum, 1987). Tricyclic antidepressants and monoamine oxidase (MAO) inhibitors are commonly used to treat anxiety disorders, whether or not MVP is present (Metcalf, 1989). More recently, serotonin-specific reuptake inhibitors (SSRIs) are being used to treat anxiety symptoms (Kaplan & Sadock, 1993), although these sometimes exacerbate anxiety in MVP patients. However, none of these drugs can be considered a "cure" and symptoms are likely to recur when drug therapy is discontinued (Rosenbaum, 1987). Furthermore, these medications can produce undesirable side effects (Dilsaver, 1989). Therefore, drug therapies may be most useful in conjunction with other treatments, particularly in the initial stages of treatment (Rosenbaum, 1986, 1987).

Surgery is rarely used for cases of congenital MVP, but is sometimes necessary when the prolapse has been caused or exacerbated by rheumatic fever. In these rare cases, the valve may be reconstructed or repaired (Spencer & Colvin, 1985). If repair is impossible, the defective valve may be replaced (Malpartida, Arcas, Alegria, Montral, & Caro, 1980), or the technique of catheter balloon valvuplasty, in which a balloon catheter is used to dilate the mitral valve, may be employed (McKay, Kawanishi, & Rahimtoola, 1987).

Mitral valve prolapse puts an individual at risk for bacterial endocarditis because of the increased turbulence in blood flow within the heart. When bacteria become trapped in turbulent blood movement within the heart, they tend to cling to the mitral valve and infection can result (Edell, 1987). Therefore, it is standard practice to give MVP patients antibiotic prophylaxis during any dental, urologic, or gastrointestinal procedures (Merrill & Swain, 1982).

Alternative Treatments for MVP

Symptoms of MVP can, in most cases, be treated successfully with alternative treatments. These treatments often make continued drug therapy unnecessary, although drugs may be used in conjunction with other interventions in the early stages of treatment. In more severe cases of MVP, continued drug therapy may still be necessary, although alternative treatments may reduce the amount of medication needed (Rosenbaum, 1986, 1987).

Diet. Frederickson (1988) outlines some dietary guidelines for MVP patients. Caffeine should be avoided, because it tends to increase heart rates and stimulates adrenalin secretion. Sugar is also to be avoided, as it stimulates the release of insulin and adrenalin. Mitral valve prolapse patients benefit from a low-fat, low-cholesterol diet, which can help prevent major cardiac problems. Because MVP patients tend to have lower than normal blood pressure and hypovolemia (low blood volume), it is important that they drink large amounts of fluid, do not try to limit their salt intake unless directed to do so by a physician, and avoid the use of diuretics. Mitral valve prolapse patients should generally avoid alcohol, as the rebound phase following initial sedation can cause anxiety in these patients (Schuckit, 1989). Iron and magnesium are particularly important supplements for MVP patients, and phosphates (found in soft drinks) should be avoided because they tend to diminish magnesium levels.

Exercise. Because exercise may bring about chest pain, fatigue, dizziness, and difficulty breathing in MVP patients, many of these patients avoid exercise and are severely deconditioned (Bashore, 1988; Frederickson, 1988). When deconditioning has occurred, MVP patients may experience exertion and uncomfortable symptoms with only small amounts of activity. Many patients mistake the elevated heart rate associated with exercise for panic and avoid exercise for this reason. Therefore, Frederickson (1988) recommends that MVP patients begin at lower levels of exertion and increase their exertion weekly, but never to the point where uncomfortable symptoms result.

Because MVP patients frequently have inflexible joints, their joints are particularly prone to injury (Frederickson, 1988; Dean, 1985). Stretching exercises are therefore recommended as part of the overall exercise program (Frederickson, 1988).

Frederickson (1988) recommends aerobic exercise, during which increased amounts of oxygen are required for prolonged periods of time, but without oxygen supplies becoming totally depleted. This exercise improves the body's ability to move air into and out of the lungs, increases the total volume of blood, and makes the tissues throughout the body better able to utilize oxygen efficiently. Aerobic exercise need not involve jogging, which is often too strenuous for MVP patients, and does not require excessive speed or athletic ability. Mitral valve prolapse patients do not need to work at exercising harder; they benefit from working at exercising longer. Walking, bicycling, and swimming, performed for 20 to 30 minutes at least three times a week, are ideal for MVP patients.

Many mitral valve prolapse patients have quite rapid heart rates, even during rest. Therefore, heart rate alone is a very poor guideline for exercise for MVP patients, as elevated heart rate alone is not sufficient to produce fitness (Frederickson, 1988).

Relaxation Techniques. Various relaxation techniques, including deep muscle relaxation, self-hypnosis, meditation, voluntary control of respiration patterns, and biofeedback are common treatments for the anxious symptoms often associated with mitral valve prolapse (Everly, 1989). These treatments reduce anxious symptoms, help shut down the sympathetic nervous system which is overly active in many MVP patients, and give patients a sense of control or mastery over their condition.

Self-Talk. Mitral valve prolapse symptoms can be terrifying, as they often cause the patient to feel as though he or she is suffocating, having a heart attack, or "going crazy." These fears, in turn, cause excessive and unnecessary anxiety in many patients. Changing the way the MVP patient talks to him or herself when symptoms occur can have tremendous impact on the process.

Anderson (1989) has developed a self-talk treatment system for anxiety disorders which is quite useful for MVP, as well. The patient and the treatment provider should thoroughly assess the anxious symptoms. Respiratory symptoms may include shortness of breath, difficulty breathing, lightheadedness, dizziness, numbness, tingling, sensation of choking, or sensation of a lump in the throat. Cardiac symptoms may include heart pounding or racing, palpitations, chest tightness, or chest pain. Psychological symptoms may include thoughts racing or jumping, depersonalization, or derealization. Other general symptoms may include trembling, shaking, tension, sweating, heat or cold, nausea, or irritability. These symptoms are characteristic of anxiety in general, but are commonly found among MVP patients.

It is important that the treatment provider help the patient to realize which fear(s) underlie these symptoms. In most cases, the fear of death by suffocation underlies respiratory symptoms; the fear of death by heart attack underlies cardiac symptoms; and the fear of "going crazy" underlies psychological symptoms.

Once the fears are identified, the patient can be helped to realize that the fears are irrational. The treatment provider should explain that the MVP symptoms just discussed do not result in death or "going crazy," and that the MVP patient may be limited in athletic areas but can essentially live a normal life.

The self-talk which the patient uses when confronted with frightening MVP symptoms should be thoroughly assessed. Then, the treatment provider can help the patient adopt new, more positive self-talk to replace any catastrophic thinking. For example, the patient who usually tells himself, "I'm suffocating" can be taught to say, instead, "Shortness of breath means I'm getting too much oxygen. I must close my mouth and slow down. I'm just anxious. I won't suffocate." The patient who usually tells herself, "I'm going crazy" can be taught to say, instead, "I'm losing concentration and thoughts are racing through my head. But this just means that I'm anxious. I won't go crazy.'' The patient who generally says, ''It will never end'' can be taught to say, instead, ''It is only temporary, and these symptoms will pass.''

It is recommended that this self-talk be practiced until it becomes habit, and practice should begin in a relatively stress-free and symptom-free situation and progress until the patient can practice it when severe symptoms occur. The positive self-talk should prevent irrational fears from exacerbating the physiological symptoms of MVP, and should allow the symptoms to naturally subside.

In some cases, anxious MVP patients can develop agoraphobia, and about 40% of agoraphobics have MVP as compared with less than 10% of the general population (Cummings & Sayama, 1995). Should the anxiety progress to the development of agoraphobia, specific psychotherapeutic techniques, such as systematic desensitization, are employed along with the treatments discussed.

SUMMARY

Although many holistic and alternative treatments remain unverified and of dubious scientific validity, others have been validated for use with particular conditions. These can be helpful, particularly as adjuncts to traditional medicine, and may augment the effectiveness of traditional treatments or reduce the need for medical treatments. Modern medicine and surgery, alternative treatments, and beliefs can together provide more effective prevention and treatment than any one of these techniques alone in many cases.

PART VI

The Epilogue

19.

A Primary Care Physician's Experience with Integrated Behavioral Health Care: What Difference Has it Made?

Steven F. Lucas, M.D., interviewed by C. J. Peek, Ph.D.

CJP: First of all, Steve, tell us a little about your practice and how you got interested in the integration of behavioral health and primary care.
SFL: My interest in integrating behavioral health with family medicine started back in residency, where a psychologist and a social worker were part of our clinic, just down the hall. Their help took two forms: They gave advice about how to manage a patient, or we could refer the patient and they would take care

Acknowledgments. Ewa Peczalska, Ph.D., a member of the Health Psychology Section of the HealthPartners Behavioral Health Division, has worked on the staff of HealthPartners primary care and oncology clinics since 1990, joining Dr. Lucas' clinic in 1995. Dr. Lucas describes their teamwork in this chapter. Dr. Peczalska earned a Ph.D. in Social and Administrative Pharmacy in 1983, and an M.A. in Counseling Psychology in 1986, both from the University of Minnesota.

HealthPartners Medical Group and Clinics is a member-governed, nonprofit health plan with more than 700,000 members in the Twin Cities. HealthPartners Medical Group and Clinics is part of the HealthPartners care delivery system, with a 100-physician Family Practice Department in a medical group of 550 physicians and 23 clinics serving approximately 275,000 members and patients.

of it. Some things were satisfying about that and some things weren't. It was satisfying to get another perspective, some advice, and a way to refer patients for better care, and my patients were more satisfied with this than with what I could do alone. But the teamwork and partnership was not as close as I would have liked.

Later I joined HealthPartners Family Practice Department where I have done full range family medicine for almost 17 years. As I did more and more family-centered care, I began to realize that mental health was a huge part of what we do; and that very often the physiologic conditions are greatly affected or caused by the emotional and social health of the patient or the family.

I began to do more and more mental health care for my patients; doing what I first called "nod therapy"; mostly just listening to their troubles and woes, being sympathetic, and trying to figure out how that was affecting their health. Then I began to be more involved in treating depression and anxiety, even before the current crop of medications that opened up new ways of treating these patients.

But medication treatment, by itself, was not that rewarding to me as a family physician, because I really wanted to base my care on a better understanding of where my patients and their symptoms were coming from. Referring patients to an offsite mental health provider rarely filled the gaps in my understanding of my patients. I often felt they were going off for "black box" treatment. I didn't have a sense of what was going on or what my role should be. The patient could have been on medication, could have been getting psychoanalytic therapy, behavior therapy, or reality therapy. I didn't know what therapy or therapeutic relationship was in play, or how this might be affecting what I saw and heard from the patient when coming to me in the clinic.

Did you know the names of the therapists you referred to?
Yes, but the "black box" phenomenon was present, even though I knew their names, the areas they specialized in, and some sense of the quality of care that they were providing. I referred based on what I had picked up over time about their

specialties and reputations. But even so, "referring out" was very unsatisfying because it brought no opportunity to really discuss or coordinate the care of my patients.

What I had always been looking for was a team member who understood what I brought to the table, and who brought complementary skills. I had been wanting someone in the clinic who was not a strictly traditional "Freudian" or other talk therapist. I wanted someone who could do ordinary "talk therapy" or counseling but who could also do specific therapies like hypnosis, biofeedback, or family interventions with chronic illnesses. I needed someone with the skills to accept medical patients as medical patients, help prepare them for care we ourselves could effectively provide, and to "groom" them for successful referral to others for specific care we didn't provide, e.g., more intensive psychotherapy or group programs.

I wanted somebody who was willing to partner with me. I never truly experienced that until Dr. Ewa Peczalska, a health psychologist, came to our clinic from the health psychology section of our Mental Health Department, as part of a 10-year demonstration of mental health integration with primary and specialty care (Peek & Heinrich, 1995, 1997).

When Dr. Peczalska (Ewa) came, it was like a breath of fresh air. I had a partner. Finally I had somebody who would come and discuss cases with me and help with the challenges of care planning. I could do biomedical evaluations, procedures, and medications. She could do "talk therapy," biofeedback, hypnosis, other "behavioral medicine" modalities, and prepare patients for therapies that would need to take place elsewhere. She would engage me with issues, problems, and suggestions for the overall care of our shared patients.

Not only did I know what she was doing but I came to know more about what I was doing. I knew which areas were specifically for me to deal with and which other areas I didn't have to directly handle. But I could reinforce the whole picture. It always felt like collaborating in our care of our patients. There was a care plan that knit together the biomedical and psychosocial aspects of care and gave us each a clear and appropriate role in it, including very effective care for patients with challenging or "borderline" personality traits. Throughout the entire process of caring for patients I felt like we were a team.

This partnership in planning and carrying out care plans has been extremely effective for patients and rewarding for me. I am no longer afraid of patients who come in with a psychosocial agenda that is outside my "comfort zone," such as great anger, chemical dependency, borderline personality traits or sociopathy (I never feel comfortable with sociopaths). I have actually started to enjoy "challenging patients" because I know that I have the tools in the clinic needed to safely and effectively engage these patients.

From the perspective of a primary care doc, what are the tough challenges?

The biggest challenge is working with patients who present with physical symptoms with strong psychosocial factors, but won't "buy" any such explanation. They may come in with multiple complaints such as gastrointestinal disturbance, chest pain, bladder problems, headaches, nausea, fatigue, or other symptoms of malaise. These patients are common in any primary care practice, and absorb a disproportionate amount of energy, time, and resources in a standard noncollaborative system. Such "somatizing" patients really do have legitimate health problems in need of treatment, yet are what I call "the overserviced and underserved." These patients are overserviced and underserved because their problems do not lend themselves to the "body–mind" dichotomy that characterizes standard medical practice.

It should be noted that "The Overserviced and Underserved" is a working title for the Mental Health Primary Care Collaboration Project at HealthPartners, initiated in 1995 to restructure the way behavioral health care is delivered in primary care, based on demonstrations such as the one discussed in this chapter. The HealthPartners Primary Care and Behavioral Health Divisions, the HealthPartners Research Foundation, and Bristol-Myers Squibb are collaborating to support the project and disseminate its findings. The first phase collected baseline data about the demonstrations of primary care/mental health integration that began in 1987. The second phase, now in progress, builds mental health capability into five primary care medical clinics not part of the previous demonstrations. Subsequent phases will focus on training, dissemination of what has been learned, and formal research to evaluate the impact of the project.

"Overserviced and underserved," a good expression.

We, as physicians, are not adequately trained to recognize the importance of body–mind splits in health care that so often lead to lots of services that do not really well serve patients and families. A primary care physician, without a way to really care for somatizing patients, typically has a couple of choices: (1) you can put them on some sort of medication, e.g., for anxiety or depression. (2) You can attempt to make a mental health referral for evaluation and treatment of any "underlying" mental health problems.

But to the patient, often neither of these alternatives solves the problem. A process of building patient self-understanding is needed to put together a care plan that combines biomedical and psychosocial interventions, correctly linked and timed. But if you are the typical primary care physician without the collaborative team I now have, you usually don't have the time or know-how to carefully unfold to the patient how the physical symptoms they feel (and you don't) are related to psychosocial factors you see (and they don't). Even if you know how to go about this sometimes delicate process of building patient self-understanding and acceptance of biopsychosocial illnesses, your clinic schedule is usually not constructed for this kind of work.

Medical consultants are unlikely to be much help with this process of building patient self-understanding either. For example, the gastroenterologist isn't going to help you treat a patient with functional bowel disease; the cardiologist isn't going to help you treat a patient with cardiac fear. They're going to see the patient, rule out serious disease, and send them back saying, "There's no problem here" or "They've got functional bowel disease," and "Take this medicine." Specialty consultants typically prefer to see patients who are really sick. They see their consult as complete when organic disease is ruled out.

And, quite frankly, traditional mental health psychologists or psychiatrists often do the same thing. If diagnosable mental illness or psychopathology is not evident, there is little to "treat" in a traditional way, and the patient comes back without a diagnosis but still with their physical symptoms entwined in psychosocial distress.

Tell us more about the challenge of making mental health referrals.

My experience is that even when you are successful at "selling" a mental health referral to a skeptical patient who is convinced they are just physically sick, your patient goes off to the mental health "black box" where you have no idea what's going on. But the patient still keeps coming back to you, their physician, with the same or similar problems. Even if the therapy is on track from a mental health perspective, the therapy or therapist often doesn't focus on my concerns as a physician, or the symptoms that bring the patient to my office. Therapy in the "black box" tends to be more concerned about whatever traditional mental health agenda has emerged. That's probably one of the most frustrating things to me as a physician.

The classic separation of medical and mental health care plans and providers is also extremely costly in care dollars. When I don't know what to do, it's like I don't have the hammer to hit this nail. So I'm going to try to define that nail better. I'm going to do an upper GI series, I'm going to do a CAT scan, and I'm going to do another treadmill. I'll do all of those tests because I want to find something that I can deal with, even if in my heart I know the answer is probably not to be found in another upper GI series.

How does a team help satisfy your need for "a finding"?

Without a "finding" to work from, primary physicians will take another pass, looking for things we can do something about. It's the way we're trained. We're trained in the model of "find and fix" (Keller & Carroll, 1994). And for us, finding mental health concerns has always been diagnosis by exclusion. If somebody comes in with a bellyache, they've got an organic bellyache until you rule out physical disease. But with the team in place, you can do more than run your patients through the same tests again when you can't answer the question by yourself. Better explanations for symptoms emerge earlier from the broad evaluations we can do together as a team than from narrow evaluations I can do as a physician. This reduces rework that we physicians often do, for lack of a better alternative.

Our health psychologist can diagnose all kinds of mental health conditions, but by and large, when I send her a patient, I think I already know what the diagnosis is. She confirms, refines, and fills in the story behind it through her interviews. This adds solidity to the picture. But it's the increased range of therapeutic options after the diagnosis that is most helpful. What the health psychologist in my clinic really provides me with is more and better therapeutic tools. A broader basis for diagnosis is only the beginning.

The biggest value of integrated behavioral health care is in expanding my range of "what to do now." Ewa and I talk about what we can do to relieve the anxiety about this chest pain, or what can we do to treat this headache in a nonmedicinal fashion. Those are extremely valuable tools that we now have, right in the clinic. We can now help patients understand physical–mental interactions, and how their particular reactions to life cause their bodies to react in certain ways they experience as medical symptoms. That's a critically important capability for any primary care clinic.

What happens to the primary care physician who runs out of things "to do" but the patient is still coming?
It becomes a transference issue. They transfer their headache and their bowel disorder to you! You get very frustrated because you know that you're not doing an effective job with the patient. And it's not satisfying for either of you to keep having visits for the same problems over and over again.

The patient gradually becomes a burden on your schedule and you don't want to see them. You become increasingly frustrated with the patient (rather than your own lack of options). I've many times seen physicians deal with this by telling the patient. "There is nothing wrong with you," that it's "all in your head." Every one of us has heard that story a million times. I think it's the physician's way of saying, "You don't have real disease; don't keep coming back to see me. I don't know what to do with someone who's not sick." Basically, that's the physician firing the patient. But it does the patient no good at all. On the other hand, if you are a physician who is willing to accept and work with those patients, you end up getting more and more of them from your colleagues. It can be burdensome if you have a whole panel of patients like that around you. All the more reason to set up a team as we have been talking about. The clinic really has no alternative but to understand its patients, even the ones who don't present with things we "like" to treat.

The other thing I see is physicians who believe their job is to turn over the biophysical stones and ignore the psycho-emotional ones. As a result, physicians cheerfully announce to the patient, "Well, we didn't find anything. You're okay." They genuinely feel their job with that patient is over. For many patients, that reassurance is all they need. They just need to know they can live life without fear of the funny feelings in their body.

But much of the time there's more to it than that. The anxiety does not dissipate with negative test results and reassurance. The reality is that for many patients the physician's job is not over, even after treadmill, angiogram, and other tests mean it is accurate to say about the chest pain, "Your heart is fine." The patient's doubts may intensify the more the physician reassures. In such an anxious person you miss the point by just doing medical tests. In the end, you have no practical option but to understand and work with all your patients, including the ones that are primarily anxious, distressed, or somatically focused. And to do that, you are going to need a team.

A physician who has turned over all the biomedical stones, eager to announce that "you check out fine," might face a disappointed patient?
Yes. You give congratulations, shake their hand, and walk out while the patient sits there numb, looking at the wall. I've been there, done that. I clearly remember occasions after I've done that when the patient asks, "But what's this pain?" I couldn't

answer it then and I probably can't answer it now. I may or may not go directly to my health psychologist, but I will certainly work with this patient's question in a variety of ways now that I know I've got someone in the clinic that I can call in as my collaborator. I'm certainly going to be much more comfortable taking the case to the next step and not "dismissing" the patient as soon as they are "well" in my book.

Can you say more about what your collaboration really looks like? When you say "call in," do you mean refer the patient, come to the exam with you, sit down at lunch and talk, or all of the above?

Certainly, I would never think of making a traditional referral to Ewa, where I write up a referral slip, the patient goes off to see her, and she does whatever she does. That just wouldn't be satisfying to either of us, and eventually the patient would catch us in a gap somehow. Sometimes we get the ball rolling "by referral" but I know that we are going to talk about the case. What I prefer to do is walk over to see Ewa for a few minutes so I can say, "Come with me, I want you to meet someone." The same goes for her, coming to see me about someone in her office at the time. But that doesn't happen as much as I would like in a busy clinical practice. But we find each other to discuss cases when we need to. Sometimes she comes down to my office, sometimes I go down to hers. We just work it out. It's hard to "preprogram" a specific communication schedule, but this is no real problem because the desire and opportunity is strong for both of us.

Does the health psychologist's office location help you connect in the clinic?

Her office is not right near mine, but she's there in the clinic among the other doctors and she's personally available to me. She has to be on-site. On days she's not in our clinic, I lose the power of the team. Fortunately, she's there at least one day when I'm there and we connect.

We don't just connect at the beginning of a case, we connect all along the length of the case too. I have an 18-year-old woman patient right now who was in a motor vehicle accident and has had persistent pain for at least a year and a half, a chronic pain syndrome. I sent her to a physiatrist to see if there were any more exercises or physiotherapy modalities needed. The physiatrist's evaluation did not point to additional physical therapy exercises or program. I made sure all those notes went to Ewa, and then we sat down and talked about the findings and created a care plan to suggest to the patient. In this case, the treatment is pretty much coming from Ewa and I, because the physical findings and treatments are already in place and the patient's challenge now is to go on with her life. After a year and a half, she's beginning to resume her life rather than search for a definitive cure for pain. She's now going through the first stages of grief.

This is the kind of care I could not provide alone, and could not have done by making a "mental health referral." Ewa's presence in the hallways of this clinic, as a normal part of the team, was essential to our clinic being able to carry this injury case beyond the acute management phases into a real recovery.

Speaking of chronic pain, can you say more about how behavioral health integration helps you with that slice of primary care?
Let's talk about headaches for example. Chronic headache treatment is one of those common primary care tasks that is often not very satisfying for physicians or effective for patients, even though medical science continues to find better and better therapies. We've got all kinds of headache medications out there. But in my view, most people have headaches for a reason; they are not just coming out of nowhere. Take migraines, for example. It is true that food or other physiological or chemical triggers exist and there can be strong hereditary predispositions. But migraines can also be triggered by emotional responses or patterns. The same goes for muscle tension headaches. Headaches can be part of an overall physical response to the psychosocial realities of a person's life.

The challenge is to help the patient understand that the headache is a little like diabetes where the task is to carefully evaluate, treat physiologically, then teach them how to manage the diabetes in the context of their own life. Headache management also requires evaluation, physiological treatment where you can, and teaching patients to understand and manage their own headaches, so they become more and more comfortable and effective in doing so. Ewa helps me teach patients how to do that. For example, she goes into the details about muscle contraction, uses biofeedback to help make habits of muscle contraction visible to patients and to help them learn to control their own muscular or other physical responses. She helps by teaching patients relaxation skills or self-hypnosis. She helps by drawing patients into careful observation of their headache patterns so they become their own "diagnostician" about what causes their headaches to occur. She helps patients work in new ways with headache factors. This really gets down to the substance of what the headache is really all about for each patient. Sometimes it's simple and sometimes it leads into complex personal areas.

Whatever the case, the goal is for the patients to understand how their headaches work, deal with it a little bit better, and to recognize that having headaches doesn't mean that they have to check out of life. Because we do this in the primary care clinic, we never have to convince the patient that their headache is "all in their head" or go to mental health to deal with it. Instead, we can help them deal with their headache as a physical reaction to a combination of physical, emotional, and behavioral factors treated by the clinic team.

To what extent has this approach to headache improved your life as a doctor?
The first thing I think of that affects "my life as a doctor" is headache patients who are drug-seeking. Quite frankly, a certain amount of discomfort comes over me when I first see them. With a team in place, I can now engage the patient in thorough discussion about what they have been through with headache care and then lead into a plan to involve Ewa in talking with the patient about how to cover all the bases with headaches, with or without medicinal therapies.

For example, I now have a patient with a physiologic disease causing body pain. This patient had been placed on Percoset some time ago. He began to experience more and more pain, became more and more intolerant of it, and became more and more demanding for more and more narcotics. This was quite uncomfortable for me. So, I discussed the case with Ewa, including my own discomfort with the current situation. We made a plan for what we were going to do about the escalating pain and demands for narcotics. My part was to deal more directly with narcotic use, its diminishing returns, and potential for abuse. The patient and I worked out a plan where every refill was for a diminishing number of pills, so that he knew that there was an end point to this. Ewa's part was to use different pain treatment modalities, hypnosis primarily. We also included a physical therapy program to improve the patient's strength, activity tolerance, and activity level. This whole plan was acceptable to the patient.

As we got further along, we discovered something that gave the plan more meaning to the patient than "substitution and withdrawal." It came to light that the patient wanted very much to do something that he had earlier given up because of pain. He had been doing metal sculpture and metalworking, but had all kinds of physical reasons why he couldn't do it anymore. Ewa and I both showed an interest in his metalworking, and his returning this activity to his life. The therapy became focused not only on "pain" but on "resuming life." One-by-one, the power of the reasons to stay away from metalworking diminished during the therapy. He got back into his sculpture shop and became a happier person. He still has good physiological cause for having pain; that's not going to go away. But I think he's focusing on it a great deal less today than before. He is focusing on what his life is about instead.

This is a good example of teamwork that improves my life as a physician, improves the life of my patients, and the life of psychologists who would otherwise have to try to treat such patients on a referral basis.

How about an example where chronic pain led to major psychosocial areas?
I remember a patient I saw one night in the After-Hours Care Center. This woman had a $2^1/_2$ inch thick chart, and it was

probably volume II. She had seen neurologists, multiple primary care providers, multiple people for chronic pain. I don't even remember now if it was headache, abdominal pain, or what part of the body was affected. I read the chart, walked into the room, and asked what she was expecting from me today. After saying she hoped to get rid of her pain, I suggested I couldn't think of any biomedical thing I could do today that she hadn't already been through. She didn't disagree with that.

So, we went about an interview. I was on a fishing trip with her, I guess. And she was very willing to come along with me. Her husband was sitting on the exam table, a rather stern-looking fellow, sitting there up higher than she and I at the desk, kind of overlooking the proceedings, intensely observing what was going on. I went into all kinds of things, like what she eats, what she does with her life, where she's working, and so on. One of the things I clearly wanted to ask about was history of physical, sexual, emotional abuse. When I got to those questions, she said, "No, this has never happened," "No, that has never happened." Then all of a sudden, out of seemingly nowhere, her husband pops up and says, "Now, just wait a minute," in kind of a stern voice, "I think you ought to tell Dr. Lucas about Uncle Tommy." And she sighed, "Oh yeah," as if a lost memory had returned to her.

The patient may not have been ready at that point in time to make a connection between Uncle Tommy and her chronic pain. But clearly, it was a whole new avenue. I knew then I couldn't do anything with it myself right then. I don't feel I'm well trained enough to take that information right then and to turn it into effective therapeutic modalities. And yet, this is a patient that I can walk down to Ewa's office and say, "Let's look at this. A new door may have been opened on this old case." The patient may not be willing to accept an abuse connection to her pain, but Ewa and the patient can find out together if there is anything to it, and if so, prepare the patient to eventually get into the right treatment, e.g., a group that helps people get past a history of abuse; and maybe eventually rid her of chronic pain.

How do you introduce the health psychologist without the patient feeling you are sending her off to mental health as "he thinks I'm nuts," or fearing she will have to expose painful secrets to a stranger for no good reason?
First of all, there is no "sending off" to do. Ewa is "one of us," part of our primary care team. In keeping with this, I do not imply that "pain" is no longer the reason for the visit, that the patient is really "mental," or that she will be pushed into a painful process of revealing secrets.

Moreover, I can tell the patient that I highly regard Dr. Peczalska as a very helpful and friendly partner to me and my patients. (Since my direct experience with Ewa is very enjoyable, helpful, professional, and based on common respect, it naturally shows when I steer a patient her way. It is easy for me to invest my credibility with patients in Ewa.)

I tell the patient that there is someone on my clinic team who helps patients explore the possibilities for helping themselves with problems like chronic pain, and helps patients look into the possible effects of personal history and life issues on medical problems. The term *health psychologist* usually creates no problem in this context, because the emphasis is on "health," and the person is a real professional. And, I emphasize to the patient that I don't know whether the "Uncle Tommy" history has anything to do with her chronic pain. I just want her willingness to explore it.

Can you say a bit more about how the clinic setup makes it safe for patients like this to see the health psychologist?
Dr. Peczalska's being a normal part of our clinic is reinforced by the clinic setup. For example, her picture is on the wall with ours, she schedules patients with the same receptionists I do, she charts in the medical charts, she works out of offices or exam rooms in the family practice areas of the clinic. Whatever copay applies to the physician applies to the health psychologist. There is no separate copay, because these visits are not categorized as mental health visits.

With all this in place, the visit to Ewa clearly does not look like a "mental health visit." It looks like a "medical" visit, in this case for chronic pain. Patients feel very comfortable with her because she doesn't switch into a mental health frame of reference by jumping right into "Uncle Tommy" and all that history. It's there, and she'll acknowledge it, but she's more interested in knowing about the headaches, what's been done before, what's worked, what hasn't worked, what the person's life is like, and the same sort of history that I had done. Eventually she'll get around to Uncle Tommy when the patient is more comfortable. I know that my patients are really quite comfortable seeing her. And yet, if I tried to write a mental health referral for many of these patients, they wouldn't go.

What's your advice for someone setting up such a system in their clinic?
First of all, position your health psychologist (or whatever behavioral health clinician you are bringing aboard) as "one of us." Do not set it up so the patient feels they are being sent to the mental health section, either off-site, or in a remote corner of your building. Clearly identify in all the subtle and not-so-subtle ways that your psychologist is a regular player with you. Give that clinician an office or exam room in the primary care section. Use the same receptionists and schedules. Don't confuse the picture with mental health charts and separate copays. Be sure the therapist and patient walk in and out of regular patient care areas, mixing with patients in for a diabetic check, fractured leg, or whatever. Be sure they know they are walking in and out of the medical side, not a psychiatric side in disguise.

The most important thing for providers is open communication. When a patient's case is complicated enough to need a team, make sure everyone knows who is on the team and what the care plan is. Communication has to be open to inquiry. It can't be hierarchical, like one person telling everyone what they have to know and do. For example, I know Ewa respects my judgments, thoughts, and theories, but she is also comfortable challenging them. And it's true the other way around; I have a great deal of confidence in how she understands things and what she thinks needs doing, but I'm not afraid to challenge these either. We keep those communication lines open so we have the benefit of our two heads. It's the proximity and the norm for open communication that makes it happen and makes it work.

How does "open communication" fit patient expectations for confidentiality? Does the patient assume that you and the psychologist are talking all the time?
Yes, we tell patients we will be talking to each other. In a medical setting, patients expect the right hand to know what the left hand is doing. Patients expect that we will talk about the care that we're giving, and stay coordinated, cooperative, and aligned around common goals.

I remember a particularly wonderful case example about the power of communication and teamwork. This was a woman who needed a new doctor. She had "borderline personality" traits, a history of chemical dependency, metastatic breast cancer, and was physically and emotionally quite ill and demanding. She tended to get all her caregivers all worked up in different directions, fragmenting her care, and impeding the development of trust. When I first started seeing this patient, she was taking a great deal of narcotic medication. She had several bottles of pain medicine stockpiled at home. The first decision I made was that I wasn't going to follow the pattern and "get fired" by this patient. That was a clear and straightforward decision I made as I stood in the hallway before I walked in to see this very ill and challenging person.

Is that to say there are certain moments a doctor can choose to "get fired" and get out from under a case like this?
Absolutely. I could have consciously or unconsciously gotten myself fired in 30 seconds.

Would anyone have known? Would it have reflected badly on you?
In a large clinic or care system, a patient like this would have gone on to see somebody else. And my being fired in that visit would have been lost in the myriad visits to multiple providers she's fired before.

So you made the conscious decision not to be fired.
Yes, and then I walked into the exam room. I listened to her side of the story. I consciously chose to act compassionately about her plight. And when she was obnoxious toward me, I recognized that this wasn't about me, it was about her. So I was able to sit there and listen, give her my opinion, and ask her to make a commitment to follow up with me.

As time went on, her behavior was often problematic. One time Ewa was trying to teach her some relaxation skills using a tape player. Her response was that she didn't have a tape recorder. So, the next time I saw her, I brought a tape recorder from home, put in fresh batteries, brought it to the clinic, and told her she could use it as long as she needed it. One time, a few months later, she came in with something brewing. She had been saying bad things about me to Ewa, saying bad things about Ewa to me. The home care nurse was wanting to retire from home care nursing, and the social worker felt like the patient's mother. There was a lot of "stuff coming down" around this patient.

When she came in on this particular day, I knew there was going to be an interesting encounter. She had a very stern look on her face and looked up at me. She put her hand on the tape recorder, slid it across the desk and said, "I don't think I'm going to need this anymore." I ignored that, and went on to talk about other things, how things were going in her relationships with the home care nurse and with her daughter (who were both subject to multiple "firings" and "rehirings"). We talked about where she was in her life. I tried to not be reactive to anything she said or did. At the end of the meeting, the one thing I remember was that I put my hand on the tape recorder and slid it back to her and said, "I think you still need this." I think the message I was trying to give was that it wasn't going to be that easy to fire me. She was "testing" to see whether I would stick with her or not. She did the same thing to the social worker who came to her home, the home visiting nurse, and the health psychologist. We all were getting the same sort of story and "test."

Soon afterward, the social worker, psychologist, and I met with her in an exam room. We talked about our roles in her care and emphasized that we were not particularly easy to get rid of. If she was successful at firing any one of us, she would be firing all of us, including her oncologist (who played a peripheral role at that point). The meeting actually went extremely well. She brightened up and her anger dissipated fairly quickly. In the end she was talkative and playful again, and we all had a good laugh. She got back on track and we didn't have any more trouble with the care plan (or with her) for at least a few weeks after that.

This woman was taking lots and lots of narcotic medication, but we extended our trust to her. Ewa, I, and the patient worked out a medication schedule together. With time, she stopped stockpiling narcotics at home. I think the patient eventually came to trust that we were going to take care of her, that we were not going to abandon her, and that we were going to be there for her when she died. If she was having pain, we were going to help her with it, and we would be predictable. A week before she died she wrote a very touching letter to Ewa that was very thankful for the care that she had gotten.

The important thing, from my perspective, was that in taking this case I knew I was walking into a hotbed. But I knew I had support and could get the help I needed. I did not have to be afraid of it. In fact, it turned out to be a good, and sometimes pleasant, experience for almost everyone involved.

The patient knew that we on our team wouldn't desert her. And I knew that the health psychologist and social worker wouldn't desert me when the going got tough. So together we dared to really take on the case. We did go through three hospice nurses before we finished. They retired from that case and wouldn't go back. But the three of us (plus the remaining hospice nurse and two members of the county welfare office who were helping the patient with medical assistance) stuck it out. After a while, it wasn't all that difficult. We had made the decision to organize ourselves as an unfirable team. It shows that you can turn some of the "worst" work into some of the best professional experiences by how you gear yourselves up for collaborative care.

Are you saying there was no way you would have handled this case alone?

There is no way that I would have tackled that one alone, and Ewa would not have either. In fact, the main thing that kept us and this case going was our care team meetings. Usually, I would get a phone call from somebody who would say, "Your patient is at it again" or "I feel like I need a vacation" or "What's all this stuff that you're doing to the patient?" The key to handling these calls was that I didn't have to answer the question posed. What I had to do was call a care team meeting. We would meet over lunch. First we ventilated and eventually figured out what was going on with us and the patient. Then we readjusted the care plan and redefined our caregiver roles accordingly. This made us all more comfortable with ourselves and clear about what we were doing individually and collectively.

This patient, because of her multiple problems and traits, could have been one that never gets good care, always gets expensive care, and dies unhappy and angry. This did not happen.

That's powerful.

Speaking of power, at the beginning, this patient would walk up to the front desk and curse everyone at the top of her voice. The staff was just absolutely petrified of this woman. After she died, I couldn't tell you the number of people who came back and commented to me about being sad that she died. People appreciated the change she had made during the process. It was highly successful. I think she died a more comfortable woman.

It sounds like this patient was a prominent figure for the entire clinic, not just for you and the team.

Yes. People in the clinic knew they could come to me or to Ewa with their concerns. They knew they wouldn't get saddled with something that they didn't know what to do with. We were always willing to take the problem on. Quite frankly, it didn't matter if I was there or not. If Ewa was there, that was fine. The perception that there was a responsible team with a care plan that reassured people even when the members of the team were away. The care plan was in place even when the team members weren't. Everybody knew that if they had a problem they could just give it to us, and we would take it as clinical data, not a "dump."

Does this example highlight that collaborative practice is also for the benefit of the providers, their peace of mind, courage, and confidence?
For sure. Let me tell an old story about this point. I don't know where this comes from, but I heard of an old experiment where you take a 5 gallon bucket, fill it half full of water and throw a rat in there. The rat swims for a certain amount of time, and then it just drowns. Then you take the same bucket and throw another rat in. If the first rat swam for 2 hours before drowning, you take the second rat out of the bucket after an hour and a half. You put the rat back into the nice warm, dry cage, give it food, and let it survive. Then if you put it back in the bucket on another day, it'll swim forever—not forever, but it will swim and swim and swim.

The lesson is that very few physicians have had success with difficult cases like this, but once you have had success, you're much more willing to go back and do it again, and will be more committed to it. Had we not been able to create a team where responsibility was distributed and I was supported by my peers, I might have gone into that room and gotten fired in 30 seconds. But I know that doesn't have to happen because the team is there and I can call them together if I get into trouble.

There were times when I did feel like firing this patient, but would call a team meeting instead. At team meetings, I would tell my story, the social worker would tell her story about how she hung drapes for the patient, walked the dog, got her mail, and we would laugh about that. This gave me perspective; it's not just me that's getting manipulated by this patient. It's all of us getting manipulated by this patient. Therefore, the problem isn't me, it's a feature of the clinical picture pulling on all of us.

With responsibility diffused throughout the team, using a care plan, are there problems figuring out who's in charge of what? I didn't see any problem in the previous case. But there were certain things we divided up. For example, I didn't deal with any of the money and payment issues. Ewa and I gave our clinical input and the social worker and county workers resolved financial matters. When the patient entered a struggle with her daughter, we would all have to deal with it, but if it got sticky and I found myself at the edge of my comfort zone, then I would say, "Let me talk to Ewa about that so that the next time you come in, you and Ewa can work something out on that." There was never any question that it was my responsibility to handle things that might involve changing drugs or monitoring biomedical conditions, e.g., watching her bladder infections and watching her for metastatic disease. She had plenty of problems. These were the last days of her life and she was quite sick. That was my job.

One time we admitted our patient to the hospital for pain management. That wasn't a decision that I made alone. At a care team meeting the agenda was "what are we going to do about pain management?" The decision of the group was to put her in the hospital for things like nerve blocks. Once that decision was made, I knew exactly what my job was. I contacted the anesthesiologist before the patient went in, discussed with him our options, and proceeded with a plan. The team participated in the process and knew how to handle any spin-off issues that resulted. I don't know if I would have been comfortable just going in this way without the team approach.

Another time I needed a psychiatric opinion on drug management. So I contacted a psychiatrist, told him the patient had terminal metastatic breast cancer, borderline personality, and that she was really quite a handful. I asked, "Please develop an opinion about what we should do with her drugs and don't let the patient fire you. Then send her back to the team and we will be perfectly happy to implement and manage the plan." I talked to the psychiatrist after the appointment (at an off-site mental health clinic) and found out that the patient had walked into the room, commenced a fight within minutes, and fired the psychiatrist. But I got my consult later when another psychiatrist came to my clinic and sat in the room while I did an interview with the patient. I learned to bring the consultant into the sanity of our team environment, rather than sending the patient to a place where she could still fight.

Was the oncologist bound by the team agreements too?
This patient had been seeing the oncologist for some time before I became involved. We attempted to involve the oncologist in the care team, but his preference was to follow independently. But he agreed to take an active role when the patient was admitted to the specialty hospital. We were trying to preserve a solid, predictable team in the hospital. I was asking the oncologist to act as her primary doctor rather than a consultant at his hospital if she needed to be admitted as an oncology patient. We already knew that the patient was capable of being disruptive when there were too many people involved in her care, and we wanted very much to avoid that situation.

The theme of having to step up to the plate is coming together across the board.
Yes. The entire team was bound by the commitment, "If she fires you, she fires me. And if she fires me, she fires you." When we agreed that we would operate that way together, the chaos of "firings" in the hospital and clinic stopped.

You built a team that provided real constraints on what the patient was able to do in the care system, but wasn't it just a financial tactic of managed care?
It turned out that it was economically sound to do things the way we did, but that wasn't the spirit behind it. The spirit was that by working together, by having a close-knit group, we are able to provide far better care, and individually we are going to be able to survive this case and be proud of our work.

What financial test does your collaborative model face in your clinic?
There's a very stringent financial test. We are "capitated," meaning that our clinic has certain financial resources to use to care for our population of patients. So the financial question isn't about generating additional fees to pay for additional

resources in the clinic. Instead, the question is about how we allocate fixed resources across the various functions and professionals needed in the clinic. The physicians in our clinic willingly shifted resources designated for physician help to pay for the health psychologist. I think that's the bottom-line test.

In other words, we need our health psychology time as much as we need more physician time. But does it pay off by saving overall costs? I don't know how much our clinic saves on an MRI here and there, or on hospital days. Clearly, we would have been at far greater financial risk with the previous patient without the team there. But I don't have any specific evidence that we saved this cost and that cost. This is under study in our organization, but our management decision was based on our clinical needs and our staffing options, not on cost-effectiveness research.

How else then should the performance of this model be evaluated?

It would be very interesting to look at total bottom-line costs (ambulatory, hospital, pharmacy, referral, specialty) and see whether or not you actually save money by doing this. I believe firmly that you improve patient care and satisfaction, and I think you save money, too. I believe you won't need that second or third upper GI, GI consult, MRI scan and extra hospital days. And I believe you won't have as many unproductive physician visits.

To begin to answer the question, a "quick and dirty" survey of the effect of the health psychologists on utilization was done (Davis, Leary, & Heinrich, 1994). It was not a rigorous study at all, but tended to confirm my impressions. It was a simple database review of total medical utilization 1-year pre- and post-health psychology intervention for about a thousand continuously enrolled patients in medical clinics. For about 250 patients who were hospitalized at some point during the two-year period, there was about a 27% reduction in hospital admissions and bed days pre and post. For the whole group of about a thousand, there was about a 9% drop in physician visits (hopefully translating into increased appointment availability), and about a 50% increase in mental health visits, not including the health psychology visits (hopefully focusing the care more sharply where it belongs). There was a big increase in referrals to hospice (perhaps coming from increased attention to personal and family issues in chronic illness). It looked like any savings that resulted were most likely coming from the inpatient area.

Whatever the savings, I have noticed that patients come back to see me less frequently and they come back with a better sense of what their problem is and who can be helpful. Whether or not my visits plus Ewa's visits is a smaller total than if she weren't there, I don't know for sure. But I do know I see them less often, with better focus, and I believe with better outcomes.

Could a person tell the care is better focused by reading the charts?
I think you can. When I read the charts of patients working with my partners and the health psychologist, I have a better sense of what's going on. I can now go to a chart on a patient with multiple complaints, and if they're seeing Ewa and one of my partners, the care plan gives me much better bearings. I can tell what my job needs to be that day. This is especially important when you're filling in or on call.

How do these "care plans" find their way into the charts?
I recommend that care plans be placed so they are easily identified in the chart. Whenever you have team-based care, you should write down what the problems are, what the care plan is, who the players are, and establish a place in the chart where it can all be found. Our care plans are there, but too often are contained in regular chart notes where it is more difficult for a new provider to find them. Put the care plan in an obvious place in the chart so everyone can work off it.

With a care plan in the chart, after-hours care, specialists, or other doctors can handle things from a better knowledge base. This makes for better care and better service, because patients usually don't feel secure when the doctor in front of them appears to know nothing about their complicated case and has to ask basic questions all over again. It is easier for other providers to look at the presenting issue, how it fits the existing care plan, and decide what their role should be. You can go on vacation and your partners can take care of much more, with much greater confidence, e.g., refilling narcotic prescriptions.

How much behavioral health time do you have in your clinic?
Dr. Peczalska is at our shop one day a week. We have nine family docs, three pediatricians, and one general internist in our practice. So we have about 12 full-time physicians and $1/5$ of a health psychologist. This proportion is way too tight. I think it should be twice that for just the health psychologist. And I personally would like to have a family therapist in our shop, working in a similar fashion, maybe one day a week.

How would you differentiate health psychology and family therapy roles in the clinic?
The health psychologist focuses on the mind–body aspects of the care. Ewa can talk to my diabetics about their diabetes, work with their cognitions and habits, and help them better deal with their diabetes. The previous cancer, headache, and chronic pain examples show this focus on mind and body. I need the person to have a comfort in biophysiology and dealing with doctors and medical patients. I think that's absolutely critical.

I don't picture the traditional family therapist dealing with physiologic disease as much. I see them dealing with family or individual dysfunction in the traditional psychological sense, where the patient understands there is an individual or family mental health issue at play. For example, I think that the patient who had a problem with Uncle Tommy might eventually need a more formal psychological approach to help with that problem. She may not see any connection and refuse any individual mental health treatment, but might be more open to an educational group or sessions with other family members. I think the transition to this form of therapy would be smoother with the therapist also in the clinic rather than off in a remote location.

How do you tell if a patient needs a family therapist, not the health psychologist?

Let me tell you about one of my failures. I took care of a family for quite a few years. I'll bet I saw someone from that family every other week. If it wasn't kids with a cold or Mom with vaginitis, it was someone else. It was always low-grade sorts of things, no episode very serious.

I knew there was something going on in this family, but I could never put my finger on it. I was in the mode of episodic care with the family, trying to create a relationship. It turned out that Mom was bulimic and had a history of sexual abuse. The kids' ear infections weren't going to get better until Mom uncovered the chronic family distress related to her bulimia and incest history. Once that happened, the kids' ears got better, she didn't get vaginitis, and the things I saw the family for became less episodic and more purposeful, e.g., school physicals, a vasectomy, and the time Mom came in just to tell me her story. I wasn't part of her discovering her distress and bulimia. She found a different pathway, I think through seeking traditional mental health. That's why I call this one of my failures. I think we could have done better care far earlier if I had had a collaborative practice at the time.

Could you have just made a referral to mental health? Or would it be better done by a clinic team member?

This person eventually found her own path to family help, but it probably would have happened far sooner with the family therapist readily accessible on the team in the clinic. In this case, the presenting symptoms just weren't going to be alleviated until we really got down to bottom-line patterns of distress in the family. When the patient had a flare-up of one of her chronic symptoms, it might be accompanied by Johnny wetting the bed. We had to deal with Johnny wetting the bed, and we certainly had to deal with Mom's perception of what that meant. I think a family therapist could do that far better than I. The bottom-line is that there's a big impact on the family when that happens, and his wetting the bed does not happen in isolation from other things going on in the family. This was a fragile family at the time.

So you would help families cope right there in the family practice clinic?

Right. It doesn't seem odd to me. For example, sometimes an out-of-control situation at home will seriously interfere with diabetes management. For adolescents, diabetes management is often as much psychosocial as physiological. Adjusting insulin may be only a temporary fix. Often I think I'm not getting to the bottom of what's going on with the patient or the family. If not, I may not be able to determine the real barriers to good diabetes care and do any more than nag or assign things they never seem to be able to do. Collaboration helps you find where to engage patients in their big picture.

And collaborative care has the effect of helping doctors cope, too?

Yes. A whole variety of situations can ruin your day if you face them alone. Here's one key: If you look at your schedule and you see a name on the schedule that, for whatever reason, makes you want to go home early, there's something wrong with the care plan or the relationship. When that happens to me, I may not know what is going on, but it definitely tells me I need someone to reflect with or collaborate with on the case.

I think there are many ways of doing this. I collaborate with our health psychologist. You could have a peer consultation or "case rounds" group if you wanted. You could do a variety of things. But practically speaking, there is no substitute for getting down to practical methods for broadly understanding our patients and what they bring to us. Arranging close and trusting collaboration with behavioral health clinicians can help us drop our own fears or resistance to engaging challenging patients outside the door before we walk in.

A closing note from Dr. Peczalska

Partnership is the right term for the working relationship Steve has described here. It is based on mutual respect, appreciation of skills and talents, and trust. A "right match" of values and personalities has also helped us work effectively and enjoyably with our patients. I am grateful that his skills, enthusiasm, and belief in integrative care have helped create the environment where effective clinical work can take place.

Not every working relationship in an integrated care setting can be so satisfying. However, it is my experience that even less optimal collaboration among providers is beneficial and rewarding for patients and clinicians. After practicing 6 years, in several clinics, using the integrated model, it is hard for me to imagine practicing "solo," not being part of the medical team. I truly believe that effective work in medical clinics depends not only on "techniques," "tests," or "therapies," but on the relationships that we model for our patients.

References

Alexander, C. N., Langer, E. J., Newman, R. I., Chandler, H. M., & Davies, J. L. (1989). Transcendental meditation, mindfulness, and longevity: An experimental study with the elderly. *Journal of Personality and Social Psychology, 57,* 950–964.

Alexander, F., & French, T. M. (1946). *Psychoanalytic therapy: Principles and applications.* New York: Ronald Press.

American Psychiatric Association (1994). *Diagnostic and statistical manual of mental disorders,* 4th ed. (DSM-IV). Washington, DC: American Psychiatric Press.

Anda, R., Williamson, D., & Jones, D. (1993). Depressed affect, hopelessness, and the risk of ischemic heart disease in a cohort of U.S. adults. *Epidemiology, 4,* 285–294.

Anderson, I., & Tomenson, B. (1995). Treatment discontinuation with selective serotonin reuptake inhibitors compared with tricyclic antidepressants: A meta-analysis. *British Medical Journal, 310,* 1433–1438.

Anderson, R., Francis, A., Lion, J., & Daughety, V. S. (1977). Psychologically related illness and health service utilization. *Medical Care, 15,* 59.

Anderson, R. O. (1989, March). How to use "self-realization" and "self-talk." *Consultant,* 69–85.

Antonovsky, A. (1987). *Unraveling the mystery of health: How people manage stress and stay well.* San Francisco: Jossey-Bass.

Auerswald, E. (1968). Interdisciplinary versus ecological approach. *Family Process, 7,* 202–215.

Azur, B. (1996, October). Intrusive thoughts proven to undermine our health. *APA Monitor, 27,* 34.

Badmaev, V., Majeed, M., & Passwater, R. (1996, July). Selenium: A quest for better understanding. *Alternative Therapies, 2,* 59–67.

Baker, N., Stuart, M., & Braddick, M. (submitted a). An evidence based approach to the treatment of minor depression and dysthymia in primary care.

Baker, N., Stuart, M., Braddick, M., & Simon, G. (submitted b). An evidence based approach to the treatment of major depression in primary care.

Balint, M. (1957). *The doctor, his patient and the illness.* New York: International Universities Press.

Bandura, A. (1977a). Self-efficacy: Toward a unifying theory of behavioral change. *Psychological Review, 84,* 191–215.

Bandura, A. (1977b). *Social learning theory.* Englewood Cliffs, NJ: Prentice-Hall.

Bandura, A. (1991). Self-efficacy mechanism in physiological activation and health-promoting behavior. In J. Madden (Ed.), *Neurobiology of learning, emotion and affect.* New York: Raven Press.

Barefoot, J. C., Helms, M. J., & Mark, D. M. (1996). Depression and long term mortality risk in patients with coronary artery disease. *American Journal of Cardiology, 78,* 613–617.

Barefoot, J. C., & Schroll, M. (1996). Symptoms of depression, acute myocardial infarction, and total mortality in a community sample. *Circulation, 93,* 1976–1980.

Barefoot, J. C., Williams, R. B., Siegler, I. C., & Schroll, M. (1995, March). *Depressive affect, hostility and socioeconomic status (SES): Interrelationships and joint effects on health.* Paper presented at the Annual Meeting of the American Psychosomatic Society, New Orleans.

Barlow, D. H., Craske, M. G., Cerny, J. A., & Klosko, J. S. (1989). Behavioral treatment of panic disorder. *Behavior Therapy, 20,* 261–282.

Barsky, A. J., Goodson, J. D., Lane, R. S., & Cleary, P. D. (1988). The amplification of somatic symptoms. *Psychosomatic Medicine, 50,* 510–519.

Bashore, T. M. (1988). Mitral valve prolapse syndrome: Dynamic changes with exercise posture. In H. Boudoulas & C. F. Wooley (Eds.), *Mitral valve prolapse and the mitral valve prolapse syndrome.* New York: Futura.

Beardslee, W. R. (1981). Self-understanding and coping with cancer. In G. P. Koocher & S. J. O'Malley (Eds.), *The Damocles syndrome: Psychosocial consequences of surviving childhood cancer* (pp. 144–163). New York: McGraw-Hill.

Beardslee, W. R. (1983). Children of parents with major affective disorders. *American Journal of Psychiatry, 140,* 825–832.

Beardslee, W. R. (1989). The role of self-understanding in resilient individuals. The development of a perspective. *American Journal of Orthopsychiatry, 59,* 226–278.

Beardslee, W. R. (1990). Development of a clinician-based preventive intervention for families with affective disorders. *Journal of Preventive Psychiatry and Allied Disciplines, 4,* 39–61.

Beardslee, W. R., & Hoke, L. A. (1992). Preventive intervention for families with parental affective disorders: Initial findings. *American Journal of Psychiatry, 149,* 1335–1340.

Beardslee, W. R., Keller, M. B., Lavori, P. W., Klerman, G. K., Dorer, D. J., & Samuelson, H. (1988). Psychiatric disorder in adolescent offspring of parents with affective disorders in a non-referred sample. *Journal of Affective Disorders, 15,* 313–322.

Beardslee, W. R., & Podorefsky, D. (1988). Resilient adolescents whose parents have serious affective and other psychiatric disorder: The importance of self-understanding and relationships. *American Journal of Psychiatry, 145,* 63–69.

Beardslee, W. R., Salt, P., Porterfield, K., Clarke Rothberg, P., Van de Velde, P., Swalting, S., Hoke, L., Moilanen, D., & Wheelock, I. (1993). Comparison of preventive interventions for families with parental affective disorder. *Journal of the American Academy of Child and Adolescent Psychiatry, 32,* 254–263.

Beardslee, W. R., Schults, L. H., & Selman, R. L. (1987). Level of social-cognitive development, adaptive functioning and DSM-III diagnosis in adolescent offspring of parents with affective disorders: Implications of the development capacity for mutuality. *Developmental Psychology, 23,* 807–815.

Beardslee, W. R., Versage, E. M., Salt, P., Gladstone, T. R. G., Wright, E., Rothberg, P. C., & Drezner, K. (1996). Examination of preventive interventions for families with depression: Evidence of change. Manuscript submitted for publication.

Beardslee, W. R., Wheelock, I. (1994). Children of parents with affective disorders. In W. M. Reynolds & H. F. Johnston (Eds.), *Handbook of depression in children and adolescents* (pp. 463–479). New York: Plenum.

Beardsley, R. S., Gardocki, G. J., Larson, D. B., & Hidalgo, J. (1988). Prescribing of psychotropic medication by primary care physicians and psychiatrists. *Archives of General Psychiatry, 45,* 1117–1119.

Beck, A. T., Steer, R. A., & Garbin, M. G. (1988). Psychometric properties of the Beck Depression Inventory: Twenty-five years of evaluation. *Clinical Psychology Review, 8,* 77–100.

Beckfield, D. F. (1994). *Master your panic and take back your life! Twelve treatment sessions to overcome high anxiety.* San Luis Obispo, CA: Impact.

Beecher, H. K. (1955). The powerful placebo. *Journal of the American Medical Association, 159,* 1602–1606.

Benson, H., & Stuart, E. M. (1992). *The wellness book: The comprehensive guide to maintaining health and treating stress-related illness.* New York: Simon & Schuster.

Berner, E. S. (1994). Performance of four computer-based diagnostic systems. *New England Journal of Medicine, 25,* 1792–1796.

Berwick, D. M. (1996). Quality comes home. *Annals of Internal Medicine,*
    125, 830–843.

Bickman, L. (1996). A continuum of care: More is not always better.
    American Psychologist, 51, 689–701.

Bird, J., & Cohen-Cole, S. A. (1983). Teaching psychiatry to non-psychia-
    trists: The application of educational methodology. *General Hospi-*
    tal Psychiatry, 5, 247–253.

Black, D. W., Warrack, G., & Winokur, G. (1985). The Iowa record-
    linkage study: Suicides and accidental death among psychiatric
    patients. *Archives of General Psychiatry, 42,* 71–75.

Blacker, C. V. R., & Clare, A. W. (1987). Depressive disorder in primary
    care. *British Journal of Psychiatry, 150,* 737–751.

Bloom, B. L. (1991). *Planned short-term psychotherapy: A clinical handbook.*
    Boston: Allyn & Bacon.

Bloom, B. L., Hodges, W. F., Kern, M. B., & McFaddin, S. C. (1985). A
    preventive intervention program for the newly separated. *Ameri-*
    can Journal of Orthopsychiatry, 55, 9–26.

Bohm, D. (1992). *Thought as a system.* New York: Rutledge.

Borkan, J., Reis, S., Hermoni, D., & Biderman, A. (1995). Talking about
    the pain: A patient-centered study of low back pain in primary
    care. *Social Science and Medicine, 40,* 977–988.

Brandenburger, A. M., & Nalebuff, B. J. (1996). *Co-opetition.* New York:
    Currency Books.

Broadhead, W. E., Leon, A. C., & Weissman, M. M. (1995). Development
    and validation of the SDDS-PC screen for multiple mental disor-
    ders in primary care. *Archives of Family Medicine, 4,* 211–219.

Bruce, M., Seeman, T. E., Merrill, S. S., & Blazer, D. G. (1994). The
    impact of depressive symptomatology on physical disability: Mac-
    Arthur Studies of Successful Aging. *American Journal of Public*
    Health, 84, 1796–1799.

Budman, S. H., & Gurman, A. S. (1988). *Theory and practice of brief*
    therapy. New York: Guilford Press.

Bultema, J. K., Mailliard, L., Getzfrid, M. K., Lerner, R. D., & Colone, M.
    (1996). Geriatric patients with depression: Improving outcomes
    using a multidisciplinary clinical path model. *Journal of Nursing*
    Administration, 1, 31–38.

Byrne, A., & Byrne, D. G. (1993). The effect of exercise on depression,
    anxiety, and other mood states: A review. *Journal of Psychosomatic*
    Research, 37, 565–574.

Callahan, C. M., Hendrie, H. C., Dittus, R. S., Brater, D. C., Hui,
    S. L., & Tierney, W. M. (1994). Improving treatment of late life
    depression in primary care: A randomized clinical trial. *Journal*
    of the American Geriatric Society, 42, 839–846.

Campbell, R. W. (1982). Arrhythmias in mitral valve prolapse. *Practical Cardiology, 8,* 124–135.

Capra, F. (1996). *Web of life.* Chicago: Anchor.

Carney, R. M., Rich, M. W., Freedland, K. E., Saini, J., TeVelde, A., Simeone, C., & Clarke, K. (1988). Major depressive disorder predicts cardiac events in patients with coronary artery disease. *Psychosomatic Medicine, 50,* 627–633.

Carson, V. B. (1993). Prayer, meditation, exercise, and special diets: Behaviors of the hardy person with HIV/AIDS. *Journal of the Association of Nurses in AIDS Care, 4,* 18–28.

Case, R. B., Moss, A. J., & Case, N. (1992). Living alone after myocardial infarction: Impact on prognosis. *Journal of the American Medical Association, 267,* 515–519.

Caudill, M., Schnable, R., Zutermeister, P., Benson, H., & Friedman, R. (1991). Decreased clinic use by chronic pain patients: Response to behavioral medicine interventions. *Clinical Journal of Pain, 7,* 305–310.

Ceci, S. J. & Bruck, M. (1995). *Jeopardy in the courtroom: A scientific analysis of children's testimony.* Washington, DC: American Psychological Association.

Celler, B. G. (1995). Remote home monitoring of health status of the elderly. *Medinfo, 1,* 615–619.

Cheung, P., & Spears, G. (1995). Illness etiology constructs, health status and use of health services among Cambodians in New Zealand. *Australian and New Zealand Journal of Psychiatry, 29,* 257–265.

Cioffi, D., & Holloway, J. (1993). Delayed costs of suppressed pain. *Journal of Personality and Social Psychology, 64,* 174–182.

Clarke, G. N., Hawkins, W., Murphy, M., Sheeber, L. B., Lewinsohn, P. M., & Seeley, J. R. (1995). Targeted prevention of unipolar depressive disorder in an at-risk sample of high school adolescents: A randomized trial of a group cognitive intervention. *Journal of the American Academy of Child and Adolescent Psychiatry, 34,* 312–321.

Cockburn, J., Thomas, R. J., McLaughlin, S. J., & Reading, D. (1995). Acceptance of screening for colorectal cancer by flexible sigmoidoscopy. *Journal of Medical Screening, 2,* 79–83.

Cohen-Cole, S. A. (1991a). Consultation-liaison research: Four selected topics. In F. K. Judd, G. D. Burrows & D. R. Lipsitt (Eds.), *Handbook of general hospital psychiatry* (pp. 79–98). Amsterdam: Elsevier.

Cohen-Cole, S. A. (1991b). *The medical interview: The three-function approach.* St. Louis, MO: Mosby-Year Book.

Cohen-Cole, S. A., & Friedman, C. P. (1983). The language problem: Integration of psychosocial variables into medical care. *Psychosomatics, 24,* 52–60.

Cohen-Cole, S. A., & Levinson, R. M. (1994). The biopsychosocial model in medical practice. In A. Stoudemire (Ed.), *Human behavior: An introduction for medical students* (pp. 22–63). Philadelphia, PA: J. B. Lippincott.

Cohen-Cole, S. A., Raju, M., & Barrett, J. (1993). Psychiatric education improves internists' knowledge: A three-year randomized, controlled evaluation. *Psychosomatic Medicine, 55,* 212–218.

Colasante, R. (in press). A behavioral treatment for temporomandibular joint syndrome. *Mind/Body Medicine.*

Cole, S. A., & Raju, M. (1996). Overcoming barriers to integration of primary care and behavioral healthcare: Focus on knowledge and skills. *Behavioral Healthcare Tomorrow, 5,* 30–37.

Cole, S. A., Saravey, S., & Steinberg, M. (1995). A model curriculum for mental disorders and behavioral problems in primary care. *General Hospital Psychiatry, 17,* 13–18.

Combrinck-Graham, L. (1990). *Giant steps: Therapeutic innovations in child mental health.* New York: Basic Books.

Cooper, K. H. (1995). *It's better to believe.* Nashville, TN: Thomas Nelson.

Cooper, M. L., Russel, M., & George, W. H. (1988). Coping, expectancies, and alcohol abuse: A test of social learning formulations. *Journal of Abnormal Psychology, 97,* 281–330.

Coyne, J., Schwenk, T. L., & Fechner-Bates, S. (1995). Non-detection of depression by primary care physicians reconsidered. *General Hospital Psychiatry, 17,* 3–12.

Cummings, N. & Sayama, M. (1995). *Focused psychotherapy: A casebook of brief intermittent psychotherapy throughout the life cycle.* New York: Brunner/Mazel.

Cummings, N. A. (1977). Prolonged (ideal) versus short-term (realistic) psychotherapy. *Professional Psychology, 8,* 491–501.

Cummings, N. A. (1979). Turning bread into stones: Our modern anti-miracle. *American Psychologist, 34,* 1119–1129.

Cummings, N. A. (1985a). Assessing the computer's impact: Professional concerns. *Computers in Human Behavior, 1,* 293–300.

Cummings, N. A. (1985b). *Biodyne training manual.* South San Francisco, CA: Foundation for Behavioral Health.

Cummings, N. A. (1986). The dismantling of our health system: Strategies for survival of psychological practice. *American Psychologist, 41,* 426–431.

Cummings, N. A. (1991a). Brief, intermittent psychotherapy throughout the life cycle. In J. K. Zeig & S. G. Gilligan (Eds.), *Brief therapy: Myths, methods and metaphors.* New York: Brunner/Mazel.

Cummings, N. A. (1991b). Arguments for the financial efficacy of psychological services in health care settings. In J. J. Sweet, R. G. Rozensky, & S. M. Tovian (Eds.), *Handbook of clinical psychology in medical settings* (pp. 113–126). New York: Plenum.

Cummings, N. A. (1993). Somatization: When physical symptoms have no medical cause. In D. Goleman & J. Gurin (Eds.), *Mind-body medicine* (pp. 221–232). Yonkers, NY: Consumer Reports.

Cummings, N. A. (1994). The successful application of medical offset in program planning and in clinical delivery. *Managed Care Quarterly, 2,* 1–6.

Cummings, N. A. (1995). Impact of managed care on employment and training: A primer for survival. *Professional Psychology: Research and Practice, 26,* 10–15.

Cummings, N. A. (1996a). Does managed mental health care offset costs relate to medical treatment? In A. Lazarus (Ed.), *Controversies in managed mental health care* (pp. 213–227). Washington, DC: American Psychiatric Press.

Cummings, N. A. (1996b). The impact of managed care on employment and professional training: A primer for survival. In N. A. Cummings, M. S. Pallak, & J. L. Cummings (Eds.), *Surviving the demise of solo practice: Mental health practitioners prospering in the era of managed care* (pp. 11–26). Madison, CT: Psychosocial Press.

Cummings, N. A. (1996c). The new structure of health care and a role for psychology. In R. A. Resnick & R. H. Rozensky (Eds.), *Health psychology through the life span* (pp. 27–37). Washington, DC: American Psychological Press.

Cummings, N. A. (in press). Approaches in prevention in the behavioral health of older adults. In P. Hartman-Stein (Ed.), *Innovative behavioral healthcare for older adults: A guide-book for changing times* (pp. 1–23). San Francisco, CA: Jossey-Bass.

Cummings, N. A., Dorken, H., Pallak, M. S., & Henke, C. J. (1991). The impact of psychological intervention on health care costs and utilization. The Hawaii Medicaid Project. *HCFA Contract Report #11-C-983344/9.*

Cummings, N. A., Dorken, H., Pallak, M. S., & Henke, C. J. (1993). The impact of psychological intervention on health care costs and utilization: The Hawaii Medicaid Project. In N. A. Cummings & M. S. Pallak (Eds.), *Medicaid, managed behavioral health and implications for public policy, Vol. 2: Healthcare and utilization cost series* (pp. 3–23). South San Francisco, CA: Foundation for Behavioral Health.

Cummings, N. A., & Follette, W. T. (1968). Psychiatric services and medical utilization in a prepaid health plan setting: Part 2. *Medical Care, 6,* 31–41.

Cummings, N. A., & Follette, W. T. (1976). Brief psychotherapy and medical utilization: An eight-year follow-up. In H. Dorken (Ed.), *The professional psychologist today* (pp. 126–142). San Francisco, CA: Jossey-Bass.

Cummings, N. A., Kahn, B. I., & Sparkman, B. (1962). *Psychotherapy and medical utilization: A pilot study.* Oakland, CA: Annual Reports of Kaiser Permanente Research Projects.

Cummings, N. A., & VandenBos, G. R. (1979). The general practice of psychology. *Professional Psychology, 1,* 430–440.

Cummings, N. A., & VandenBos, G. R. (1981). The twenty year Kaiser-Permanente experience with psychotherapy and medical utilization: Implications for national health policy and national health insurance. *Health Policy Quarterly, 1,* 159–175.

Cykert, S., Kissling, G., Layson, R., & Hansen, C. (1995). Health insurance does not guarantee access to primary care: A national study of physicians' acceptance of publicly insured patients. *Journal of General Internal Medicine, 10,* 345–348.

Davanloo, H. (1978). *Basic principles and techniques in short-term dynamic psychotherapy.* New York: Spectrum.

Davis, T. F., Leary, D., & Heinrich, R. L. (1994). Data appearing in "The over-serviced and under-served: The mental health / primary care collaboration project, profile analysis report, phase I, May, 1996," unpublished manuscript, HealthPartners.

Dean, G. A. (1985, September). Mitral valve prolapse. *Hospital Practice,* 75–82.

Dede, C., & Fontana, L. (1995). Transforming health education via new media. In L. M. Harris (Ed.), *Health and the new media* (pp. 163–183). Mahwah, NJ: Lawrence Erlbaum.

DeGenova, M. K., Patton, D. M., Jurich, J. A., & MacDermid, S. M. (1994). Ways of coping among HIV-infected individuals. *Journal of Social Psychology, 134,* 655–663.

deKooning, D., Debets, W., Blom, C., & Sandfort, T. G. (1993). Evaluation of a small scale AIDS prevention activity for men with homosexual contacts. *International Conference on AIDS, 2,* 746.

Depression Guideline Panel (1993a). *Depression in primary care: Vol. 1. Detection and diagnosis. Clinical practice guideline, Number. 5.* Rockland, MD: U.S. Department of Health and Human Services, Public Health Service, Agency for Health Care Policy and Research, AHCPR Publication No. 93-0550.

Depression Guideline Panel (1993b). *Depression in primary care: Vol. 2: Treatment of major depression. Clinical Practice Guideline, Number 5.* Rockland, MD: U.S. Department of Health and Human Services, Public Health Service, Agency for Health Care Policy and Research, AHCPR Publication No. 93-0551.

Descartes, R. (1650). *Passions of the Soul,* Part I, Article XXXIV.

DeShazer, S. (1982). *Patterns of brief family therapy: An ecosystemic approach.* New York: Guilford.

Diehr, P., Williams, S., Martin, D., & Price, K. (1984). Ambulatory mental health services utilization in three provider plans. *Medical Care, 22,* 1–13.

Dilsaver, S. C. (1989, June). Panic disorder. *American Family Physician, 39,* 167–172.

Docherty, J. P. (1996). Disease management strategy. *Behavioral Healthcare Tomorrow, 1,* 51–53.

Doherty, W., & Baird, M. (1983). *Family therapy and family medicine.* New York: Guilford.

Doherty, W. J., McDaniel, S. H., & Baird, M. A. (1996). Five levels of primary care/behavioral healthcare collaboration. *Behavioral Healthcare Tomorrow, 5,* 25–27.

Downey, G., & Coyne, J. C. (1990). Children of depressed parents: An integrative review. *Psychology Bulletin, 108,* 50–76.

Dowrick, C., & Buchan, I. (1995). Twelve month outcome of depression in general practice: Does detection or disclosure make a difference? *British Medical Journal, 311,* 1274–1277.

Dym, B., & Berman, S. (1986). The primary health care team: Family physician and family therapist in joint practice. *Family Systems Medicine, 4,* 9–12.

Eddy, D. (1993). Three battles to watch in the 1990s. *Journal of the American Medical Association, 270,* 520–526.

Eddy, D. (1994). Health care system reform: Will controlling costs require rationing services? *Journal of the American Medical Association, 272,* 324–328.

Edell, D. S. (1987, June/July). Mitral valve prolapse. *The People's Medical Journal.*

Edelman, G. (1992). *Bright air, brilliant fire.* New York: Basic Books.

Engel, G. E. (1993). The need for a new medical model: A challenge for biomedicine. *Science, 196,* 129–136.

Epstein, A. L., Budd, M. A., & Cole, S. A. (1995). Behavioral disorders: An unrecognized epidemic with implications for providers. *HMO Practice, 9,* 53–56.

Erickson, M. H. (1980). *Collected papers* (Vols. 1–4), E. Rossi (Ed.). New York: Irvington.

Everly, G. S. (1989). *A clinical guide to the treatment of the human stress response.* New York: Plenum.

Fawzy, F. I. (1995). A short-term psychoeducational intervention for patients newly diagnosed with cancer. *Supportive Care in Cancer, 3,* 235–238.

Fawzy, F. I., Fawzy, N. W., & Hyun, C. S. (1993). Malignant melanoma: Effects of an early structured psychiatric intervention, coping, and affective state on recurrence and survival 6 years later. *Archives of General Psychiatry, 50,* 681–689.

Ferguson, T. (1995). Consumer health informatics. *Healthcare Forum Journal, 1,* 29–32.

Fiedler, J. L., & Wright, R. B. (1989). *The medical offset effect and public policy.* New York: Praeger.

Follette, W. T., & Cummings, N. A. (1967). Psychiatric services and medical utilization in a prepaid health plan setting. *Medical Care, 5,* 25–35.

Ford, C. V. (1983). *The somatizing disorders: Illness as a way of life.* New York: Elsevier.

Ford, C. V. (1986). The somatizing disorders. *Psychosomatics, 27,* 327–337.

Forehand, R., & McCombs, A. (1988). Unraveling the antecedent-consequence conditions in maternal depression and adolescent functioning. *Behavioral Research and Therapy, 26,* 399–405.

Fraser, J. S. (1996). All that glitters is not always gold: Medical offset effects and managed behavioral health care. *Professional Psychology: Research and Practice, 27,* 335–344.

Frasure-Smith, N., Lesperance, F., & Talajic, M. (1993). Depression following myocardial infarction: Impact on 6-month survival. *Journal of the American Medical Association, 270,* 1819–1825.

Frasure-Smith, N., & Prince, R. (1985). The Ischemic Heart Disease Life Stress Monitoring Program: Impact on mortality. *Psychosomatic Medicine, 47,* 431–445.

Freda, M. C., Damus, K., Andersen, H. F., Brustman, L. E., & Merkatz, I. R. (1990). A "PROPP" for the Bronx: Preterm birth prevention education in the inner city. *Obstetrics and Gynecology, 76,* 93S–96S.

Frederickson, L. (1988). *Confronting mitral valve prolapse.* San Marcos, CA: Slawson Communications, Inc.

Freud, S. (1955). Group psychology and the analysis of the ego. In J. Strachey (Ed.), *The standard edition of the complete psychological works of Sigmund Freud* (Vol. 18, pp. 63–143). London: Hogarth. (Original work published 1921)

Friedman, H. S., & Booth-Kewley, S. B. (1987). The "disease prone personality": A meta-analytic view of the construct. *American Psychologist, 42,* 539–555.

Friedman, M., Thoresen, C. E., & Gill, J. J. (1986). Alteration of type A behavior and its effect on cardiac recurrences in post myocardial infarction patients: Summary results of the Recurrent Coronary Prevention Project. *American Heart Journal, 112,* 653–665.

Friedman, R., Sobel, D., Myers, P., Caudill, M., & Benson, H. (1995). Behavioral medicine, clinical health psychology, and cost offset. *Health Psychology, 14,* 1–10.

Friedman, R., Sobel, D., Myers, P., Caudill, M., & Benson, H. (1996). Behavioral medicine, clinical health psychology and cost offset. *Medical Cost Offset,* Fall, 25–45.

Fulop, G., Strain, J. A., & Fahs, M. C. (1989). Medical disorders associated with psychiatric comorbidity and prolonged length of stay. *Hospital Community Psychiatry, 40,* 80–82.

Gerber, P. D., Barrett, J., Barrett, J., Manheimer, E., Whiting, R., & Smith, R. (1989). Recognition of depression by internists in primary care: A comparison of internist and "gold standard" psychiatric assessments. *Journal of General Internal Medicine, 4,* 7–13.

Gershwin, M. E., & Beach, R. S. (1985). *Nutrition and immunity.* New York: Academic Press.

Glick, M. (in press). A study of group treatment for irritable bowel syndrome. *Mind/Body Medicine.*

Glazer, W. (1993, June-July). Approaching hidden psychiatric illness in PPOs: The "medical offset" effect. *AAPPO Journal,* 15–21.

Glazer, W., & Bell, N. (1993). *Mental health benefits: A purchaser's guide.* Brookfield, WI: International Foundation of Employee Benefits Plans Press.

Glenn, M. (1987). *Collaborative health care: A family-oriented model.* New York: Praeger.

Goldberg, I., Allen, G., Kessler, L. G., Carey, J. F., Locke, B. Z., & Cook, W. A. (1981). Utilization of medical services after short-term psychiatric therapy in a prepaid health plan setting. *Medical Care, 19,* 672–686.

Goldberg, I. D., Krantz, G., & Locke, B. Z. (1970). Effect of a short-term outpatient psychiatric benefit on the utilization of medical services in a prepaid group practice medical program. *Medical Care, 8,* 419–428.

Goldberg, I. D., Krantz, G., & Locke, B. Z. (1979). Effect of short-term outpatient benefit and the utilization of health care. *Medical Care, 17,* 118–124.

Goldensohn, S., & Fink, R. (1979). Mental health services for Medicaid enrollees in a prepaid group practice plan. *American Journal of Psychiatry, 136,* 160–164.

Goleman, D., & Gurin, J. (1993). *Mind-body medicine.* New York: Consumer Reports Books.

Gonzales, J. J., Magruder, K. M., & Keith, S. L. (1994). Mental disorders in primary care services: An update. *Public Health Reports, 109,* 251–258.

Gordon, D., Burge, D., & Hammen, C. (1989). Observations of interactions in depressed women with their children. *American Journal of Psychiatry, 146,* 50–55.

Gordon, J. H., Walerstein, S. J., & Pollack, S. (in press). The advanced clinical skills program in medical interviewing: A block curriculum for residents in medicine. *General Hospital Psychiatry.*

Greenberg, L. S., & Safran, J. D. (1989). Emotion in psychotherapy. *American Psychologist, 44,* 19–29.

Greenberg, P. D., Stiglin, L. E., Findelstein, S. N., & Berndt, E. R. (1993). Depression: A neglected major illness. *Journal of Clinical Psychiatry, 54,* 419–424.

Greenleaf, R. (1977). *Servant leadership.* Boston: Paulist Press.

Griffin, K. (1996, October). The new doctors of natural medicine. *Health, 10,* 61–68.

Griffin, K., & Gallagher, D. (1995, October). Hands on healing. *Health, 9,* 59–63.

Gross, M., DeJong, W., Lamab, D., Enos, T., Mason, T., & Weitzman, E. (1994). "Drugs and AIDS—reaching for help": A videotape on AIDS and drug abuse prevention for criminal justice populations. *Journal of Drug Education, 24,* 1–20.

Groth-Marnat, G., & Edkins, G. (1996). Professional psychologists in general health care settings: A review of the financial efficacy of direct treatment intervention. *Professional Psychology: Research and Practice, 27,* 161–174.

Hammen, C. (1988). Self-cognitions, stressful events, and the prediction of depression in children of depressed mothers. *Journal of Abnormal Child Psychology, 16,* 347–360.

Hammen, C., Burge, D., Burney, E., & Adrian, C. (1990). Longitudinal study of diagnoses in children of women with unipolar and bipolar affective disorder. *Archives of General Psychiatry, 47,* 1112–1117.

Handley, M., & Stuart, M. (1994). An evidence-based approach to evaluating and improving clinical practice: Guideline development. *HMO Practice, 8,* 10–19.

Handley, M., Stuart, M., & Kirz, H. (1994). An evidence-based approach to evaluating and improving clinical practice: Implementing practice guidelines. *HMO Practice, 8,* 75–83.

Hankin, J., Kessler, L. G., Goldberg, I. D., Steinwachs, D. M., & Starfield, B. H. (1983). A longitudinal study of offset in the use of nonpsychiatric services following specialized mental health care. *Medical Care, 21,* 1099–1110.

Hankin, J., Steinwachs, D. M., & Eldes, C. (1980). The impact of utilization of a copayment increase for ambulatory psychiatric care. *Medical Care, 18,* 807–815.

Hardy, A. (1970). *The Terrap manual for the treatment of agoraphobia.* Menlo Park, CA: Terrap.

Harris, L. M. (1995). Differences that make a difference. In L. M. Harris (Ed.), *Health and the new media* (pp. 3–18). Mahwah, NJ: Lawrence Erlbaum.

Harvard Medical School (1995, September). Acupuncture. *Harvard Women's Health Watch, 3,* 4–5.

Hau, L. (1996, December 2). HCIS firms may rebound from shakeout. *Wall Street Journal,* p. B12C.

Hayes, S. (1994). Content, context, and the types of psychological acceptance. In S. Hayes, N. Jacobson, W. Follette, & M. Dougher (Eds.), *Acceptance and change: Content and context in psychotherapy* (pp. 13–35). New York: Guilford.

Hayes, S., & Strosahl, K. (1997). *Acceptance and commitment therapy: Understanding and treating human suffering.* New York: Guilford.

Hayes, S. C. (1987). A contextual approach to therapeutic change. In N. Jacobson (Ed.), *Psychotherapists in clinical practice: Cognitive and behavioral perspectives* (pp. 327–387). New York: Guilford.

Hayes, S. C., & Gifford, E. V. (in press). The trouble with language: Experiential avoidance, rules, and the nature of verbal events. *Psychological Science.*

Hayes, S. C., & Wilson, K. G. (1993). Some applied implications of a contemporary behavior, analytic account of verbal behavior. *The Behavior Analyst, 16,* 283–301.

Hayes, S. C., Wilson, K. G., Gifford, E. V., Follette, V. M., & Strosahl, K. (1996). Experiential avoidance and behavioral disorders: A functional dimensional approach to diagnosis and treatment. *Journal of Consulting and Clinical Psychology, 64,* 1152–1168.

Heidegger, M. (1962). *Being and time.* New York: Harper & Row.

Hellman, C., Budd, M., Borysenko, J., McClelland, D. C., & Benson, H. (1990). A study of the effectiveness of two group behavioral medicine interventions for patients with psychosomatic complaints. *Behavioral Medicine, 8,* 165–173.

Hengeveld, M. W., Ancion, F. A. J. M., & Rooihans, H. M. G. (1988). Psychiatric consultations with depressed medical inpatients: A randomized controlled cost-effectiveness study. *International Journal of Psychiatric Medicine, 18,* 33–43.

Henk, H., Katzelnick, D. J., Kobak, K. A., Greist, J. H., & Jefferson, J. W. (1996). Medical costs attributed to depression among patients with a history of high medical expenses in a health maintenance organization. *Archives of General Psychiatry, 53,* 899–904.

Hepworth, J., & Jackson, M. (1985). Health care for families: Models of collaboration between family therapists and family physicians. *Family Relations, 34,* 123–127.

Herskovits, E. (1995). Struggling over subjectivity: Debates about the "self" and Alzheimer's disease. *Medical Anthropology Quarterly, 9,* 146–164.

Herzlinger, R., & Freeman, M. (1996). Reclaiming behavioral healthcare: How consumer-centered technologies can shape the marketplace. *Behavioral Healthcare Tomorrow, 4,* 99–104.

Higgins, E. S. (1994). A review of unrecognized mental illness in primary care: Prevalence, natural history, and efforts to change the course. *Archives of Family Medicine, 3,* 908–917.

Hinshaw, A., & DeLeon, P. (1995). Toward achieving multidisciplinary professional collaboration. *Professional Psychology: Research and Practice, 26,* 115–116.

Hirsh, B. J., Moos, R. H., & Reischi, T. M. (1985). Psychosocial adjustment of adolescent children of a depressed, arthritic, or normal parent. *Journal of Abnormal Psychology, 94,* 154–164.

House, J. S., Landis, K. R., & Umberson, D. (1988). Social relationships and health. *Science, 241,* 540–545.

Howard, K. I. (1992). The psychotherapeutic service delivery system. *Psychotherapy Research, 2,* 164–180.

Hoyt, M. F. (1995). *Brief psychotherapy and managed care.* San Francisco: Jossey-Bass.

Institute of Medicine. (1989). *Research on children and adolescents with mental, behavioral, and developmental disorders.* Washington, DC: National Academy Press.

Ireland, S. J., McMahon, R. C., Malow, R. M., & Kouzekanani, K. (1994). Coping style as a predictor of relapse to cocaine abuse. In L. S. Harris (Ed.), *Problems of drug dependence, 1993: Proceedings of the 55th Annual Scientific Meeting* (p. 58). National Institute of Drug Abuse Monograph Series No. 141. Washington, DC: U.S. Government Printing Office.

Jacobs, D. G., Kopans, B. S., & Reizes, J. M. (1995). Reevaluation of depression: What the general practitioner needs to know. *Mind/Body Medicine, 1,* 7–22.

Jameson, J., Shuman, L. J., & Young, W. W. (1978). The effects of outpatient psychiatric utilization on the costs of providing third-party coverage. *Medical Care, 16,* 383–399.

Jaycox, L. H., Reivich, K. J., Gillham, J., & Seligman, M. E. P. (1994). Prevention of depressive symptoms in school children. *Behaviour Research and Therapy, 32,* 801–816.

Jeresaty, R. M. (1984). Mitral valve prolapse: Complications, prognosis, and treatment. *Practical Cardiology, 10,* 136–140.

Jeresaty, R. M. (1985). Mitral valve prolapse: An update. *Clinical Cardiology, 254,* 793–795.

Johnston, M. E. (1994). Effects of computer-based clinical decision support systems on clinician performance and patient outcome: A critical appraisal of research. *Annals of Internal Medicine, 2,* 135–142.

Joint National Committee on Detection, Evaluation, and Treatment of High Blood Pressure: The Fifth Report (JNC V) (1993). *Archives of Internal Medicine, 153,* 154–183.

Jones, K. R., & Vischi, T. R. (1979). The impact of alcohol, drug abuse, and mental health treatment on medical care utilization: A review of the research literature. *Medical Care, 17* (suppl.), 43–131.

Jones, K. R., & Vischi, T. R. (1980). *The Bethesda Consensus Conference on Medical Offset. Alcohol, drug abuse, and mental health administration report.* Rockville, MD: Alcohol, Drug Abuse, and Mental Health Administration.

Kabat-Zinn, J., Massion, A. O., Kristeller, J., Peterson, L. G., Fletcher, K. E., Pbert, L., Lenderking, W. R., & Santorelli, S. F. (1992). Effectiveness of a meditation-based stress reduction program in the treatment of anxiety disorders. *American Journal of Psychiatry, 149,* 936–943.

Kaiser, J. D., & Donegan, E. (1996). Complementary therapies in HIV disease. *Alternative Therapies in Health and Medicine, 2,* 42–46.

Kaplan, G. A. (1995). Where do shared pathways lead? Some reflections on a research agenda. *Psychosomatic Medicine, 57,* 208–212.

Kaplan, H. I., & Sadock, B. J. (1993). *Pocket handbook of psychiatric drug treatment.* Baltimore, MD: Williams & Wilkins.

Karpel, M. (1986). *Family resources: The hidden partner in family therapy.* New York: Guilford.

Kashner, T. M., Rost, K., & Cohen, B. (1995). Enhancing the health of somatization disorder patients: Effectiveness of short-term group therapy. *Psychosomatics, 36,* 462–470.

Katon, W., Robinson, P., VonKorff, M., Lin, E., Bush, T., Ludman, E., Simon, G., & Walker, E. (1996). A multifaceted intervention to improve treatment of depression in primary care. *Archives of General Psychiatry, 53,* 924–932.

Katon, W., & Sullivan, M. D. (1990). Depression and chronic medical illness. *Journal of Clinical Psychiatry, 51*(6 supplemental), 3–11.

Katon, W., VonKorff, M., Lin, E., Bush, T., Lipscomb, P., & Russo, J. (1992). A randomized trial of psychiatric consultation with distressed high utilizers. *General Hospital Psychiatry, 14,* 86–98.

Katon, W., VonKorff, M., Lin, E., Bush, T., & Ormel, J. (1992). Adequacy and duration of antidepressant treatment in primary care. *Medical Care, 30,* 67–76.

Katon, W., VonKorff, M., Lin, E., Lipscomb, P., Russo, J., Wagner, E., & Polk, E. (1990). Distressed high utilizers of medical care: DSM-III-R diagnoses and treatment needs. *General Hospital Psychiatry, 12,* 355–362.

Katon, W., VonKorff, M., Lin, E., Walker, E., Simon, G., Bush, T., Robinson, P., & Russo, J. (1995). Collaborative management to achieve treatment guidelines: Impact in primary care. *Journal of the American Medical Association, 273,* 1026–1031.

Katzelnick, D. J., Koback, K. A., Greist, J. H., Jefferson, J. W., & Henk, H. J. (1997). Effect of primary care treatment of depression on service use by patients with high medical expenditures. *Psychiatric Services, 48,* 59–64.

Keitner, G. I., & Miller, I. W. (1990). Family functioning and major depression. *Journal of Clinical Psychiatry, 147,* 1128–1137.

Keller, M. B., Lavori, P. W., Beardslee, W. R., Wunder, J., Dils, D. L., & Samuelson, H. (1988). Course of major depression in non-referred adolescents: A retrospective study. *Journal of Affective Disorders, 15,* 235–243.

Keller, V. F., & Carroll, J. G. (1994). A new model for physician–patient communication. West Haven, CT: Miles Institute for Health Care Communication (400 Morgan Lane, West Haven, CT).

Kemeny, M. E. (1996a, February 2). *The immune system: Minding the body and embodying the mind.* Presented at Mind Matters Seminar, Phoenix, Arizona.

Kemeny, M. E. (1996b, November 1). *Psychobiology of mental control.* Presented at Mind Matters Seminar, Phoenix, Arizona.

Kemmer, F. W., Bisping, R., Steingruber, H. J. (1986). Psychological stress and metabolic control in patients with type 1 diabetes mellitus. *New England Journal of Medicine, 314,* 1078–1084.

Kent, J., Coates, T., Pelletier, K. & O'Regan, B. (1989). Unexpected recoveries: Spontaneous remission and immune functioning. *Advances, 6,* 66–73.

Kessler, L., Cleary, P. & Burke, J. (1985). Psychiatric disorders in primary care. *Archives of General Psychiatry, 42,* 583–587.

Kessler, L. G., Burns, B. J., Shapiro, S., Tischler, G. I., George, L. K., Hough, R. L., Bodison, D., & Miller, R. H. (1987). Psychiatric diagnoses of medical services users: Evidence from the Epidemiologic Catchment Area program. *American Journal of Public Health, 77,* 18–24.

Kessler, R., Nelson, C., McGonagle, K., Liu, J., Swartz, M., & Blazer, D. (1994). Lifetime and 12 month prevalence of DSM-III-R psychiatric disorders in the United States. *Archives of General Psychiatry, 51,* 8–19.

Kiesler, C., & Silbulkin, A. (1987). *Mental hospitalization: Myths and facts about a national crisis.* Beverly Hills, CA: Sage.

Klein, R. H., & Carroll, R. (1986). Patient characteristics and attendance patterns in outpatient group psychotherapy. *International Journal of Group Psychotherapy, 36,* 115–132.

Kleinman, A. (1988). *The illness narratives: Suffering, healing and the human condition.* New York: Basic Books.

Klerman, G. I., Lavori, P. W., & Rice, J. (1985). Birth cohort trends in rates of major depressive disorder among relatives of patients with affective disorder. *Archives of General Psychiatry, 42,* 689–693.

Kobasa, S., Maddi, S., & Kahn, S. (1982). Hardiness and health: A prospective study. *Journal of Personality and Social Psychology, 42,* 168–177.

Kochanska, G., Kuczynski, L., & Radke-Yarrow, M. (1987). Resolutions of control episodes between well and affectively ill mothers and their young children. *Journal of Abnormal Child Psychology, 15,* 441–456.

Kolata, G. (1996, September 18). Experts are at odds on how best to tackle risk in teenagers' drug use. *New York Times,* p. A17.

Kotler, P. (1997). *Marketing management* (9th ed.). Englewood Cliffs, NJ: Prentice-Hall.

Kotter, P. (1996). *Leading change.* Boston: Harvard Business School Press.

Kovacs, M., Gatsonis, C., Paulauskas, S. L. & Richards, C. (1989). Depressive disorders in childhood: A longitudinal study of comorbidity with and risk for anxiety disorders. *Archives of General Psychiatry, 46,* 776–782.

Kroenke, K. (1989). Common symptoms in ambulatory care. *Journal of the American Medical Association, 86,* 262–265.

Kroenke, K., & Mangelsdorff, D. (1989). Common symptoms in ambulatory care: Incidence, evaluation, therapy, and outcome. *The American Journal of Medicine, 86,* 262–266.

Kroner-Herwig, B., Hebing, G., van Rijn-Kalkmann, U., Frenzel, A., Schikowsky, G., & Esser, G. (1995). The management of chronic tinnitus: Comparison of a cognitive-behavioral group training with yoga. *Journal of Psychosomatic Research, 39,* 153–165.

Kuhn, T. (1962). *Structure of scientific revolutions.* Chicago: University of Chicago Press.

Landau-Stanton, J., & Clements, C. (1993). AIDS, health, and mental health professional teams: Prevalence and feasibility. *Family Systems Medicine, 12,* 37–45.

Langford, H., Davis, B., & Blaufox, M. (1991). Effect of drug and diet treatments of mild hypertension on diastolic blood pressure. *Hypertension, 17,* 210–217.

Langone, J. (1996, Fall). Alternative therapies: Challenging the mainstream. *Time, 148,* 40–43.

Leitenberg, H., Greenwald, E., & Cado, S. (1992). A retrospective study of long-term methods of coping with having been sexually abused during childhood. *Child Abuse and Neglect, 16,* 399–407.

Levenson, J. L., Hamer, R., & Silverman, J. J. (1986). Psychopathology in medical inpatients and its relationship to length of stay: A pilot study. *International Journal of Psychiatry in Medicine, 16,* 231–236.

Lewinsohn, P. M. (1987). The coping-with-depression course. In R. F. Munoz (Ed.), *Depression prevention: Research directions* (pp. 159–170). New York: Hemisphere.

Lin, E., Katon, W., Simon, G., VonKorff, M., Bush, T., Rutter, C., Saunders, K., & Walker, E. (in press). Achieving guidelines for the treatment of depression in primary care: Is physician education enough? *Medical Care.*

Lin, E., VonKorff, M., Katon, W., Bush, T., Simon, G. E., Walker, E., & Robinson, P. (1995). The role of the primary care physician in patients' adherence to antidepressant therapy. *Medical Care, 33,* 67–74.

Litman, R. E. (1995). Suicide prevention in a treatment setting. *Suicide and Life Threatening Behavior, 25,* 134–142.

Loftus, E. F. (1993). The reality of repressed memories. *American Psychologist, 48,* 518–537.

Lorig, K., & Fries, J. (1990). *Arthritis helpbook* (3rd ed.). Reading, MA: Addison-Wesley.

Luborsky, L., Crits-Christorph, P., & Mintz, J. (1988). *Who will benefit from psychotherapy: Predicting therapeutic outcomes.* New York: Basic Books.

Lustman, P. S., Griffith, L. S., & Clouse, R. E. (1986). Psychiatric illness in diabetes mellitus: Relationship to symptoms and glucose control. *Journal of Nervous and Mental Diseases, 174,* 736–742.

MacLachlan, M., Nyirenda, T., & Nyando, C. (1995). Attributions for admission to Zomba Mental Hospital: Implications for the development of mental health services in Malawi. *International Journal of Social Psychiatry, 41,* 79–87.

Magruder-Habib, K., & Zung, W. W. (1990). Improving physicians' recognition and treatment of depression in general medical care: Results from a randomized clinical trial. *Medical Care, 28,* 239–250.

Malan, D. H. (1976). *The frontiers of brief psychotherapy: An example of the convergence of research and clinical practice.* New York: Plenum.

Malpartida, F., Arcas, R., Alegria, E., Montral, F., & Caro, D. M. (1980). Surgical treatments for chest pain in mitral valve prolapse. *Chest, 17,* 101–104.

Manning, W., Wells, K., & Benjamin, B. (1987). Use of outpatient mental health services over time in a health maintenance organization and fee-for-service plans. *American Journal of Psychiatry, 144,* 283–287.

Manning, W., Wells, K. B., Duan, N., Newhouse, J. P., & Ware, J. E. (1986). How cost sharing affects the use of ambulatory mental health services. *Journal of the American Medical Association, 256,* 1930–1934.

Matarazzo, J. D. (1994). Health and behavior: The coming together of science and practice in psychology and medicine after a century of benign neglect. *Journal of Clinical Psychology in Medical Settings, 1,* 7–41.

Mathias, S., Fifer, S. K., Mazonson, P. D., Lubeck, D. P., Buesching, D. P., & Patrick, D. L. (1994). Necessary but not sufficient: The effect of screening and feedback on outcomes of primary care patients with untreated anxiety. *Journal of General Internal Medicine, 9,* 606–615.

Maturana, H. (1972). *Autopesis and cognition.* Boston: Reidel.

Maturana, H. (1987). *Tree of knowledge.* Santiago, Chile: Shambala.

McClelland, D. (in press). Psychologic changes induced by a behavioral medicine intervention. *Mind/Body Medicine.*

McDaniel, S., Campbell, T., & Seaburn, D. (1990). *Family-oriented primary care: A manual for medical providers.* New York: Springer-Verlag.

McGee, R., & Tangalos, E. G. (1994). Delivery of health care to the underserved: Potential contributions of telecommunications technology. *Mayo Clinic Proceedings, 12,* 1131–1136.

McGinnis, J. M., Deering, M. J., & Patrick, K. (1995). Public health information and the new media: A view from the Public Health Service. In L. M. Harris (Ed.), *Health and the new media* (pp. 127–141). Mahwah, NJ: Lawrence Erlbaum.

McKay, C. R., Kawanishi, D. T., & Rahimtoola, S. H. (1987). Catheter balloon valvuplasty of the mitral valve in adults using a double-balloon technique. *Journal of the American Medical Association, 257,* 1753–1761.

McLachlan, M., Nyirenda, T., & Nyando, C. (1995). Attributions for admission to Zomba Mental Hospital: Implications for the development of mental health services in Malawi. *International Journal of Social Psychiatry, 41,* 79–87.

McLeod, C. (in press). Treatment of somatization in primary care. *Journal of General Hospital Psychiatry.*

McNamara, D. M. (1994): Health-oriented telecommunications: A community resource. *Nursing Management, 12,* 40–41.

Mechanic, D. (1966). Response factors in illness: The study of illness behavior. *Social Psychiatry, 1,* 52–73.

Mechanic, D. (1991). Strategies to integrating public mental health services. *Hospital and Community Psychiatry, 42,* 780–797.

Meijer, A. M., & Oppenheimer, L. (1995). The excitation-adaptation model of pediatric chronic illness. *Family Process, 34,* 441–454.

Melek, S. P. (1996). Behavioral healthcare risk-sharing and medical cost offset. *Behavioral Healthcare Tomorrow, 5,* 39–46.

Melek, S. P., & Pyenson, B. (1995). *Capitation handbook.* Washington, DC: American Psychiatric Association.

Meredith, L., Wells, K. B., Kaplan, S. H., & Mazel, R. M. (1996). Counseling typically provided for depression: Role of clinician specialty and payment system. *Archives of General Psychiatry, 53,* 905–912.

Merrill, A. J., & Swain, L. (1982). Evaluation of the systolic click: When does the mitral valve prolapse? *Practical Cardiology, 8,* 136–145.

Mertens, J. R., Moos, R. H., & Brennan, P. L. (1996). Alcohol consumption, life context and coping predict mortality among late-middle-aged drinkers and former drinkers. *Alcoholism, Clinical and Experimental Research, 10,* 313–319.

Metcalf, H. L. (1989). Anxiety: Finding the right treatment approach. *The Female Patient, 14,* 105–111.

Mintz, J., Mintz, L. I., Arruda, M. J., & Hwang, S. S. (1992). Treatments of depression and the functional capacity to work. *Archives of General Psychiatry, 49,* 761–768.

Miranda, J., Hohmann, A., Attkisson, C., & Larson, D. (Eds.) (1994). *Mental disorders in primary care.* San Francisco: Jossey-Bass.

Mumford, E., Schlesinger, H. J., & Glass, G. V. (1982). The effects of psychological intervention on recovery from surgery and heart attacks: An analysis of the literature. *American Journal of Public Health, 72,* 141–151.

Mumford, E., Schlesinger, H. J., Glass, G. V., Patrick, C., & Cuerdon, T. (1984). A new look at evidence about reduced cost of medical utilization following mental health treatment. *American Journal of Psychiatry, 141,* 1145–1158.

Munoz, R. F., Hollon, S. D., McGrath, E., Rehm, L. P., & VandenBos, G. R. (1994). On the AHCPR depression in primary care guidelines: Further considerations for practitioners. *American Psychologist, 49,* 42–61.

Munoz, R. F., & Ying, Y. W. (1993). *The prevention of depression: Research and practice.* Baltimore, MD: Johns Hopkins University Press.

Munstedt, K., Kirsch, K., Milch, W., Sachsse, S., & Vahrson, H. (1996). Unconventional cancer therapy: Survey of patients with gynecological malignancy. *Archives of Gynecology and Obstetrics, 258,* 81–88.

Mynors-Wallis, L. M., Gath, D. H., Lloyd-Thomas, A. R., & Tomlinson, D. (1995). Randomized controlled trial comparing problem solving treatment with amitriptyline and placebo for major depression in primary care. *British Medical Journal, 310,* 441–445.

Narrow, W., Reiger, D. A., Rae, D. S., Manderscheid, R., & Locke, B. Z. (1993). Use of services by persons with mental and addictive disorders: Findings from the National Institute of Mental Health Epidemiologic Catchment Area Program. *Archives of General Psychiatry, 50,* 95–107.

National Institute of Mental Health. (1993). *The prevention of mental disorders: A national research agenda.* Bethesda, MD: National Institute of Mental Health.

Neaton, J., Grimm, R., & Prineas, R. (1993). Treatment of mild hypertension study: Final results. *Journal of the American Medical Association, 270,* 713–724.

Nielson, A. C., & Williams, T. A. (1980). Depression in ambulatory medical patients: Prevalence by self-report questionnaire and recognition by nonpsychiatric physicians. *Archives of General Psychiatry, 37,* 999–1004.

Newman, R. (1996, September 27). *Primary care physician collaboration and interface.* Presented at Managing Anxiety and Depressive Disorders Conference, NMHCC.

Newton-John, T. R., Spence, S. H., & Schotte, D. (1995). Cognitive–behavioral therapy versus EMG biofeedback in the treatment of chronic low back pain. *Behaviour Research and Therapy, 33,* 691–697.

Nicholson, A. (1996). Diet and the prevention and treatment of breast cancer. *Alternative Therapies in Health and Medicine, 2,* 32–38.

Norquist, G., & Wells, K. B. (1991). How do HMOs reduce outpatient mental health care costs. *American Journal of Psychiatry, 148,* 96–101.

Novack, D. H., Dube, C., & Goldstein, M. G. (1992). Teaching medical interviewing: A basic course on interviewing and the physician-patient relationship. *Archives of Internal Medicine, 152,* 1814–1820.

O'Brien, A. (1996, Winter). Mind matters. *Vim & Vigor,* 46–50.

O'Donohue, W., & Krasner, L. (1995). *Handbook of psychological skills training.* Needham Heights, MA: Allyn & Bacon.

O'Koon, M., & Morrow, S. (1995). When rheumatology meets psychology. *Arthritis Today,* November/December, 28–33.

Olfson, M., & Klerman, G. L. (1992). Depressive symptoms and mental health service utilization in a community sample. *Social Psychiatry and Psychiatric Epidemiology, 27,* 161–167.

Ormel, J., Koeter, M. W., VanDenBrink, W., & VandeWillige, G. (1991). Recognition, management, and course of anxiety and depression in general practice. *Archives of General Psychiatry, 48,* 700–706.

Ormel, J., VonKorff, M., Ustun, T. B., Pini, S., Korten, A., & Oldehinkel, T. (1994). Common mental disorders and disability across cultures. *Journal of the American Medical Association, 272,* 1741–1748.

Ormel, J., VonKorff, M., VanDenBrink, W., Katon, W., Brilman, E., & Oldehinkel, T. (1993). Depression, anxiety, and social disability show synchrony of change in primary care patients. *American Journal of Public Health, 83,* 385–390.

Ornish, D. M., Brown, S. E., & Scherwitz, L. W. (1990). Can lifestyle changes reverse coronary heart disease? The Lifestyle Heart Trial. *Lancet, 2,* 129–133.

Padgett, D., Patrick, C., Burns, B. J., & Schlesinger, H. J. (1994). Ethnicity and the use of outpatient mental health services in a national insured population. *American Journal of Public Health, 84,* 222–226.

Pagano, R. (1995). Recognizing the developmental stages of managed care in a medical community. *Managed Care Medicine,* July/August, 44–51.

Pallak, M. S., & Cummings, N. A. (1992). Inpatient and outpatient psychiatric treatment: The effect of matching patients to appropriate level of treatment on psychiatric and medical-surgical hospital days. *Applied and Preventive Psychology, 1,* 83–87.

Pallak, M. S., Cummings, N. A., Dorken, H., & Henke, C. J. (1994). Medical costs, Medicaid, and managed mental health treatment: The Hawaii study. *Managed Care Quarterly, 2,* 64–70.

Pallak, M. S., Cummings, N. A., Dorken, H., & Henke, C. J. (1995). Effect of mental health treatment on medical costs. *Mind/Body Medicine, 1,* 7–12.

Patel, V., Musara, T., Butau, T., Maramba, P., & Fuyane, S. (1995). Concepts of mental illness and medical pluralism in Harare. *Psychological Medicine, 25,* 485–493.

Payor, L. (1988). *Medicine and culture.* New York: Penguin.

Peek, C. J., & Heinrich, R. L. (1995). Building a collaborative healthcare organization: From idea to invention to innovation. *Family Systems Medicine, 13,* 327–342.

Peek, C. J., & Heinrich, R. L. (1997). Developing primary care/behavioral health collaborations in healthcare organization: From pilot to mainstream. In A. Blount (Ed.), *Integrated primary care: The future of medical and mental health collaboration* (pp. 67–89). New York: Norton.

Peele, S. (1978, September). Addiction: The analgesic experience. *Human Nature,* 26–36.

Pelletier, K. R. (1993). Between mind and body: Stress, emotions and health. In D. Goleman & J. Gurin (Eds.), *Mind/body medicine* (pp. 19–38). Yonkers, NY: Consumer Reports.

Peterson, C., & Bossio, L. M. (1993). Healthy attitudes: Optimism, hope, and control. In D. Goleman & J. Gurin (Eds.), *Mind/body medicine* (pp. 351–366). Yonkers, NY: Consumer Reports.

Philbrick, J., Connelly, J. E., & Wofford, A. B. (1996). The prevalence of mental disorders in rural office practice. *Journal of General Internal Medicine, 11,* 9–15.

Pickering, T. (1994). Blood pressure measurement and detection of hypertension. *Lancet, 344,* 31–35.

Pigott, H. E. (1996). Information technology: Changing the equation for entrepreneurial innovation. *Behavioral Health Management, 16,* 6–8.

Pigott, H. E., Alter, G., & Heggie, D. (in press). Linking expert systems to outcomes analysis in behavioral healthcare. In P. L. Spath (Ed.), *Creative advancements in patient care management.* Chicago: American Hospital Publishing.

Pigott, H. E., & Broskowski, A. (1995). Outcomes analysis: Guiding beacon or bogus science? *Behavioral Health Management, 15,* 22–24.

Pigott, H. E., & Trott, L. (1993). Translating research into practice: The implementation of an in-home crisis intervention, triage and treatment service in the private sector. *American Journal of Medical Quality, 8,* 138–144.

Pincus, T., & Callahan, L. F. (1995). What explains the association between socioeconomic status and health: Primarily access to medical care or mind-body variables? *Advances, 11,* 4–36.

Poche, C., Yoder, P., & Miltenberger, R. (1988). Teaching self-protection to children using television techniques. *Journal of Applied Behavior Analysis, 21,* 253–261.

Pomerleau, O. F. (1979). Behavioral medicine: The contribution of the experimental analysis of behavior to medical care. *American Psychologist, 34,* 654–663.

Price, R. H., van Ryn, M., & Vinokur, R. P. (1992). Impact of preventive job search intervention on the likelihood of depression among the unemployed. *Journal of Health and Social Behavior, 33,* 158–167.

Primary Care Weekly. (1995, September 4). Curriculum touts interdisciplinary team in primary care. *Primary Care Weekly, 1,* 1, 3–4.

Quirk, M., Strosahl, K., Todd, J., Fitzpatrick, W., Casey, M., Hennessey, S., & Simon, G. (1995). Quality and customers: Type 2 change in mental health delivery within health care reform. *Journal of Mental Health Administration, 22,* 414–425.

RAND Corporation. (1987). *A report on the changing practice patterns of primary care physicians in geographical areas with too many physicians.* Santa Monica, CA: RAND Corporation.

Rapee, R. M., Craske, M. G., Brown, T. A., & Barlow, D. H. (1996). Measurement of perceived control over anxiety-related events. *Journal of Cognitive and Behavioral Practice, 3,* 279–291.

Regier, D. A., Goldberg, I. D., & Taube, C. A. (1978). The de facto U.S. mental health services system: A public health perspective. *Archives of General Psychiatry, 35,* 685–693.

Regier, D. A., Narrow, W. E., Rae, D. S., Manderscheid, R. W., Locke, B. Z., & Goodwin, F. K. (1993). The de facto U.S. mental and addictive disorders service system: Epidemiologic Catchment Area prospective 1-year prevalence rates of disorders and services. *Archives of General Psychiatry, 50,* 85–94.

Robinson, P. (1996). *Living life well: New strategies for hard times.* Reno, NV: Context.

Robinson, P., Bush, T., VonKorff, M., Katon, W., Lin, E., Simon, G., & Walker, E. (1995). Primary care physician use of cognitive behavioral techniques with depressed patients. *Journal of Family Practice, 40,* 352–357.

Robinson, P., Del Vento, A., & Wischman, C. (1997). Integrated care for the frail elderly: The group care clinic. In A. Blount (Ed.),

Integrated primary care: The future of medical and mental health collaboration (pp. 123–141). New York: Norton.

Robinson, P., Katon, W., VonKorff, M., Bush, T., Ludman, E., Simon, G., Lin, E., & Walker, E. (n.d.) Effects of a combined treatment for depressed primary care patients on behavioral change and process of care variables. Manuscript submitted for publication.

Robinson, P., Wischman, C., & Del Vento, A. (1996). *Treating depression in primary care: A manual for primary care and mental health providers.* Reno, NV: Context Press.

Rogers, W. H., Wells, K. B., Meredith, L. S., Strum, R., & Burnam, A. (1993). Outcomes for adult outpatients with depression under prepaid or fee-for-service financing. *Archives of General Psychiatry, 50,* 517–525.

Rosenbaum, J. F. (1986, August). Panic disorder. *Drug Therapy,* 113–142.

Rosenbaum, J. F. (1987). Proper drug selection in anxiety disorders. *Modern Medicine, 55,* 101–108.

Roter, D. L. (1995). Improving physicians' interviewing skills and reducing patients' emotional distress: A randomized clinical trial. *Archives of Internal Medicine, 155,* 1877–1884.

Rutan, J. S., & Stone, W. N. (1984). *Psychodynamic group psychotherapy.* Lexington, MA: Callamore Press.

Rutter, M. (1986). The developmental psychopathology of depression: Issues and perspectives. In M. Rutter, C. E. Izard & P. B. Read (Eds.), *Depression in young people: Developmental and clinical perspectives.* New York: Guilford Press.

Rutter, M. (1990). Commentary: Some focus and process considerations regarding effects of parental depression on children. *Developmental Psychology, 26,* 60–67.

Sachs, M. H. (1993). Exercise for stress control. In D. Goleman & J. Gurin (Eds.), *Mind/Body Medicine* (pp. 315–327). Yonkers, NY: Consumer Reports.

Samowitz, P., Levy, P., Levy, J., & Jacobs, R. (1989). A video AIDS prevention training program for people who are mentally retarded/developmentally disabled. *International Conference on AIDS, 5,* 700.

Sato, T., Takeichi, M., Shiranhama, M., Fukui, T., & Gude, J. K. (1995). Doctor-shopping patients and users of alternative medicine among Japanese primary care patients. *General Hospital Psychiatry, 17,* 115–125.

Schlesinger, H. J., Mumford, E., Glass, G. V., Patrick, C., & Sharfstein, S. (1983). Mental health treatment and medical care utilization in a fee-for-service system: Outpatient mental health treatment following the onset of a chronic disease. *American Journal of Public Health, 73,* 422–429.

Schneider, P. (1997). Telemedicine: Helping the underserved at home and abroad. *Healthcare Informatics, 1,* 17–18.

Schuckit, M. A. (1989). *Drug and alcohol abuse.* New York: Plenum Medical.

Schulberg, H. C., Block, M. R., Madonia, M. J., Scott, C., Rodriguez, E., Imber, S., Perel, J., Lave, J., Houck, P., & Coulehan, J. L. (1996). Treating major depression in primary care practice: Eight-month clinical outcomes. *Archives of General Psychiatry, 53,* 913–919.

Schulberg, H. C., McClelland, M., & Gooding, W. (1987). Six-month outcomes for medical patients with major depressive disorders. *Journal of General Internal Medicine, 2,* 312–317.

Schulberg, H. D., Saul, M., McClelland, M., Ganguli, M., Christy, W., & Frank, R. (1985). Assessing depression in primary medical and psychiatric practices. *Archives of General Psychiatry, 42,* 1164–1170.

Schwartz, M. S., & Schwartz, N. M. (1993). Biofeedback: Using the body's signals. In D. Goleman & J. Gurin (Eds.), *Mind/body medicine* (pp. 301–313). Yonkers, NY: Consumer Reports.

Scott, J., & Robertson, B. (1996). Kaiser Colorado's cooperative health care clinic: A group approach to patient care. In P. Box, & T. Fama (Eds.), *Managed care and chronic illness* (pp. 125–132). Gaithersburg, MD: Permagon.

Seaburn, D., Landau-Stanton, J., & Horowitz, S. (1995). Core techniques in family therapy. In R. Mikesell, D. Lusterman & S. McDaniel (Eds.), *Integrating family therapy: Handbook of family psychology and systems theory* (pp. 5–26). Washington, DC: American Psychological Association Press.

Seaburn, D., Lorenz, A., Gunn, W., Gawinski, B., & Mauksch, L. (1996). *Models of collaboration: A guide for mental health professionals working with health care practitioners.* New York: Basic Books.

Seligman, M. E. P. (1975). *Helplessness: On depression, development, and death.* San Francisco: W. H. Freeman.

Seligman, M. E. P. (1994). *What you can change and what you can't.* New York: Alfred A. Knopf.

Semmens, J., & Peric, J. (1995). Children's experience of a parent's chronic illness and death. *Australian Journal of Advanced Nursing, 13,* 30–38.

Shaffer, D. (1989). Prevention of psychiatric disorders in children and adolescents: A summary of findings and recommendations from project prevention. In D. Shaffer, I. Phillips & N. B. Enzer (Eds.), *Prevention of mental disorders, alcohol and other drug use in children and adolescents.* U.S. Department of Health and Human Services, OSAP Prevention Monograph 2.

Shapiro, A. K., & Morris, L. A. (1978). The placebo effect in medical and psychological therapies. In S. L. Garfield & A. E. Bergin (Eds.), *Handbook of psychotherapy and behavior change* (2nd. ed.). New York: Wiley.

Shapiro, D. E., & Koocher, G. P. (1996). Goals and practical considerations in outpatient medical crisis intervention. *Professional Psychology: Research and Practice, 27,* 109–120.

Sifneos, P. E. (1987). *Short-term dynamic psychotherapy: Evaluation and technique* (2nd. ed.). New York: Plenum.

Simon, G., Grothaus, L., Durham, M., VonKorff, M., & Pabiniak, C. (1996). Impact of visit copayments on outpatient mental health utilization by members of a health maintenance organization. *American Journal of Psychiatry, 153,* 331–338.

Simon, G., Lin, E., Katon, W., Saunders, K., VonKorff, M., Walker, E., Bush, T., & Robinson, P. (1995). Outcomes of "inadequate" antidepressant treatment in primary care. *Journal of General Internal Medicine, 10,* 663–670.

Simon, G., Ormel, J., VonKorff, M., & Barlow, W. (1995). Health care costs associated with depressive and anxiety disorders in primary care. *American Journal of Psychiatry, 152,* 352–357.

Simon, G., Ustun, T. B., & VonKorff, M. (1996). *Depressive disorders: Recognition and outcome in the WHO collaborative survey of psychological problems in general health care.* Presented at NIMH Mental Health Services Research Conference.

Simon, G., & VonKorff, M. (1995a). Recognition, management, and outcomes of depression in primary care. *Archives of Family Medicine, 4,* 99–105.

Simon, G., & VonKorff, M. (1995b). Results from the Seattle centre. In T. Ustun & N. Sartorius (Eds.), *Mental illness in general health care.* New York: Wiley.

Simon, G., VonKorff, M., & Barlow, W. (1995). Health care costs associated with depressive and anxiety disorders in primary care. *Archives of General Psychiatry, 52,* 850–856.

Simon, G., VonKorff, M., Barlow, W., Pabiniak, C., & Wagner, E. (1996). Predictors of chronic benzodiazepine use in a health maintenance organization sample. *Journal of Clinical Epidemiology, 49,* 1067–1073.

Simon, G., VonKorff, M., & Durham, M. L. (1994). Predictors of outpatient mental health utilization in an HMO primary care sample. *American Journal of Psychiatry, 151,* 908–913.

Simon, G., VonKorff, M., Heiligenstein, J. H., Revicki, D. A., Grothaus, L., Katon, W., & Wagner, E. H. (1996). Initial antidepressant selection in primary care: Effectiveness and cost of fluoxetine vs. tricyclic antidepressants. *Journal of the American Medical Association, 275,* 1897–1902.

Simon, G., VonKorff, M., Wagner, E. H., & Barlow, W. (1993). Patterns of antidepressant use in community practice. *General Hospital Psychiatry, 15,* 399–408.

Sleek, S. (1995, December). Rallying the troops inside our bodies. *APA Monitor, 26, 1,* 24–25.

Smith, R., Monson, R., & Ray, D. (1986). Psychiatric consultation in somatization disorder. *New England Journal of Medicine, 314,* 1407–1413.

Smith, R., Rost, K., & Kashner, M. (1995). A trial of the effect of a standardized psychiatric consultation on health outcomes and costs in somatizing patients. *Archives of General Psychiatry, 52,* 238–243.

Smith, T. W. (1992). Hostility and health: Current status of a psychosomatic hypothesis. *Health Psychology, 11,* 139–150.

Sobel, D. (1995a, November). *Beyond mental illness and mental health services.* Lecture given at the Behavioral Medicine Series. Boston: Pilgrim Health Care.

Sobel, D. (1995b). Rethinking medicine: Improving health outcomes with cost-effective psychosocial interventions. *Psychosomatic Medicine, 57,* 234–244.

Soffa, V. M. (1996, March). Alternatives to hormone replacement for menopause. *Alternative Therapies, 2,* 34–39.

Solomon, G. (1985). Psychoneuroimmunology. In G. Adelman (Ed.), *The encyclopedia of neuroscience* (pp. 164–192). Cambridge, MA: Brinkhauser.

Spencer, F. C., & Colvin, S. B. (1985, May). The NYU experience with the Carpenter techniques of mitral valve reconstruction. *Surgical Rounds,* 88–94.

Spiegel, D. (1993). Social support: How friends, family, and groups can help. In D. Goleman & J. Gurin (Eds.), *Mind/body medicine* (pp. 331–349). Yonkers, NY: Consumer Reports.

Spiegel, D. (1995). Social support and cancer. In N. R. S. Hall, F. Altman, & S. J. Blumenthal (Eds.), *Mind–body interactions and disease.* Tampa, FL: Health Dateline.

Spiegel, D., Bloom, J. R., & Kraemer, H. C. (1989). Effect of psychosocial treatment on survival of patients with metastatic breast cancer. *Lancet, 2,* 888–890.

Spitzer, R., Kroenke, K., Linzer, M., Hahn, S. R., Williams, J. B. W., deGruy, F. V., Brody, D., & Davies, M. (1995). Health-related quality of life in primary care patients with mental disorders. *Journal of the American Medical Association, 274,* 1511–1517.

Spitzer, R., Williams, J. B. W., Kroenke, K., Linzer, M., deGruy, F. V., Hahn, S. R., Brody, D., & Johnson, J. G. (1994). Utility of a new procedure for diagnosing mental disorders in primary care: The PRIME-MD 1000 study. *Journal of the American Medical Association, 272,* 1749–1756.

Sprenkle, D., & Bischof, G. (1994). Contemporary family therapy in the United States. *Journal of Family Therapy, 16,* 5–23.

Steinberg, M., Cole, S. A., & Saravay, S. M. (1996). Consultation-liaison psychiatry fellowship in primary care. *International Journal of Psychiatry in Medicine, 26,* 135–145.

Stone, W. N., & Rutan, J. S. (1984). Duration of group psychotherapy. *International Journal of Group Psychotherapy, 32,* 29–47.

Strain, J. (1986). The role of psychiatry in the training of primary care physicians. *General Hospital Psychiatry, 8,* 372–385.

Strain, J. J. (1993). Psychotherapy and medical conditions. In D. Goleman & J. Gurin (Eds.), *Mind/body medicine* (pp. 367–383). Yonkers, NY: Consumer Reports Books.

Strain, J., Hammer, J. S., & Fulop, G. (1994). APM Task Force on Psychosocial Interventions in the General Hospital Inpatient Setting: A review of cost-offset studies. *Psychosomatics, 35,* 253–262.

Strosahl, K. (1994a). Entering the new frontier of managed mental health care: Gold mines and land mines. *Cognitive and Behavioral Practice, 1,* 5–23.

Strosahl, K. (1994b). New dimensions in behavioral health primary care integration. *HMO Practice, 8,* 176–179.

Strosahl, K. (1995). Behavior therapy 2000: A perilous journey. *The Behavior Therapist, 18,* 130–133.

Strosahl, K. (1996a). Primary mental health care: A new paradigm for achieving health and behavioral health integration. *Behavioral Healthcare Tomorrow, 5,* 93–96.

Strosahl, K. (1996b). Confessions of a behavior therapist in primary care: The Odyssey and the ecstasy. *Cognitive and Behavioral Practice, 3,* 1–28.

Strosahl, K. (in press). Integration of primary care and behavioral health services: The primary mental healthcare model. In A. Blount (Ed.), *Integrative primary care: The future of medical and mental health collaboration* (pp. 43–66). New York: Norton.

Strosahl, K., & Sobel, D. (1996). Behavioral health and medical cost offset effect: Current status, key concepts and future applications. *HMO Practice, 10,* 156–162.

Stuart, M., Handley, M., Chamberlain, M., Wallach, R., Penna, A., & Stergachis, A. (1991). Successful implementation of a guideline program for the rational use of lipid lowering drugs. *HMO Practice, 5,* 198–204.

Stuart, M., Handley, M., Thompson, R., Conger, M., & Timlin, D. (1992). Clinical practice and new technology: Prostate-specific antigen (PSA). *HMO Practice, 6,* 5–11.

Sturm, R., & Wells, K. B. (1995). How can care for depression become more cost effective? *Journal of the American Medical Association, 273,* 51–58.

Telch, M. J., Miller, L. M., Killen, J. D., Cooke, S., & Maccoby, N. (1990). Social influences approach to smoking prevention: The effects of videotape delivery with and without same-age peer leader participation. *Addictive Behavior, 15,* 21–28.

Tiemens, B., Ormel, J., & Simon, G. E. (1996). Occurrence, recognition, and outcomes of psychological disorders in primary care. *American Journal of Psychiatry, 153,* 636–644.

Trussolini, C. P., & The Pew-Fetzer Task Force. (1994). *Health professions education and relationship centered care.* San Francisco, CA: Pew Health Professions Commission.

Troy, W. G., & Shueman, S. A. (1996). Program redesign for graduate training in professional psychology: The road to accountability in a changing professional world. In N. A. Cummings, M. S. Pallak, & J. L. Cummings, (Eds.), *Surviving the demise of solo practice: Mental health practitioners prospering in the era of managed care* (pp. 55–79). Madison, CT: Psychosocial Press.

University of California at Berkeley. (1995, September). Investigating homeopathy. *Wellness Letter,* 4–5.

Unutzer, J., Patrick, D., Simon, G., Grembowski, D., Walker, E., & Katon, W. (1996). *Depression, quality of life, and use of health services in primary care patients over 65: A four-year prospective study.* Presented at American Psychiatric Association, 148th Annual Meeting.

U.S. Department of Health and Human Services, Public Health Service. (1991). *Healthy people 2000: National disease prevention and health promotion objectives.* Washington, DC: Government Printing Office.

Van Blerkom, L. M. (1995). Clown doctors: Shaman healers of Western medicine. *Medical Anthropology Quarterly, 9,* 462–475.

VandenBos, G., & DeLeon, P. (1984). The use of psychotherapy to improve physical health. *Psychotherapy, 25,* 335–343.

Van Hammond, T., & Deans, C. (1995). A phenomenological study of families and psychoeducation support groups. *Journal of Psychosocial Nursing and Mental Health Services, 33,* 7–12.

Vega, W. A., Valle, R., Kolodoy, B., & Hough, R. (1987). The Hispanic social network prevention intervention study: A community-based randomized trial. In R. F. Munoz (Ed.), *Depression prevention: Research directions* (pp. 217–231). New York: Hemisphere.

Vickery, D., Kalmer, H., & Lowry, D. (1983). Effect of a self-care education program on medical visits. *The Journal of the American Medical Association, 250,* 2952–2956.

VonKorff, M., Katon, W., Lin, E., Saunders, K., Simon, G., Walker, E., Robinson, P., & Bush, T. (1994). *Evaluation of cost and cost offset of collaborative management of depressed patients in primary care.* Presented at Eighth Annual NIMH Research Conference on Mental Health Problems in the General Health Care Sector.

VonKorff, M., Ormel, J., Katon, W. J., & Lin, E. H. B. (1992). Disability and depression among high utilizers of health care. *Archives of General Psychiatry, 49,* 91–100.

VonKorff, M., Shapiro, S., Burke, J. D., Teitlebaum, M., Skinner, E. A., German, P., Turner, R. W., Klein, L., & Burns, B. (1987). Anxiety and depression in a primary care clinic: Comparison of Diagnostic Interview Schedule, General Health Questionnaire, and practitioner assessments. *Archives of General Psychiatry, 44,* 152–156.

VonKorff, M., & Simon, G. (1996). The prevalence and impact of psychological disorders in primary care: HMO research needed to improve care. *HMO Practice, 10,* 150–155.

Ware, J. E. (1996). Patient-based assessment: Tools for monitoring and improving healthcare outcomes. *Behavioral Healthcare Tomorrow, 3,* 87–88.

Waters, D., & Lawrence, E. (1992). *Competence, courage and change.* New York: Norton.

Webster-Stratton, C. (1994). Advancing videotape parent-training: A comparison study. *Journal of Consulting and Clinical Psychology, 62,* 583–593.

Weissman, M. M., Leif, P., & Bruce, M. L. (1987). Single parent women. *Social Psychiatry, 22,* 29–36.

Wells, K. B., Golding, J. M., & Burnham, M. A. (1988). Psychiatric disorder in a sample of the general population with and without chronic medical conditions. *American Journal of Psychiatry, 145,* 976–981.

Wells, K. B., Katon, W., Rogers, B., & Camp, P. (1994). Use of minor tranquilizers and antidepresssant medication by depressed outpatients: Results from the Medical Outcomes Study. *American Journal of Psychiatry, 151,* 694–700.

Wells, K. B., Stewart, A., Hays, R., Burnam, M., Rogers, W., Daniels, M., Berry, S., Greenfield, S., & Ware, J. (1989). The functioning and well-being of depressed patients: Results from the Medical Outcome Study. *Journal of the American Medical Association, 262,* 914–919.

White, M., & Epston, D. (1990). *Narrative means to therapeutic ends.* New York: Norton.

Wickramasekera, I. (1989). Somatizers, the health care system, and collapsing the psychological distance that the somatizer has to travel for help. *Professional Psychology: Research and Practice, 29,* 105–111.

Wiggins, J. (1994). Would you want your child to be a psychologist? *American Psychologist, 49,* 485–492.

Wiggins, J. G. (1997). Medical cost-offset: Psychology's great give-away. *The National Psychologist, 1,* 17.

Will, G. (1989, January 8). Cocaine: A trickle-down affliction. *Washington Post,* p. C7.

Williams, R. B. (1994). Neurobiology, cellular and molecular biology, and psychosomatic medicine. *Psychosomatic Medicine, 56,* 308–315.

Williams, R. B., Barefoot, J. C., & Califf, R. M. (1992). Prognostic importance of social and economic resources among medically treated patients with angiographically documented coronary artery disease. *Journal of the American Medical Association, 267,* 520–524.

Williams, R. B., Feaganes, J., & Suarez, E. C. (1996, March). *Stress management training boosts social support in married working mothers.* Paper presented at the Annual Meeting, Society of Behavioral Medicine, Washington, DC.

Williams, R. B., & Gentry, W. D. (Eds.). (1997). *Behavioral approaches to medical treatment.* Cambridge: Ballenger Press.

Williams, R. B., & Williams, V. P. (1994). *Anger kills: Seventeen strategies for controlling the hostility that can harm your health* (Original work published 1993). New York: Harper Perennial.

Williams, R. B., & Williams, V. P. (1995). *Anger kills.* New York: Harper.

Winett, R. A., Anderson, E. S., Moore, J. F., Taylor, C. D., Hook, R. J., Webster, D. A., Neubauer, T. E., Harden, M. C., & Mundy, L. L. (1993). Efficacy of a home-based human immunodeficiency virus prevention video program for teens and parents. *Health Education Quarterly, 20,* 555–567.

Wingrod, T. (1986). *Understanding computers and cognition.* Boston: Ablex.

Zahn-Waxler, C., Kochanska, G., Krupnick, J., & McKnew, D. H. (1990). Patterns of guilt in children of depressed and well mothers. *Developmental Psychology, 26,* 51–59.

Zamarra, J. W., Schneider, R. H., Besseghini, I., Robinson, D. K., & Salerno, J. W. (1996). Usefulness of the transcendental meditation program in the treatment of patients with coronary artery disease. *American Journal of Cardiology, 77,* 867–870.

Zettler, A., Duran, G., Waadt, S., Herschback, P., & Strain, F. (1995). Coping with fear of long-term complications in diabetes mellitus: A model clinical program. *Psychotherapy and Psychosomatics, 64,* 178–184.

Zohar, D. (1990). *The quantum self.* New York: Morrow.

Zuckerman, B. S. & Beardslee, W. R. (1987). Maternal depression: A concern for pediatricians. *Pediatrics, 79,* 110–117.

Zung, W. K., Broadhead, E., & Roth, M. E. (1993). Prevalence of depressive symptoms in primary care. *The Journal of Family Practice, 37,* 337–344.

Name Index

Subject Index